COMPUTERIZED TOMOGRAPHY IN NEURO-OPHTHALMOLOGY

Computerized Tomography in Neuro-Ophthalmology

I.F. Moseley
BSc, MD, MRCP, FRCR

Radiologist to the National Hospital for Nervous Diseases, Queen Square, London

M.D. Sanders
FRCP, FRCS

Consultant Ophthalmologist, the National Hospital for Nervous Diseases, Queen Square, London

Consultant Ophthalmologist, St. Thomas' Hospital, London

Consultant Adviser in Ophthalmology to the Royal Air Force

W. B. Saunders Company
Philadelphia · Toronto

First published 1982
by Chapman and Hall Ltd
11 New Fetter Lane, London EC4P 4EE

Distribution rights in the United States and Canada
assigned to W.B. Saunders Company, West Washington Square,
Philadelphia, Pa. 19105

Printed in the United States of America

ISBN 0-7216-6579-9 (Saunders)
LOC 81-48599

IN SPERE VENIAE
HOC LIBRUM DEDICAMUS
AD MARY ET THALIA

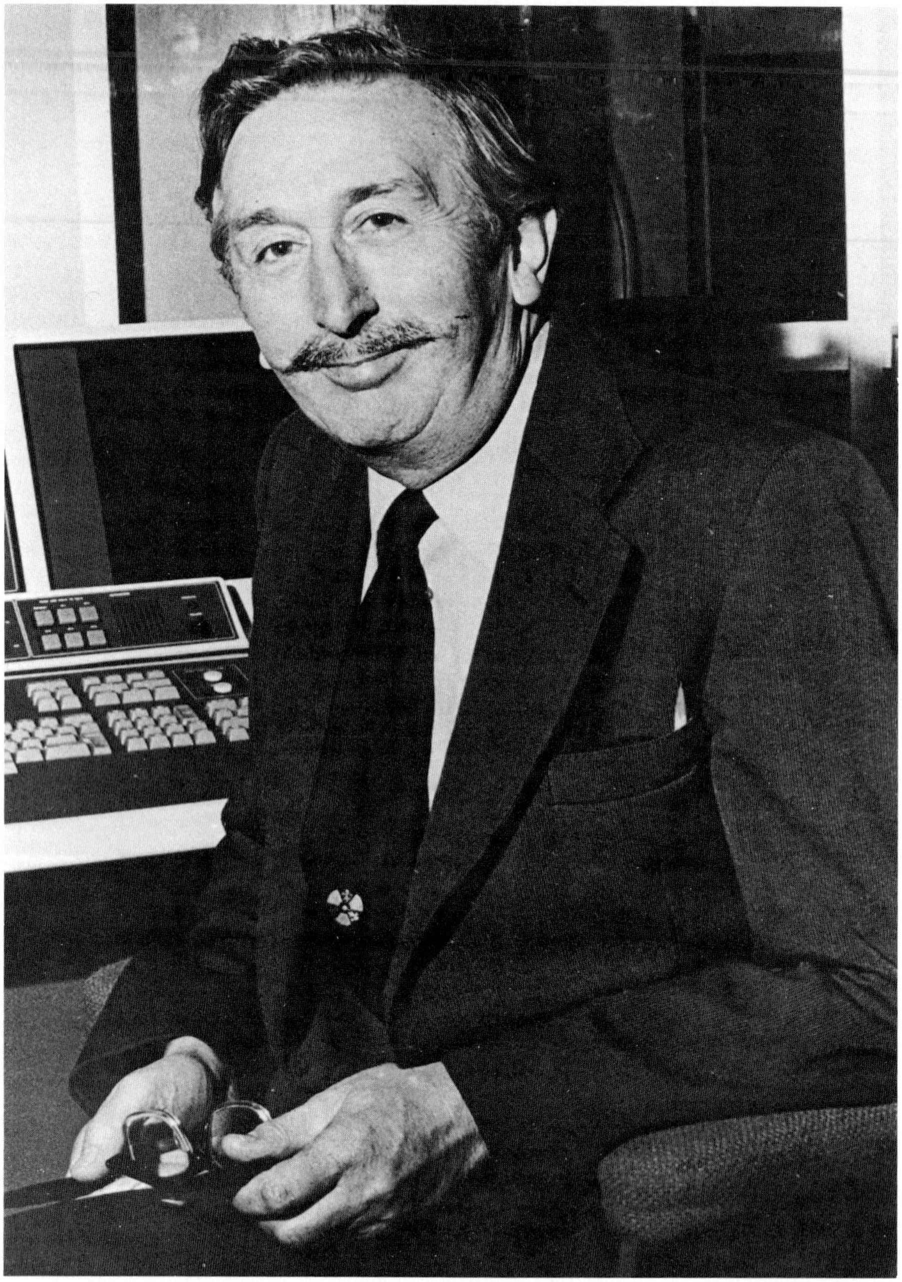

Sir Godfrey Hounsfield FRS

Contents

Preface

'Any fool may write a valuable book' observed the eighteenth century poet Thomas Gray 'if he will only tell us what he heard and saw with veracity'. Accepting this advice we have largely described our personal experience of computerized tomography (CT) in relation to clinical neuro-ophthalmology. The need for this book evolved with the recognition that the clinician could now recognize the anatomical and pathological substrate of the CT slices, and the radiologist was equipped with a more powerful tool for examining small areas and needed greater clinical appreciation. This book is therefore intended to provide sufficient clinical information for the ophthalmologist or neurologist to relate this accurately to the CT appearances, and for the radiologist to perform his duties closely attuned to the clinical environment.

The text is aimed to cover general aspects of neuro-ophthalmology with emphasis on special areas of relevance to CT. The bibliography is similarly defined. We recommend the well established textbooks by Walsh and Hoyt (*Clinical Neuro-ophthalmology* Williams and Wilkins), by Jones and Jakobiec (*Diseases of the Orbit*, Harper and Row), and by Glaser (*Neuro-opthalmology*, Harper and Row) as supplying complementary information. Illustrations have been profuse and range from common to extremely rare disorders, for which we have provided detailed descriptions. These elaborate case histories are aimed at involving the reader in the complexity of neuro-ophthalmic diagnosis and to provide a firmer foundation for this book, as advancing technology will inevitably supersede the current CT scans.

The clinical material has largely been referred to the Department of Neuro-Ophthalmology at the National Hospital and the Department of Ophthalmology at St. Thomas' Hospital. We are grateful to those who allowed us to use their patients and in particular Dr C.J. Earl, Dr R.W. Ross Russell, Professor W.I. McDonald and Mr D.S.I. Taylor at the National Hospital and Mr J. Winstanley and Mr T.J. ffytche at St. Thomas' Hospital. Radiological colleagues have been generous with time and material and we are indebted to Professor G. du Boulay, Dr B. Kendall and Dr D. Sutton at the National Hospital. Other departments or individuals may have assisted, but their recognition is associated with the material supplied, though D.S.I. Taylor, D. Spalton and T. Buchanan reviewed some of the chapters.

Special credit and an essential ingredient of this book is due to the photographic skill of Mr Rolf Sennhenn, and to the secretarial and organizational help of Miss Josephine Lace. Additional help was provided by Mrs P. Byrne, Miss J. Cox and Mrs G. Jurewicz. The CT studies were performed by a group of skilled radiographers in the Lysholm Department or Radiology, and we are indebted to Miss V. Fullom for her special interest.

We are grateful to the publishers for organizing the large number of illustrations, and particularly to Dr Barry Shurlock for his encouragement.

1 · Introduction

1.1 HISTORICAL

The first practical technique for computerized tomography (CT) was developed by Sir Godfrey Hounsfield, working in the laboratories of Electrical and Musical Industries in England and this achievement was recognized by the award of the Nobel Prize for Medicine in 1979. The most suitable region for study by this revolutionary method was the head, since immobility was necessary for several minutes, and a water surround which was more or less cylindrical and symmetrical, facilitated reconstruction of the images.

The first clinical apparatus was installed in 1972 at Atkinson Morley's Hospital in Wimbledon, South London, and other machines were soon operating in the Mayo Clinic, in Manchester and at the National Hospital for Nervous Diseases, Queen Square. Very quickly it was noted that, in addition to the intracranial structures, both normal and pathological, the orbits and their contents could be seen on the computed tomograms in a way which had previously been quite impossible (Gawler *et al*., 1974).

Since the introduction of computerized tomography the trend has been to increase the spatial and contrast resolution and to decrease the scanning time. Hounsfield's bench model required several days for scanning a brain section and computing the results, and the first production models gave a picture composed of elements (pixels), representing blocks of tissue 3 × 3 × 13mm in size (voxels). Current machines can be used to produce sections with elements as small as 0.375 × 0.375 × 2mm in a few seconds, without major increase in radiation dose.

1.2 THE PHYSICAL PRINCIPLES OF COMPUTERIZED TOMOGRAPHY

When a beam of X-rays transverses any structure, attentuation occurs, to a degree with is related to: (a) the atomic number of the element of which the structure is composed, or the effective atomic number of a complex structure and (b) the concentration of the substances forming that structure. Thus, the density of electrons, or effective electron density, determines the degree to which a given beam of X-rays will be attenuated. X-ray beams are, however, composed of X-rays of different energies: the greater the effective energy of a particular beam, the less attenuation occurs on passing through a given structure.

These facts are made use of in classical radiography by placing an X-ray or photosensitive film alongside the object to be radiographed, so that it lies perpendicular to the incident rays (Fig. 1.1). The large majority of X-rays emerging from the object will also be perpendicular to the film, but some are scattered; their influence may be reduced by the use of grids designed to prevent non-perpendicular rays reaching the film. Photographic emulsions are, however, relatively insensitive to modulation of the beam intensity by biological tissues, and it has been estimated that they register in a useful form only about 1% of the information potentially extractable from the emergent beam.

If all the information contained in the beam emerging from the skull, for example, were registered on the film, the overlapping of the many different tissue planes would render the picture virtually uninterpretable. The technique of tomography is used to render one plane sharply defined by blurring out adjacent planes. This is usually achieved by causing the X-ray source and

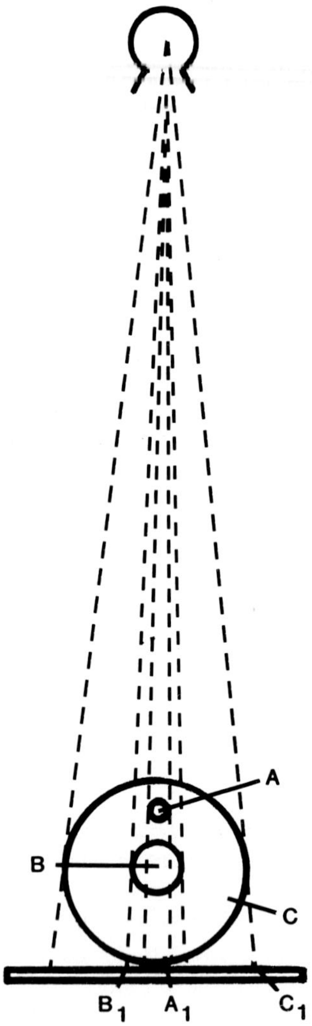

Fig. 1.1 Conventional radiography. The shadows A_1, B_1, C_1, of the elements, A,B,C, of the body being examined are completely superimposed on the final image.

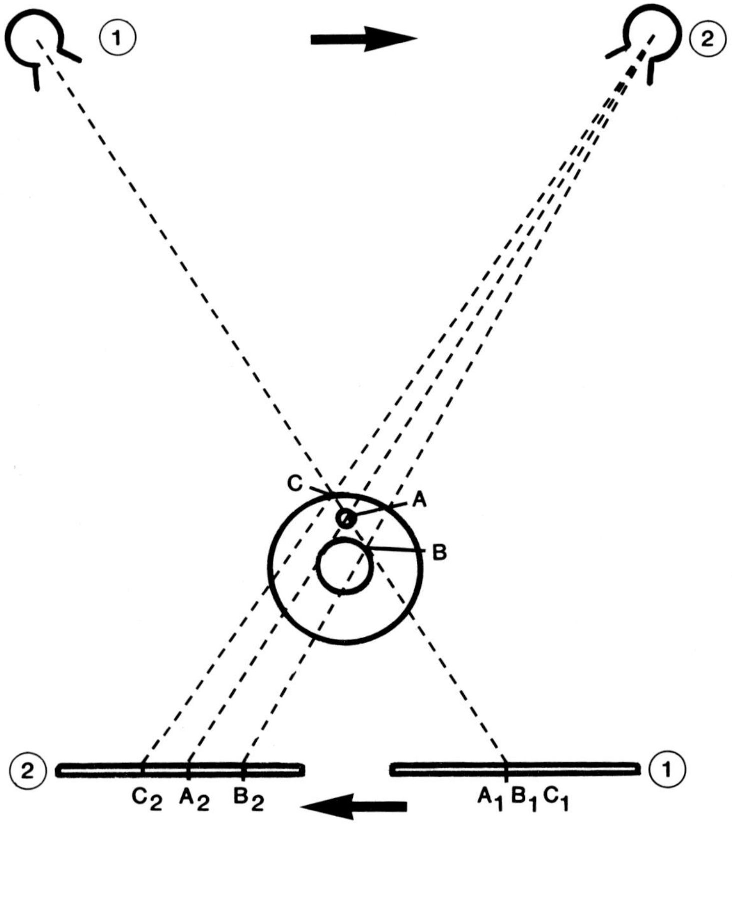

Fig. 1.2 Conventional X-ray tomography. If A is the structure under study, it is isolated from adjacent structures by being made the pivotal plane of the movement of tube and film during the exposure. (1) Initial positions; (2) final positions. Whereas the image of A (A_1, A_2) is projected on the same spot on the film throughout the exposure, the images of B and C, initially superimposed (B_1, C_1), are blurred out by being projected over a wide area ($B_1 - B_2$, $C_1 - C_2$).

film to move relative to the patient during a prolonged exposure, such that the pivotal point of the movement is the plane which is desired to be defined clearly (Fig. 1.2). There is no relative motion between the X-ray source and the film during the exposure. Examples of conventional tomograms obtained in this way are seen on p.113.

In autotomography, an alternative system of tomography, the object being radiographed oscillates about the desired plane during the exposure, the other elements, i.e. X-ray tube and film, remaining stationary. A sophisticated version of autotomography permits examination of planes at right angles to the long axis of the body and this is termed axial tomography.

Computerized axial tomography is similar only in that movement is used to isolate a plane within the body for radiographic purposes. The two fundamental innovations which make it possible are that sensitive emulsion is no longer used for recording the modulations of intensity of the emergent beam, and that the image is reconstructed by a computer.

In the most basic 'translate-rotate' system (Fig. 1.3), of which many currently available techniques are developments, one or more highly sensitive X-ray detectors (sodium iodide crystals, Xenon tubes etc.) are rigidly connected to a finely collimated or 'focused' source of X-rays. The detectors and tube scan across on either side of the object to be examined, the detectors recording a series of X-ray beam intensities. By reference to a detector which monitors the incident beam, the degree of X-ray attenuation can be measured. The angle at which the X-ray beam enters the object is then altered, in steps of 1°, by rotating the detector/X-ray tube assembly (the gantry) around the object. The passage across the object is then repeated, and a similar series of readings is obtained. This procedure is repeated until a given number of series, usually at least 180, has been recorded. It is then relatively simple for the computer to reconstruct from these series a plan of the object through which the scans were made. Several different mathematical procedures are used, which are beyond the scope of the present description.

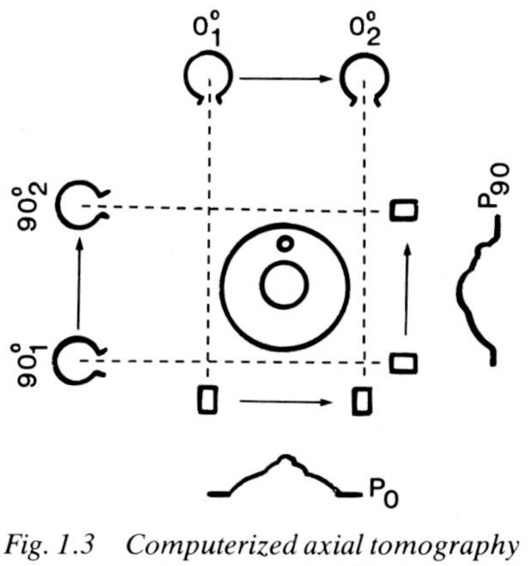

Fig. 1.3 Computerized axial tomography (translate–rotate system). The body being examined is similar to that in Fig. 1.1. and 1.2. In the initial position (0_1°) the rays from the tube are directed at the detector (d); the two then traverse the body together (to 0_2°). Po = profile of X-ray *attenuation* during this traverse. This is repeated (usually 180 times), giving 180 profiles at one degree angles; 90_1° – 90_2°; traverse after indexing 90°; P_{90} corresponding profile. The data from the profiles is then used to reconstruct an axial section in the plane of the page. See text for a further explanation.

The reconstruction takes the form of a number of data points to each of which a capacity for attenuation of the X-ray beam can be assigned. Since, however, the beam of X-rays is of finite depth at right angles to the axial plane which has been scanned, each of these data points, or pixels (picture elements) represents the scanned X-ray attenuation coefficient of a volume of tissue (the voxel or volume element), the dimensions of which will depend on the individual machine. On the original commercially available EMI Scanner, the reconstruction was on a matrix of 80 × 80 pixels, each representing a voxel 3 mm × 3 mm in a plane 13 mm deep. In practice, the machine was constructed to scan two adjacent 13-mm planes simultaneously.

The attenuation coefficient of that pixel is given in terms of an

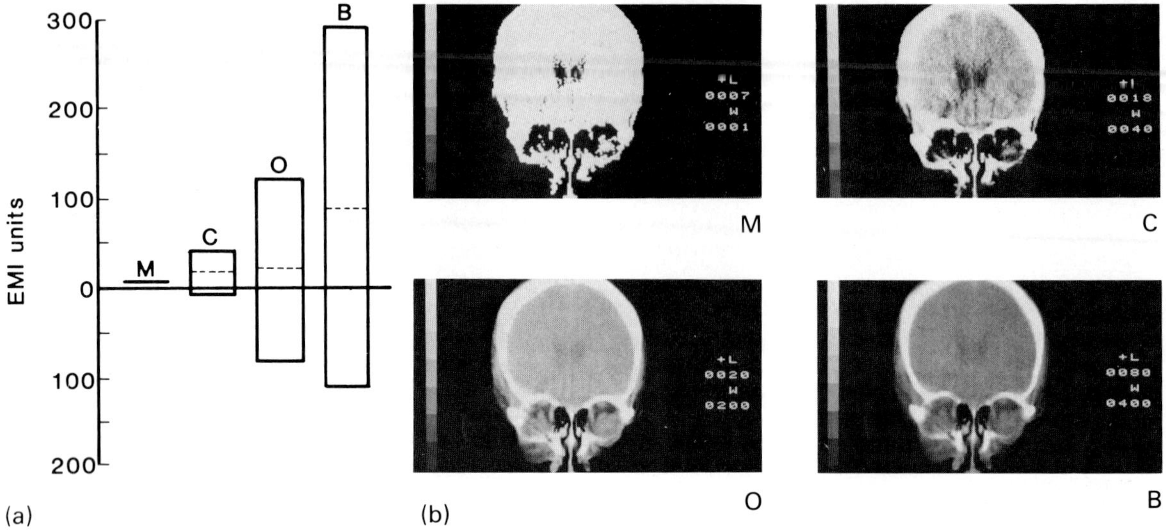

Fig. 1.4 Effect of window level and width on CT image. (a) Graph showing level (dotted line) and range of EMI numbers covered by grey scale at various width settings; (b) coronal section imaged in the same way; M: measure (window level 7 EMI units, window width 1 EMI unit) showing in this example the ventricular CSF and the orbital fat (EMI numbers below 7) in black; C: level 18, width 40 for brain imaging; O: level 20, width 200 for the orbits; B: level 80, window width 400 for bone detail.

arbitrary scale: for the original EMI scanner this was on the basis of air = −500 EMI units; water = 0 EMI units and dense bone = approximately +500 EMI units. Some subsequent machines from the same company have used Hounsfield units, which are half the value of EMI units, such that air = −1000 Hounsfield units, etc. It should be remembered that all such systems are arbitrary, that the attenuation coefficient of a given pixel may represent a voxel with greatly differing structures within it, and that the term 'density' often used in connection with computerized tomograms is correct only if it is understood to refer to electron density, and not to density in the generally accepted sense; 'attenuation coefficient' is therefore preferable. It must be emphasized that in the purely physical sense, the linear relationship between EMI or other numbers and the concentration of a given salt (e.g. calcium) is very close.

A digital/analogue converter is then employed to convert the numerical matrix into a picture for diagnostic purposes, usually by relating the attentuation coefficients to a suitably graduated grey scale, which is displayed on a cathode ray tube (CRT). An important aspect of the CT picture is that it is not a single immutable object, like the conventional X-ray film. The CRT display can be modified at will so that the extremes of the grey scale represent pixels having a difference of attenuation coefficient of only 1 EMI unit, or of several hundred units; this variation of grey scale extent is referred to as 'window width'. Similarly, the attenuation coefficient which lies at the central point of the grey scale can also be altered, throughout the entire range of coefficients which the apparatus can determine; this is referred to as 'window level'.

Typical window width and level settings for routine work are (in EMI units) for the orbits: width 200, level 20; for the intracranial structures: width 40, level 18; and for the skull base: width 400, level 80 (Fig. 1.4).

Many of the CT images reproduced in this book have been made with a modification of the translate-rotate system, which enables more rapid examination. Instead of a single detector and finely collimated beam, a fan beam is directed at an array of approximately ten angled detectors; each traverse of the X-ray tube/detector array is thus equivalent to ten traverses of the system described above, and only 18 traverses are required to scan the full 180°. 'High resolution' scans referred to in the text are obtained by decreasing the voxel size by more rapid switching of the detectors, without increase in X-ray dosage to the patient.

Descriptions of more advanced systems – rotate only, fixed detector, nutating, etc. – are to be found in standard texts.

1.3 CONDUCT OF THE EXAMINATION

Patient preparation

No special preparation is required, although most patients find the examination more tolerable after a sympathetic explanation. Some children and uncooperative adults will require sedation or general anaesthesia (the latter undoubtedly being preferable for children).

All accoutrements such as wigs, hair pieces, ear-rings and spectacles should be removed, as should false teeth with metallic components and ocular prostheses. When the orbits are being scanned, the patient should be instructed to keep the eyes in the primary position or to direct the gaze at a certain object. (Slight elevation is an advantage for optic nerve imaging.) It should be noted that, should the scan be carried out under general anaesthesia, the eyes may be slightly divergent.

Plane of section

Planes of section are usually described relative to the orbitomeatal line, which is drawn from the outer canthus of the eye to the external auditory meatus. The plane can be changed by flexion (OM+) or extension (OM−) of the head and neck or, in some machines, by angulation of the whole X-ray tube/detector assembly (the gantry).

For examination of the *orbit*, the head is extended such that the plane of section is at approximately 10° to the orbito-meatal (OM) line. This OM−10° position gives a plane which passes through the lens, optic nerve and canal region. Van Damme *et al.* (1977) suggested that this 'neuro-ocular plane' was reliably indicated by the lower orbital margin and the upper border of the external auditory meatus. For the *intracranial structures*, angulation of between OM+0° to OM+25° are employed, the former being preferred for the sellar region, and OM+10−15° for sections of the cerebrum; the latter gives a better view of the structures in the posterior cranial fossa. Some workers simply perform all scans in the orbito-meatal plane. This plane is probably the most suitable for examination of the sella turcica and suprasellar region, being parallel to the plane of the chiasmatic cistern. However, the inclination of the chiasm and intracranial optic nerves is sufficiently variable to render any given plane of section unsatisfactory in many cases. Although some standardization of position is desirable, the radiologist controlling the CT study should choose those positions and planes which appear to produce optimal demonstration of anticipated sites of abnormality.

Sections in the coronal plane can be obtained in a variety of ways: in the prone position, by resting the head on the chin; in the supine position by letting the head fall backwards, to rest on the vertex; in the sitting position, with the neck slightly extended. The latter is the easiest position for older patients who may be suffering from spondylosis, but is not possible on many machines, where the couch on which the patient normally lies cannot be separated from the gantry. Angulation of the gantry is particularly useful in these elderly patients.

Coronal sections are particularly helpful in the assessment of orbital and parasellar lesions. However, dental fillings may cause unacceptable artefacts on such sections, and it is often necessary to choose a plane which is not strictly orthogonal to the axial plane in order to avoid such degradation of the images.

Oblique sections can be obtained in many planes, by appropriate positioning of the head, but they are of limited value because of problems in interpretation. A coronal oblique plane, the head turned at approximately 45°, will demonstrate the relationship of the lateral rectus muscle to the lateral wall of the orbit on the side away from which the head is turned. These structures are sectioned very obliquely in the usual coronal sections. On some whole body scanners, the head aperture is large enough to accept the head in the lateral position, giving a direct sagittal plane. With other machines direct sagittal sections may be rendered possible, e.g. in the lateral decubitus position, with lateral flexion of the neck and angulation of the gantry.

Section thickness (Fig. 1.5)

The choice of section thickness is governed by two opposing factors. Firstly, the thinner the section, the more homogeneous

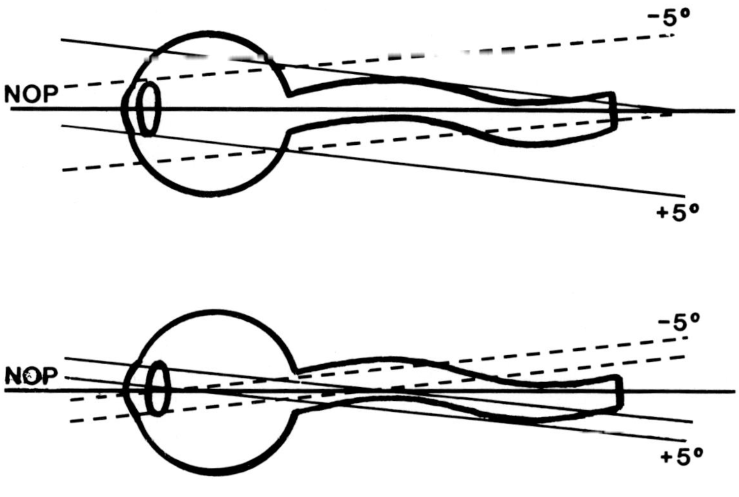

Fig. 1.5 The effects of section thickness on images of a normally undulating optic nerve. (Top) 13-mm sections; (bottom) 3-mm sections, correctly centred on the optic nerve head, but with +5° (solid lines) or −5° (dotted lines) angulation to the neuro-ocular plane (NOP). Even with this slight degree of angulation, much of the optic nerve is excluded from the thin sections. The disadvantage of the 13-mm sections is the inclusion of a relatively large proportion of orbital fat in the sections which demonstrate the nerve.

the voxel, and therefore the more truly representative the pixel. Thus, if a scan of the orbits is carried out using a section thickness of 13 mm, the optic nerve will occupy considerably less than half the height of the section; the pixels which show it will therefore represent more than 50% orbital fat. If the thickness is reduced to 3–5 mm, the section which passes through the equator of the nerve will have voxels composed almost entirely of optic nerve. Secondly, to obtain such thin sections in which the attenuation coefficients are reliable, it is necessary to increase the radiation dose. The principal reason for this is that in thin sections the electronic 'noise' is increased. Also, the shape of the section is such that, if small volumes of tissue are not to be excluded from adjacent sections these must overlap slightly, and with thinner sections this overlap is proportionately more significant.

It is therefore desirable to use the thickest section which will not degrade the anatomical detail or diagnostic potential of the CT examination. Section thickness of 3–5 mm for the orbits, 5–8 mm for the sellar region and 10–13 mm for the cerebrum would appear to represent suitable compromises.

Such thin sections can be 'piled up' by the computer, and sections in other planes reconstructed. In this way, sagittal images can be obtained, which although inferior in quality to direct sagittal sections, are nevertheless of diagnostic utility in the orbit and, particularly, the parasellar region.

Radiation dosage with most CT scanners is comparable to that resulting from plain radiographs, and considerably less than that from conventional multidirectional tomography. Furthermore, it is not spread over a wide area. However, the most radiosensitive structure in the orbit is the lens, and this cannot be excluded from many of the sections. A substantial reduction in dose (of the order of 85%) can however be achieved using translate-rotate machines if it is ensured that the X-ray tube passes across the back of the head, so that the lens is exposed to an already attenuated beam. Some translate-rotate scanners, e.g. the EMI CT 1010 and 5005 machines, have the tube above the patient, but in such cases the scan can be carried out, without considerable extra difficulty, with the patient lying prone; some modification to the head-rest may be helpful (i.e. a slit to accommodate the nose). The prone position is probably preferable in cases of proptosis, since displacement of the globe may then be maximal. In some patients a Valsalva manoeuvre sustained during the scan may also render pathological changes more apparent (e.g. orbital varices).

Contrast media as adjuncts to CT

There is little or no evidence that the use of intravenous iodinated contrast media adds to the detection rate in CT examinations (Moseley, 1977), apart from in certain well-recognized conditions, such as recent cerebral infarction and arteriovenous malformations. The injection of contrast medium adds to the discomfort, risk, duration, radiation dose and overall cost of the study. Nevertheless, there is no doubt that the *differential diagnostic yield* and *anatomical information* are substantially increased by the use of intravenous contrast medium. This is particularly true of intracranial disorders, where disturbances of the blood–brain barrier produce a higher concentration of contrast medium in the abnormal tissues. In the orbit, however, the blood–brain barrier is insignificant and contrast medium provides a lower diagnostic yield and is less useful in differential diagnosis.

From the foregoing it is evident that intravenous contrast media should be used whenever necessary, but that *routine*, pre- and post-contrast medium scans are not essential, particularly when the orbit is being examined. Specific indications will be indicated in the following chapters.

REFERENCES

Gawler, J., Sanders, M.D., Bull, J.W.D., du Boulay, G. and Marshall, J. (1974), Computer assisted tomography in orbital disease. *Br. J. Ophthal.*, **58** (6), 571–87.

Moseley, I.F. (1977), The use of contrast media as an adjunct to CT scanning. *In*: *Computer Assisted Tomography*, (ed. W.J. Kuhler), Exerpta Medica, Amsterdam, pp.26–45.

Van Damme, W., Kosmann, P. and Wackenheim, C. (1977), A standardized method for computed tomography of the orbits. *Neuroradiology*, **13**, 139–40.

2 · Anatomy

2.1 THE ORBIT (Tadmor and New, 1978) (Fig. 2.1)

The orbital walls

The medial wall of the orbit, the lamina papyracea, is extremely thin and is formed largely by the ethmoid bone, which is normally slightly convex towards the orbit. Loss of this convexity may suggest expansion of the orbit. Despite the ease with which the thin bone is displaced, it does not show the defects due to absorptive changes which may be seen in the orbital roof in later life. Anteriorly, the lacrimal fossa may be identified as a rounded depression in the medial wall about 5 mm deep, bounded by the anterior and posterior lacrimal crests.

The lateral wall is thicker than the medial, particularly anteriorly and in its mid portion. The orbit expands behind the thick orbital rim and is widest about 1.5 cm behind its margin, with a focal expansion superolaterally accommodating the lacrimal gland. The superior orbital fissure is seen as a defect in the superomedial part of the lateral wall, while above and medial to this, the medial and lateral walls form the borders of the optic canal, which runs posteromedially at an angle of about 35°; its lateral border is the better defined. Since the optic canal is only about 5 mm in diameter, precision is necessary in obtaining the CT section which passes exactly through it, and the superior orbital fissure may be mistaken for the canal. The anterior clinoid process, which lies above it, may obscure visualization of the canal, but the latter may be seen if the window width and level are adjusted.

Neither the short floor nor the roof of the orbit can be assessed adequately in axial sections. It is important to note the irregularity of the latter in relation to the frontal cerebral convolutions; this may cause it to appear discontinuous or to show as isolated areas of high attenuation which appear to lie within the frontal lobes. The floor is traversed in the anteroposterior direction by the infraorbital sulcus and canal, which may also produce apparent discontinuity. The floor slopes downwards from the medial to the lateral side, so that in sections through the inferior part of the orbit, the subjacent maxillary antrum may appear to bulge into the orbit from the medial aspect. These features are well demonstrated on coronal scans.

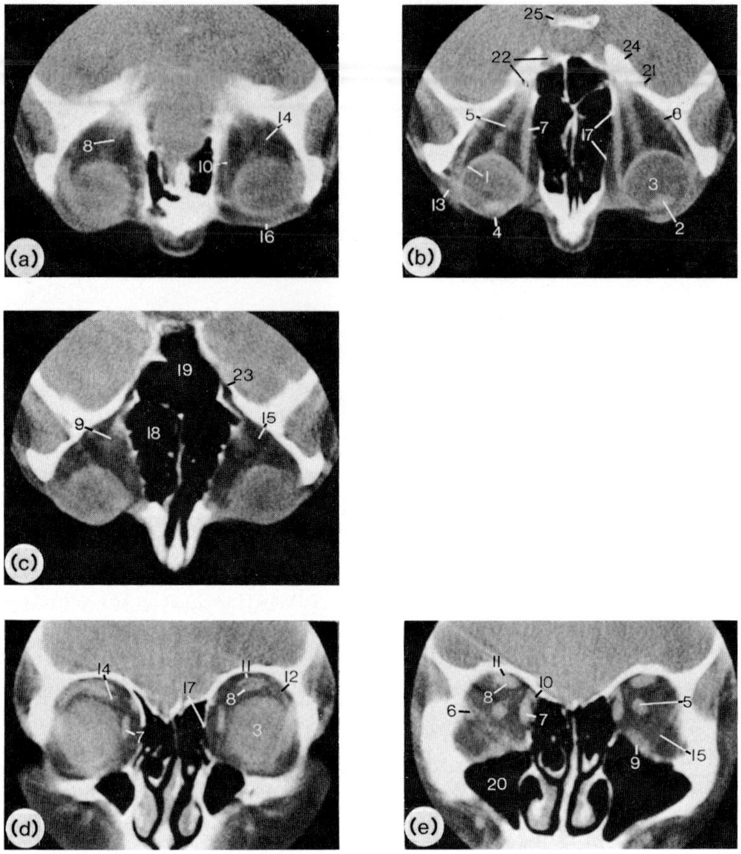

Fig. 2.1 Normal orbits. (a, b, c) Upper, mid-orbit and lower axial sections; (d, e) anterior and retrobulbar coronal sections. (1) Dense outer layer of globe, formed principally by sclera; (2) lens; (3) vitreous; (4) anterior chamber; (5) optic nerve; (6) lateral rectus muscle; (7) medial rectus muscle; (8) superior rectus muscle; (9) inferior rectus muscle; (10) superior oblique muscle; (11) levator palpebrae superioris muscle; (12) intermuscular septum; (13) lacrimal gland; (14) superior ophthalmic vein; (15) orbital fat; (16) eyelid; (17) lamina papyracea; (18) ethmoid sinuses; (19) sphenoid sinuses; (20) maxillary antrum; (21) region of superior orbital fissure; (22) optic canal; (23) inferior orbital fissure; (24) anterior clinoid process; (25) dorsum sellae.

The globe and optic nerve

The eye occupies only about 20% of the volume of the orbit. Its normal position can be defined in the axial plane relative to a line passing between the lateral orbital margins on either side. However, minor asymmetry of positioning in the scanner, or of the face, can cause considerable variation in the apparent position of the globe, so that CT measurement of proptosis is of limited value. The equatorial diameter of the eye in the anteroposterior plane is between 21–26 mm, the transverse and vertical diameters varying between 23–25 mm, while at birth the anteroposterior diameter is 16–17 mm. A fine high attenuation line is seen around the globe, to which the sclera is probably the main contributor. The lens lies between a small area of lower attenuation anteriorly, representing the anterior chamber and the slightly higher attenuation of the main portion of the globe, representing the vitreous. The lens is approximately 3.5 × 6.5 mm in size in newborn infants and 4.5 × 9.0 mm in adults. There is considerable variation in size and shape during accommodation, and the posterior surface is relatively flattened.

The optic nerve runs backwards and medially in the orbit at an angle of about 35° to the sagittal plane, passing posteriorly from the globe to the optic canal. In the primary position, the optic nerve head lies 3 mm medial to the posterior pole of the eye (and just above it), but there is obviously a considerable variation in both the position and form of the optic nerves depending on the direction of gaze (Fig. 2.2). When the nerves are found at CT to be asymmetrical in form or position, the location of the lenses may be used as an indicator of the direction of the visual axis. It is also desirable to confirm that the section traverses the plane of lens, optic nerve and optic canal (the 'neuro-ocular plane') on both sides.

Measurement of the size of the optic nerve is complicated by its undulating form, which means that any given axial or coronal CT sections either may not pass through its maximum diameter or may pass obliquely through the nerve, thus increasing its apparent size. Furthermore, significant differences in size may not be detectable without high resolution scans. When coronal scans are under-tilted, as is often the case because of limited extension of the neck, the nerve may be seen lying apparently *above* the globe. Reconstruction of sections is facilitated by more recent machines (Fig. 2.3).

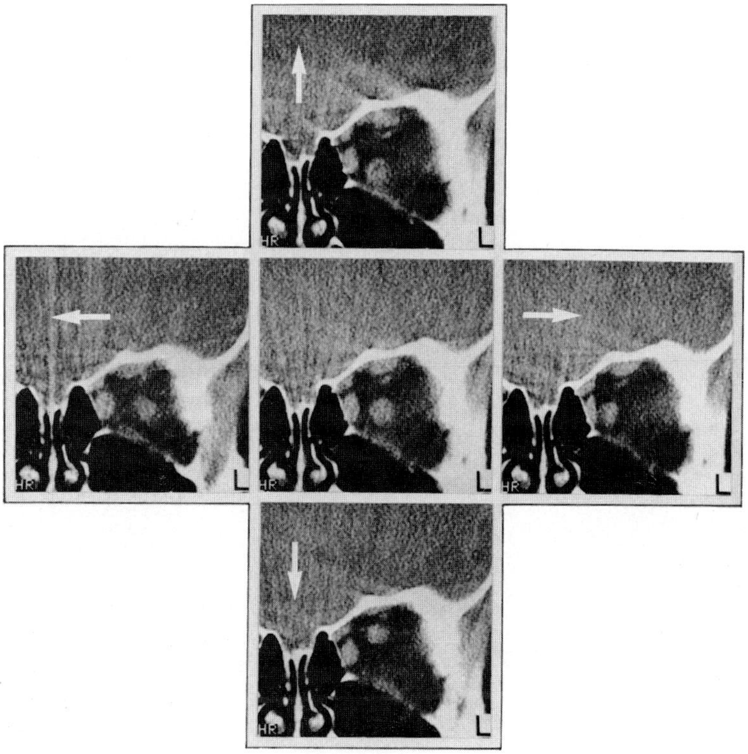

Fig. 2.2 Variations in optic nerve position and extraocular muscles with voluntary eye movements. Coronal sections: (Centre) primary position. Gaze direction indicated by arrows. Note (1) optic nerve does not enter inferolateral portion of orbit; (2) variations in muscle bulk: compare levator palpebrae and superior rectus in upgaze and downgaze, or medial rectus in abduction and adduction.

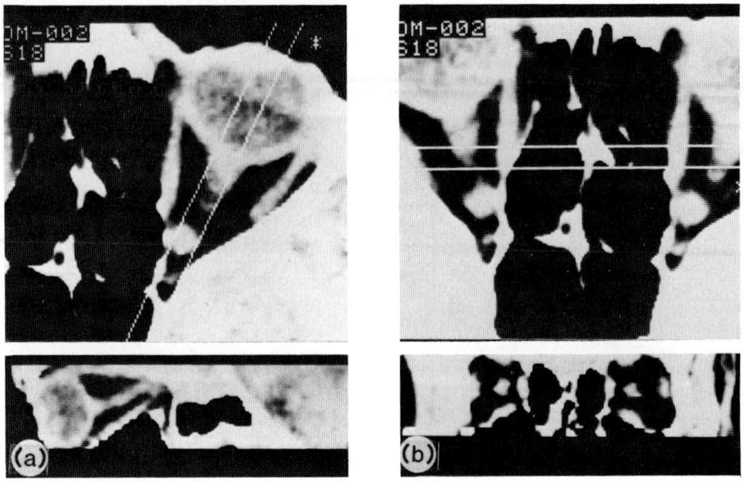

Fig. 2.3 Paraxial (a) and coronal (b) reconstruction of normal orbits from 1½ mm axial sections.

Magadur (quoted by Salvolini *et al.*, 1978) proposed a neuro-ocular index, obtained by dividing the width of the optic nerve at the midpoint of its orbital course by the width of the globe at its equator, expressing the result as a percentage. However, the normal range varies from 12–18, so that minor differences cannot be detected; furthermore, although such indices compensate for magnification and for individual variation, they compound errors in mensuration. The mean diameter of the optic nerve as assessed at CT is 3.6 mm, the normal range being from 2.4–4.3 mm. The optic nerve varies in length from 35–55 mm and can be divided into an intraocular portion (1.0 mm), intra-orbital (25 mm), intracanalicular (4–10 mm) and intracranial (10 mm).

In axial cuts, the superior rectus muscle may be confused with the subjacent optic nerve; however, it appears to fade out anteriorly, and does not join the posterior surface of the globe.

Measurement of attenuation coefficients in the orbit are rendered difficult by the small size of the structures involved. This is indicated by the results of Salvolini and his co-workers (1978) who found the range of attenuation coefficients corresponding to the optic nerve to be −10 to +19 EMI units. These figures clearly indicate the effects of a variable amount of low attenuation orbital fat in each voxel.

The extraocular muscles

The four rectus muscles arise from the tendinous annulus of Zinn at the orbital apex, encircling the orbital end of the optic canal and the medial portion of the superior orbital fissure. The vertical rectus muscles are projected at an angle of 23° with the sagittal diameter of the globe.

The medial rectus is the largest of the four (41 mm long) and arises from the annulus and the medial parts of the superior and inferior orbital tendons. At its tendinous insertion to the globe it is approximately 1 cm across. Between these two points it runs forward, parallel with the lamina papyracea, from which it may be seen at CT to be separated by a thin strip of fat. It is the most consistently visualized of the extraocular muscles; without high resolution scans, it cannot usually be separated from the proximal portion of the superior oblique.

The lateral rectus (40.5 mm long) arises from a curved origin, comprising the annulus and the lateral ends of the superior and inferior orbital tendons, and runs along the lateral border of the orbit, from which it is separated anteriorly by fat and the lacrimal gland. It is slightly smaller than the medial rectus.

The superior rectus (41 mm long) arises from the annulus and superior orbital tendon immediately below the levator palpebrae superioris. On axial scans it is poorly distinguished from the latter, but on good quality coronal scans a thin low-attenuation line representing fat separates the rectus from the wider and thinner levator above. As noted previously, the superior rectus should not be mistaken for the optic nerve in axial sections.

The inferior rectus muscle (40 mm long) is the shortest of the four, and, although usually visible on axial cuts as a rather broad, featureless mass just above the orbital floor, it is often rather poorly defined on coronal sections.

The superior oblique muscle is the longest of the extraocular muscles, comprising a direct portion to the trochlea of 40 mm, and an indirect portion from the trochlea to the point of insertion on the globe of 20 mm. On axial scans it can sometimes be identified running forwards above the medial rectus, while on coronal scans the distinction between the two muscles is usually clear. The indirect portion is poorly defined, passing posterolaterally beneath the distal portion of the superior rectus and becoming tendinous 10 mm behind the trochlea.

The inferior oblique muscle also runs posterolaterally from a short tendon attached to a shallow depression in the orbital plate of the maxilla in the anteromedial corner of the floor of the orbit. It is rarely seen clearly.

The levator palpebrae superioris lies just below the roof of the orbit, separating it from the superior rectus, as noted above.

Orbital fat

Fat is of lower attenuation than water and this results in excellent visualization of the orbital structures at CT, because of the high contrast between them and the fat.

The orbital fat is divided into two portions: that within the cone formed by the four recti, and that outside it. This division is reinforced by the intermuscular septum, which may be seen on

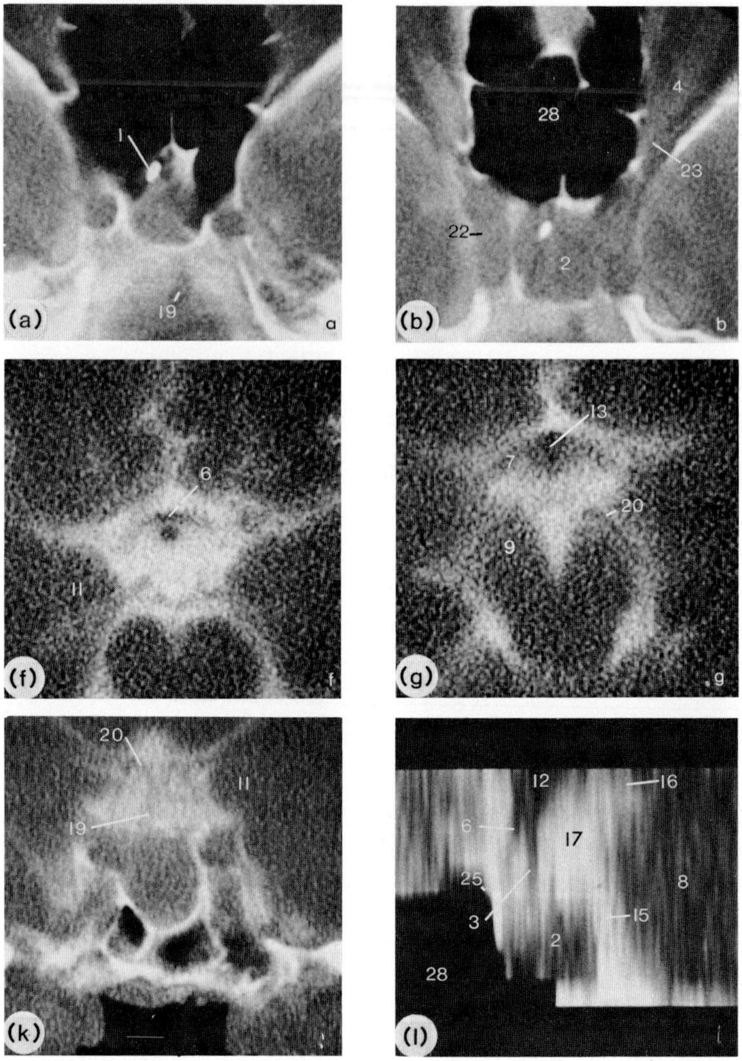

Fig. 2.4 Sellar region. This young woman presented with infertility and galactorrhoea; she was found to have marked hyperprolactinaemia and an expanded sella turcica. Despite implantation of yttrium seeds and treatment with bromocryptine, the hyperprolactinaemia persisted. Metrizamide CT cisternography was carried out prior to operation, showing that there was no suprasellar tumour (a–h: axial sections from base to pituitary fossa to third ventricle; i–k: coronal sections through pituitary fossa; l: computer reconstruction of midline sagittal section, from axial sections). (1) Yttrium seed, at base of sella, near the midline, i.e. very eccentrically placed in pituitary gland (2); (3) infundibulum (note central low attenuation corresponding to infundibular recess, in (e); (4) orbital portion of optic nerve; (5) intracranial optic nerve; (6) chiasm; (7) optic tract; (8) pons; (9) cerebral peduncle; (10) frontal lobe (gyrus rectus); (11) temporal lobe (uncus); (12) third ventricle; (13) chiasmatic recess; (14) cerebellopontine angle cistern; (15) pontine cistern; (16) interpeduncular fossa; (17) chiasmatic cistern; (18) ambient cistern; (19) basilar artery; (20) posterior cerebral artery (lying in crural cistern); (21) internal carotid artery; (22) position of cavernous sinus; (23) orbital opening of optic canal; (24) cranial opening of optic canal; (25) tuberculum sellae; (26) anterior clinoid process; (27) dorsum sellae; (28) sphenoid sinus. Note also a depression in the upper surface of the tumour (arrows in (c) and (i)), possibly the result of involution due to radiotherapy.

coronal sections as a fine white line, often apparently incomplete, joining the rectus muscles.

A further membrane covers the anterior surface of the globe and muscle cone; fat anterior to this is limited by the fine orbital septum. The anterior component may be augmented in proptosis, due to herniation of fat through the 'orifices adipeux' of Charpy in the intervening membrane. Anterior to the orbital septum, and often rendering it invisible at CT, are the eyelids. Occasionally, small zones of greatly reduced attenuation representing tiny air bubbles may be seen between the globe and the eyelids.

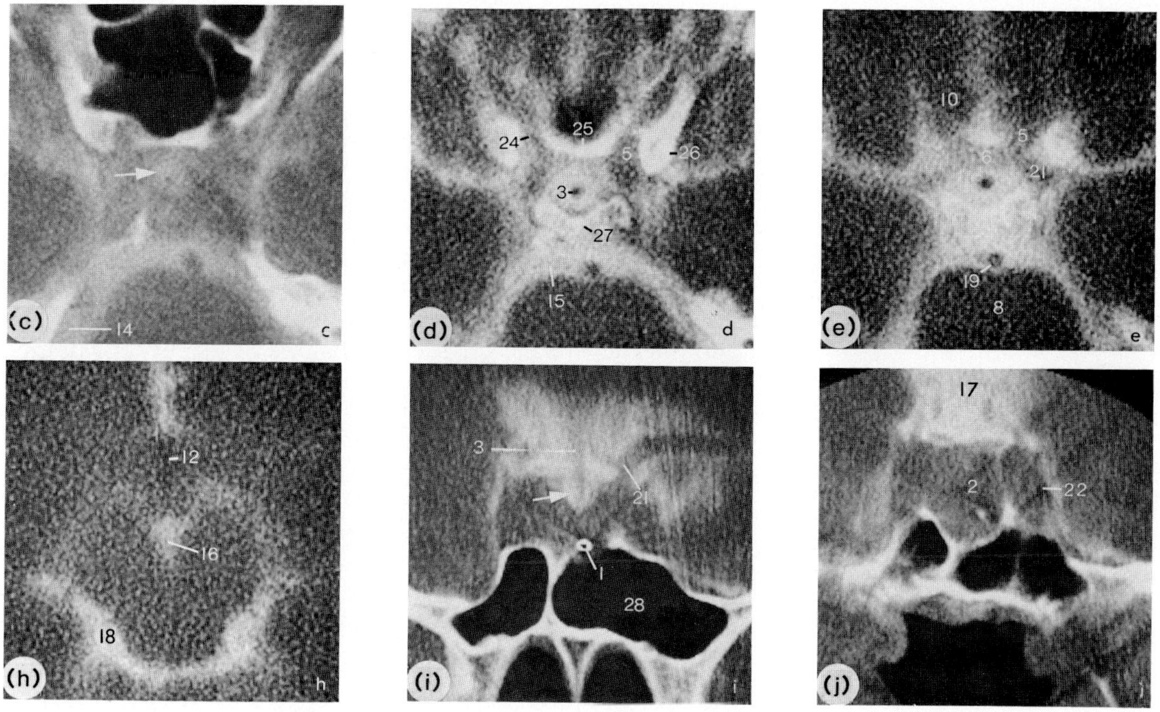

Other intraorbital structures

The superior ophthalmic vein can be seen in many normal cases, lying just above the optic nerve. It runs posterolaterally, and then turns more medially towards the medial end of the superior orbital fissure. Less frequently, the ophthalmic artery can be seen as a fine linear structure winding around the proximal portion of the optic nerve. Both these structures are seen more consistently and with greater clarity following intravenous contrast medium.

The lacrimal gland is often seen, but rarely clearly defined, as a soft tissue attenuation area overlying the insertion of the lateral rectus muscle.

2.2 THE SELLAR REGION (Fig. 2.4)

The region of the seall turcica is of extreme interest in neuro-ophthalmology, not only because the optic chiasm lies directly above the sella, but also because many different pathological processes arise specifically in this region, giving rise to visual sensory or ocularmotor disturbances.

The sella turcica lies above and behind the sphenoid sinus, the exact relationship varying between individuals. It is bounded posteriorly by the dorsum sellae, which may also be pneumatized. Anterolaterally on either side lie the anterior clinoid processes, which, if the head is slightly tilted to one side, may simulate a dense lesion. The contents of the sella are of the same attenuation values as brain tissue, but these values may be masked in thick CT sections by the air in the sphenoid sinus below, and the cerebrospinal fluid in the cisterns above.

The subarachnoid cisterns

Directly above the sella turcica lies the chiasmatic cistern, which is continuous behind with the interpenduncular cistern. The visibility of the former at CT depends on its size, and the plane and thickness of the CT section. Failure to identify the normal cisterns on overlapping sections of the suprasellar region in a patient with a clinical suspicion of chiasmal compression is strongly suggestive of a lesion in this situation.

The classical form of the interpenduncular fossa (which is not however seen in every case, but depends on the individual anatomy and the plane of section) is a pentagon, the base of which is formed by the anterior surface of the brain stem (pons and/or cerebral peduncles), the lower lateral border by the medial surface of the uncus, and the concave upper lateral border by the posterior extremity of the gyrus rectus on either side. Potentially visible within the cisterns are the following:

1. The pituitary stalk, as a small central point of soft tissue density.
2. The mamillary bodies, as paired paramedian soft tissue structures.
3. The optic chiasm, as a thin transverse band of soft tissue.

With intravenous contrast medium, a variable portion of the circle of Willis and its major branches becomes visible; the middle cerebral artery may be seen as far laterally as its trifurcation. It should be noted that the vessels which encircle the brain stem represent both the posterior cerebral and superior cerebellar arteries and their accompanying veins. The cavernous sinuses, which are paired and seen on either side of the sella, show considerable increase in attenuation, but are less clearly defined than the other vessels.

2.3 THE RETROCHIASMAL OPTIC PATHWAYS

The optic tract is rarely identified as it passes posterolaterally between the uncus and the cerebral peduncle, unless the tract is thickened as by an infiltrative glioma. The tract may also be rendered visible by contrast opacification of the cerebrospinal fluid (Fig. 2.5).

From the optic tract 80% of the fibres pass to the lateral geniculate body and the remainder to the superior corpora quadrigemina and pretectal region. Recognition of these synaptic

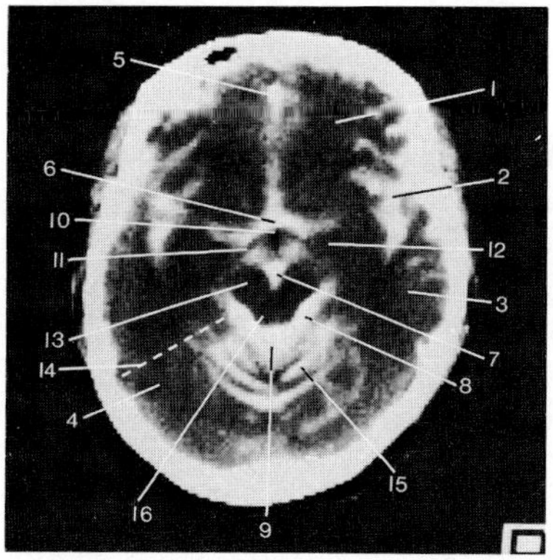

Fig. 2.5 Metrizamide cisternogram, midcranial section showing cerebral anatomy. (1) Frontal lobe, separated by (2) Sylvian fissure, from (3) temporal lobe; (4) occipital lobe; (5) interhemispheric fissure; (6) chiasmatic cistern; (7) interpeduncular fossa; (8) ambient cistern; (9) quadrigeminal cistern; (10) optic chiasm; (11) optic tract, running between (12) uncus of temporal lobe and (13) cerebral peduncle; (14) position of tentorium; (15) cerebellar sulci; (16) tectum of midbrain – quadrigeminal plate.

areas is easier than recognition of the tracts. Thus, the former is seen as a slight prominence on the posterolateral aspect of the pulvinar of the thalamus, projecting into the lateral portion of the wing of the ambient cistern, while the latter appears as a paired swelling on either side of the midline on the posterior surface of the mesencephalon. Although the nuclei of the superior corpora quadrigemina are larger than those of the inferior, the latter are more prominent; it is difficult to be sure which pair is in the plane of the section.

From the lateral geniculate bodies, the visual radiations pass through the posterior limb of the internal capsule, which is clearly visible as a fine band of relatively low attenuation between the thalamus medially and the lentiform nucleus laterally. Their course to the cortex represents a continuum, though the vertical positioning allows clinical separation into two main fibre bundles: an upper, which runs directly to the visual cortex, and a lower, which passes around the temporal horn of the lateral ventricle and beneath the occipital horn, before also arriving in the striate cortex. These fibre tracts are not identifiable *per se* at CT, but form part of the deep, periventricular, cerebral white matter (Fig. 2.6).

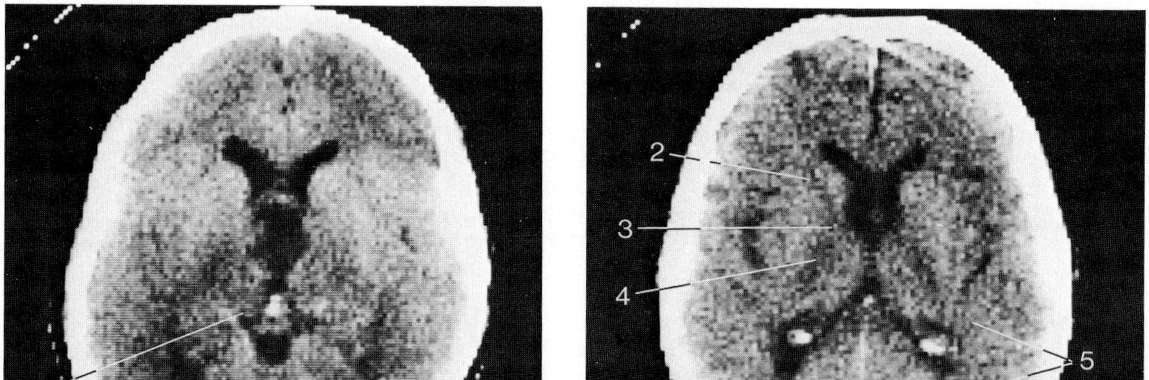

Fig. 2.6 Postchiasmal optic pathways. (1) Position of lateral geniculate body (patient with craniopharyngioma); (2) anterior limb; (3) genu and (4) posterior limb of internal capsule; (5) deep white matter, including radiations; (6) occipital cortex; (7) occipital horn of lateral ventricle.

The primary visual cortex, Brodman's area 17, occupies the medial aspect of the occipital lobe above, below and in the depths of the calcarine fissure. A small and variable extension around the occipital pole is important because it represents the cortical projection of the macula. The remaining fibres project topographically, so that the anterior part of the striate cortex represents the peripheral field. The fissure is angled forwards and upwards, so that in those cases in which the plane of section does not correspond with the plane of the fissure, the macular area tends to be shown on a lower section than the more anterior peripheral field.

The latter point was emphasized by McAuley and Ross Russell (1977), who sectioned cadaver brains in 13-mm slices in the plane usually employed for CT scanning. They found that the region they took to represent the striate cortex was present in at least two sections, and sometimes in as many as four. The section passing through the pineal gland generally contained the greatest length of the calcarine fissure. These workers noted however, that there is considerable variation between individuals, and even between the two hemispheres in a given subject. The boundaries of the visual cortex can only be loosely inferred from the CT images (Salamon, Lecaque, Hall and Corbaz, 1974). Questions are often best resolved by consideration of pathological cases, and the reader is referred to the section on the occipital lobe in Chapter 4.

It is important to note than in the planes customarily employed for CT, the two occipital lobes are separated by the tentorium cerebelli, with the medial portions of the superior cerebellar cistern and the superior vermis below. This separation is often considerably reduced in postmortem specimens, and the apex of the tentorium may reach as high as the pineal gland. The plane of the tentorium is sufficiently oblique to the CT section for the tentorium itself to be invisible in most cases, though after intravenous contrast medium it is frequently seen. In the section which passes through the quadrigeminal cistern, the tentorium runs posterolaterally from the lateral portion of the cistern at an angle of approximately 45°.

REFERENCES

McAuley, D.L.F. and Ross Russell, R.W. (1977), Vascular disease of the visual radiations and cortex. *In*: *First European Seminar on Computerised Axial Tomography in Clinical Practice*. (eds. G.H. Du Boulay and I.F. Moseley), Springer, Berlin, pp.243–8.

Salamon, G., Lecaque, G., Hall, K. and Corbaz, J.M. (1977), CAT scanning: correlation with vascular and topographical anatomy. *In*: *First European Seminar on Computerised Axial*

Tomography in Clinical Practice. (eds. G.H. Du Boulay and I.F. Mosely). Springer, Berlin, pp.17–23.

Salvolini, U., Cabanis, E.A., Rodallec, A., Menichelli, F., Pasquini, U. and Iba-Zizen, M.T. (1978), Computed tomography of the optic nerve. Part I: Normal results. *J. Comput. Assist. Tomogr.* **2**, 141–9.

Tadmor, R. and New, P.F.J. (1978), Computed tomography of the orbit with special emphasis on coronal sections. Part 1: Normal anatomy. Part 2: Pathological anatomy. *J. Comput. Assist. Tomogr.* **2**, 24–34; 35–44.

3 · Diseases of the orbit

This chapter deals with acquired diseases of the eye, adnexa, orbital and periorbital tissues. Abnormalities of the optic nerve are discussed in Chapter 5, and developmental anomalies in Chapter 7.

Published data on the incidence of orbital conditions reflect the interest and subspecialty of the authors and the nature of their institutions. Thus, ophthalmologists working in paediatric hospitals will produce a different profile from those working in conjunction with a radiotherapy unit or a major neurological hospital. Analysis of published series led Jakobiec and Jones (1979) to the following conclusions concerning the relative frequency of orbital diseases.

Adults	*Children*
1. Cellulitis	1. Capillary haemangioma
2. Sequelae of trauma	2. Dermoid cyst
3. Thyroid ophthalmopathy	3. Cellulitis
4. Pseudotumour	4. Haematoma
5. Lymphoma	5. Pseudotumour
6. Cavernous haemangioma	6. Thyroid ophthalmopathy
7. Lacrimal gland tumour	7. Craniostenosis
8. Peripheral nerve tumour	8. Rhabdomyosarcoma
9. Meningioma	9. Neuroblastoma and sarcoma
10. Mucocoele	10. Leukaemia
11. Metastatic tumour	11. Neurofibroma
	12. Optic nerve glioma

Orbital disease will be considered here under four main headings: 1. inflammatory disease; 2. tumours; 3. vascular lesions, and finally, 4. disorders of the periorbital tissues.

In this and other chapters, traumatic lesions are dealt with only where appropriate in other contexts, for two reasons: firstly, in the acute phase, they are frequently the domain of the ophthalmologist and faciomaxillary surgeon rather than the neuro-ophthalmologist and secondly because, working in a neurological and

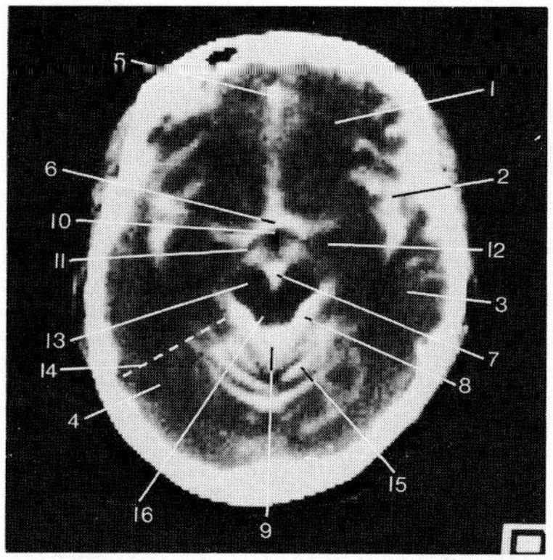

Fig. 2.5 Metrizamide cisternogram, midcranial section showing cerebral anatomy. (1) Frontal lobe, separated by (2) Sylvian fissure, from (3) temporal lobe; (4) occipital lobe; (5) interhemispheric fissure; (6) chiasmatic cistern; (7) interpeduncular fossa; (8) ambient cistern; (9) quadrigeminal cistern; (10) optic chiasm; (11) optic tract, running between (12) uncus of temporal lobe and (13) cerebral peduncle; (14) position of tentorium; (15) cerebellar sulci; (16) tectum of midbrain – quadrigeminal plate.

areas is easier than recognition of the tracts. Thus, the former is seen as a slight prominence on the posterolateral aspect of the pulvinar of the thalamus, projecting into the lateral portion of the wing of the ambient cistern, while the latter appears as a paired swelling on either side of the midline on the posterior surface of the mesencephalon. Although the nuclei of the superior corpora quadrigemina are larger than those of the inferior, the latter are more prominent; it is difficult to be sure which pair is in the plane of the section.

From the lateral geniculate bodies, the visual radiations pass through the posterior limb of the internal capsule, which is clearly visible as a fine band of relatively low attenuation between the thalamus medially and the lentiform nucleus laterally. Their course to the cortex represents a continuum, though the vertical positioning allows clinical separation into two main fibre bundles: an upper, which runs directly to the visual cortex, and a lower, which passes around the temporal horn of the lateral ventricle and beneath the occipital horn, before also arriving in the striate cortex. These fibre tracts are not identifiable *per se* at CT, but form part of the deep, periventricular, cerebral white matter (Fig. 2.6).

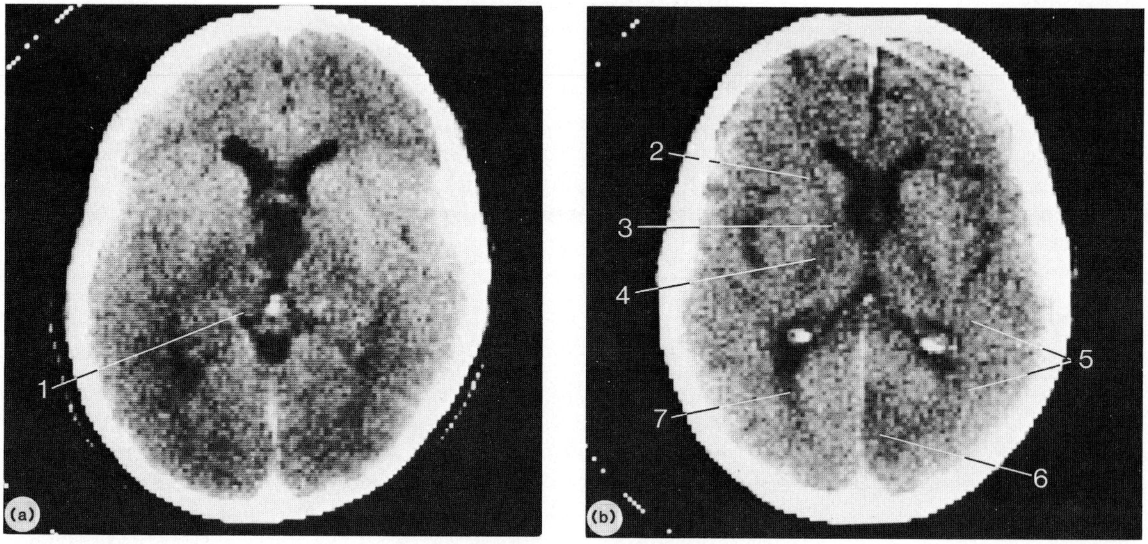

Fig. 2.6 Postchiasmal optic pathways. (1) Position of lateral geniculate body (patient with craniopharyngioma); (2) anterior limb; (3) genu and (4) posterior limb of internal capsule; (5) deep white matter, including radiations; (6) occipital cortex; (7) occipital horn of lateral ventricle.

The primary visual cortex, Brodman's area 17, occupies the medial aspect of the occipital lobe above, below and in the depths of the calcarine fissure. A small and variable extension around the occipital pole is important because it represents the cortical projection of the macula. The remaining fibres project topographically, so that the anterior part of the striate cortex represents the peripheral field. The fissure is angled forwards and upwards, so that in those cases in which the plane of section does not correspond with the plane of the fissure, the macular area tends to be shown on a lower section than the more anterior peripheral field.

The latter point was emphasized by McAuley and Ross Russell (1977), who sectioned cadaver brains in 13-mm slices in the plane usually employed for CT scanning. They found that the region they took to represent the striate cortex was present in at least two sections, and sometimes in as many as four. The section passing through the pineal gland generally contained the greatest length of the calcarine fissure. These workers noted however, that there is considerable variation between individuals, and even between the two hemispheres in a given subject. The boundaries of the visual cortex can only be loosely inferred from the CT images (Salamon, Lecaque, Hall and Corbaz, 1974). Questions are often best resolved by consideration of pathological cases, and the reader is referred to the section on the occipital lobe in Chapter 4.

It is important to note than in the planes customarily employed for CT, the two occipital lobes are separated by the tentorium cerebelli, with the medial portions of the superior cerebellar cistern and the superior vermis below. This separation is often considerably reduced in postmortem specimens, and the apex of the tentorium may reach as high as the pineal gland. The plane of the tentorium is sufficiently oblique to the CT section for the tentorium itself to be invisible in most cases, though after intravenous contrast medium it is frequently seen. In the section which passes through the quadrigeminal cistern, the tentorium runs posterolaterally from the lateral portion of the cistern at an angle of approximately 45°.

REFERENCES

McAuley, D.L.F. and Ross Russell, R.W. (1977), Vascular disease of the visual radiations and cortex. *In*: *First European Seminar on Computerised Axial Tomography in Clinical Practice*. (eds. G.H. Du Boulay and I.F. Moseley), Springer, Berlin, pp.243–8.

Salamon, G., Lecaque, G., Hall, K. and Corbaz, J.M. (1977), CAT scanning: correlation with vascular and topographical anatomy. *In*: *First European Seminar on Computerised Axial*

Tomography in Clinical Practice. (eds. G.H. Du Boulay and I.F. Mosely). Springer, Berlin, pp 17–23

Salvolini, U., Cabanis, E.A., Rodallec, A., Menichelli, F., Pasquini, U. and Iba-Zizen, M.T. (1978), Computed tomography of the optic nerve. Part I: Normal results. *J. Comput. Assist. Tomogr.* **2**, 141–9.

Tadmor, R. and New, P.F.J. (1978), Computed tomography of the orbit with special emphasis on coronal sections. Part 1: Normal anatomy. Part 2: Pathological anatomy. *J. Comput. Assist. Tomogr.* **2**, 24–34; 35–44.

3 · Diseases of the orbit

This chapter deals with acquired diseases of the eye, adnexa, orbital and periorbital tissues. Abnormalities of the optic nerve are discussed in Chapter 5, and developmental anomalies in Chapter 7.

Published data on the incidence of orbital conditions reflect the interest and subspecialty of the authors and the nature of their institutions. Thus, ophthalmologists working in paediatric hospitals will produce a different profile from those working in conjunction with a radiotherapy unit or a major neurological hospital. Analysis of published series led Jakobiec and Jones (1979) to the following conclusions concerning the relative frequency of orbital diseases.

Adults	*Children*
1. Cellulitis	1. Capillary haemangioma
2. Sequelae of trauma	2. Dermoid cyst
3. Thyroid ophthalmopathy	3. Cellulitis
4. Pseudotumour	4. Haematoma
5. Lymphoma	5. Pseudotumour
6. Cavernous haemangioma	6. Thyroid ophthalmopathy
7. Lacrimal gland tumour	7. Craniostenosis
8. Peripheral nerve tumour	8. Rhabdomyosarcoma
9. Meningioma	9. Neuroblastoma and sarcoma
10. Mucocoele	10. Leukaemia
11. Metastatic tumour	11. Neurofibroma
	12. Optic nerve glioma

Orbital disease will be considered here under four main headings: 1. inflammatory disease; 2. tumours; 3. vascular lesions, and finally, 4. disorders of the periorbital tissues.

In this and other chapters, traumatic lesions are dealt with only where appropriate in other contexts, for two reasons: firstly, in the acute phase, they are frequently the domain of the ophthalmologist and faciomaxillary surgeon rather than the neuro-ophthalmologist and secondly because, working in a neurological and neurosurgical reference centre, the authors have limited personal experience in this field.

3.1 INFLAMMATORY DISEASE OF THE ORBITS

Endocrine: thyroid eye disease

Thyroid ophthalmopathy is the most common cause of orbital disease and continues to present an interesting enigma to the immunologist. The condition should be considered in any patient with proptosis, monocular elevator palsy, lid lag, unusual ocular movements with tethering, or even when one muscle is limited in action or exhibits reduced saccadic velocity. Hyperthyroidism or Graves' disease represents an immunological stimulation of the thyroid stimulating hormone (TSH) receptors on the thyroid cell membrane. TSH receptors are found on retro-ocular fat cells but it is of interest that no TSH receptors are found in the ocular muscles. Instead, the muscles seem to contain a high concentration of thyroglobulin-antithyroglobulin complexes, which produce the sequence of histological events seen with immune complex disease. This includes muscle injury, histamine release, leucocyte attraction, increased vascular permeability, and the production of glycosaminoglycans by fibroblasts. This inflammatory process finally results in atrophy of muscles. It would appear that two processes occur: (a) myositis and (b) fat and connective tissue proliferation. The ophthalmopathy may be seen with hyperthyroidism, hypothyroidism or normal thyroid function tests, and the clinician's antennae should be tuned to the detection of other autoimmune diseases such as myasthenia gravis, pernicious anaemia, diabetis mellitus, vitiligo etc.

Diagnosis of thyroid disease

The diagnosis of thyroid disease depends on clinical suspicion and biochemical tests. The main investigations include measurement of serum T_3 and T_4 and of the thyroid stimulating hormone (TSH) after an intravenous injection of thyrotrophin releasing hormone (TRH). Thyroid antibodies may help to confirm the diagnosis if other tests are negative, though in a small percentage of cases all tests may be negative initially, but become positive later in the disease.

CT is of value diagnostically and furthermore:

1. Serves to exclude an orbital tumour.
2. Confirms thickening of the ocular muscles which, when bilateral, is almost certainly due to thyroid ophthalmopathy.
3. Provides information on the efficacy of therapy, either medical or surgical.

The main finding at CT is enlargement of the extraocular muscles; in severe cases the muscles may be more than 1 cm in

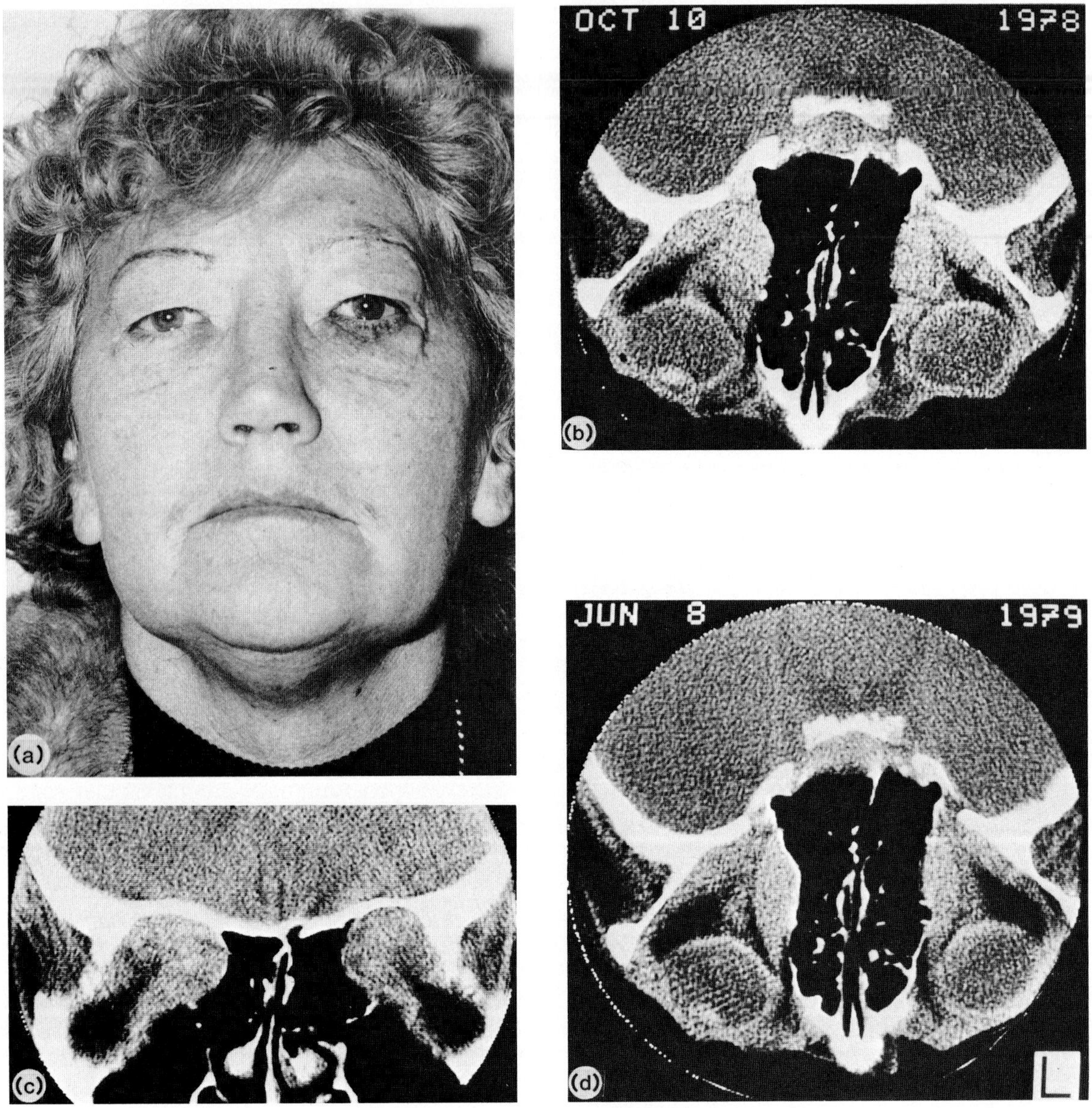

Fig. 3.1 *Thyroid eye disease with visual loss.* This 37-year old woman with known thyroid disease, developed visual loss, which progressed to counting fingers in each eye. The orbits were tense, there was proptosis, and eye movements were limited in all directions (a). CT (10.10.78) showed marked enlargement of the rectus muscles, with expansion of the orbits (b, c). Dramatic clinical improvement followed prednisolone 100 mg/day, with restoration of vision to 6/9 bilaterally in one week. CT (8.6.79) confirmed a reduction in size of the muscles (d) but this was considerably less striking than the clinical recovery; an increase in orbital fat is also demonstrated. (CT (10.10.78) reproduced with kind permission of the Royal Society of Medicine; previously published in the *J. R. Soc. Med., 1980,* **73** (April).

diameter (Fig. 3.1). Most reports have stressed the increased thickness of the rectus muscles, but coronal scans in severely affected patients clearly show thickening of the superior oblique and levator palpebrae superioris muscles in addition. Enzmann *et al*. (1976b) stated that the medial and lateral rectus muscles were the most frequently involved, which is not in accordance with clinical data. However, a subsequent survey of 116 patients by the same workers (Enzmann *et al*., 1979) showed that the inferior rectus was affected in almost 80% of cases, the medial rectus in 75%, and the superior and lateral recti in 50% (Fig. 3.2). The latter muscles also tended to be affected less severely. In 10% of cases, the inferior rectus was the only muscle involved (Fig. 6.37); when more than one muscle was abnormal, the pattern was very variable, but enlargement of all the recti was seen in 30%. These findings were similar to those of Trokel and Hilal (1979).

Unilateral proptosis is a not uncommon finding in Graves' disease. In the series of Enzmann *et al*. (1979), bilateral abnormalities were present at CT in half of the 12% of patients with clinically unilateral involvement, while the corresponding figures for the series of Trokel and Hilal (1979) were 95% of the 43% with apparently unilateral disease. Such a disparity presumably reflects different clinical or CT criteria for abnormality. Nevertheless, the demonstration of bilateral changes in a patient with proptosis of unknown cause makes thyroid disease even more likely.

A small number of patients with normal CT scans will show slight but definite clinical signs, while up to 40% of patients with thyroid disease, but no evidence of ophthalmopathy, have been shown to have abnormal CT studies; however, it is not clear why these patients were examined (Enzmann *et al*., 1979). Nine of the patients with abnormal scans in the series were euthyroid. There was no correlation between the severity of the CT changes and the degree of disturbance of thyroid function or serum antibody concentrations. There was, however, a roughly linear correlation between the size of the medial and inferior recti and the clinical severity of the ophthalmopathy.

The enlargement of the muscles in thyroid disease affects mainly the belly, but is often particularly prominent at the orbital apex, where several thickened muscles apparently become confluent and may simulate a tumour, so that a number of unnecessary diagnostic orbitotomies have been performed. This error should be avoided with improved scans, particularly including coronal sections. Wing *et al.* (1979) found that direct sagittal sections were useful for identifying the superior and, particularly, the inferior rectus muscles, but their results, based on a small population, do not suggest that a real diagnostic benefit accrues from adding a third projection to orbital CT.

Intravenous contrast medium produces marked enhancement

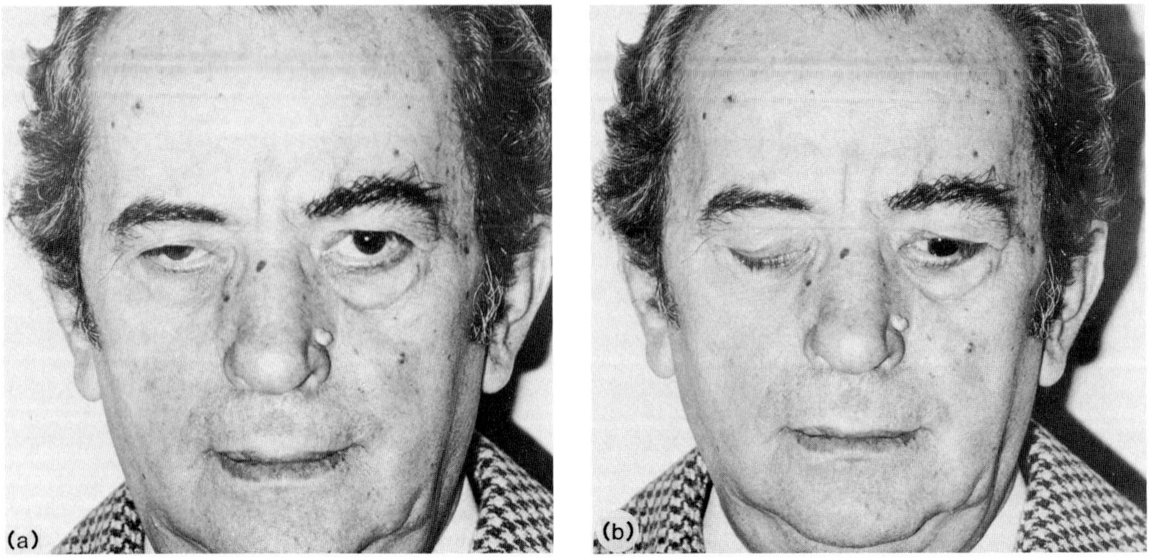

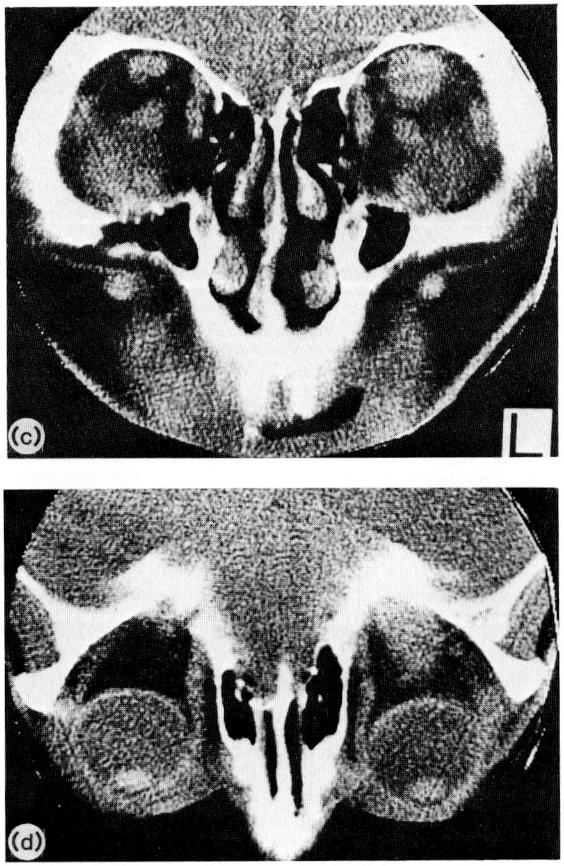

Fig. 3.2 Thyroid eye disease. This 55-year old man gave a three-year history of retraction of the left upper lid (a). There was failure of inhibition of the levator palpebrae on down gaze (b) and eye movements showed impaired elevation with evidence of tethering. TRH and thyroid antibody tests were positive. CT (c, d): there is swelling of the levator palpebrae and/or superior rectus on the left which may be depressing the optic nerve (c).

of the involved muscles. This may indicate hypervascularity, although, unlike the brain, the muscles have no blood–tissue barrier.

Prominence of the lids and fullness of the orbit in thyroid ophthalmopathy are due to prolapse of the orbital fat through the 'orifices adipeux' of Charpy (Chapter 2). This is particularly marked in the superomedial angle of the orbit, where the skin can be seen to be stretched over the extruded, low attenuation fat. The attentuation coefficients of the orbital fat are normally low in thyroid disease, an observation which aids in the distinction from orbital granuloma. In many patients the fat volume appears increased; Enzmann *et al.* (1979) noticed that in these cases the ophthalmopathy was relatively inactive (Fig. 3.3).

The optic nerve may appear elongated and of decreased diameter in severe ophthalmopathy, and these changes are sometimes marked in patients with optic nerve compression and optic atrophy (Fig. 3.3). In patients without evidence of compression, similar appearances probably represent loss of the normal tortuosity of the nerve. Several groups of workers have, however, noted *increased* diameter of the optic nerve; it was found by Trokel and Hilal (1979) to be constant in patients with visual loss, and to occur in 40% of those with corneal ulceration. Swelling of the optic disc in thyroid ophthalmopathy may be associated with reduced vision, and this has been attributed to reduced perfusion of the optic disc and retrolaminar optic nerve, but whether the optic nerve may show axonal, epineural or sheath changes when perfusion is grossly reduced is speculative. There is some evidence from ultrasound studies that apparent enlargement of the nerve represents distension of the dural sheath rather than dilatation of the nerve, possibly due to obstruction of the sheath at the orbital apex (Skalka, 1978). It should be noted, however, that Alper (1979) saw no evidence of optic nerve changes, other than stretching, nor did Enzmann *et al.* (1979) in their much larger series. Early reports of irregular thickening of the nerve were probably due to confusion with adjacent rectus muscles, and partial volume effects.

Chronic gross thickening of the extraocular muscles leads to expansion of the orbits, which may affect not only the thinner portions of the walls, such as the lamina papyracea, but later the roofs and floors, and eventually the normally more resistant lateral walls. Thickening of the muscles in the orbital apex may also produce optic nerve compression with a normal optic disc.

Management of thyroid disease

Management of thyroid ophthalmopathy consists of normalization of the thyroid status and suppression of the immunological response in the orbits by means of steroids, often in very high dosage, supported if necessary by other immunosuppressive

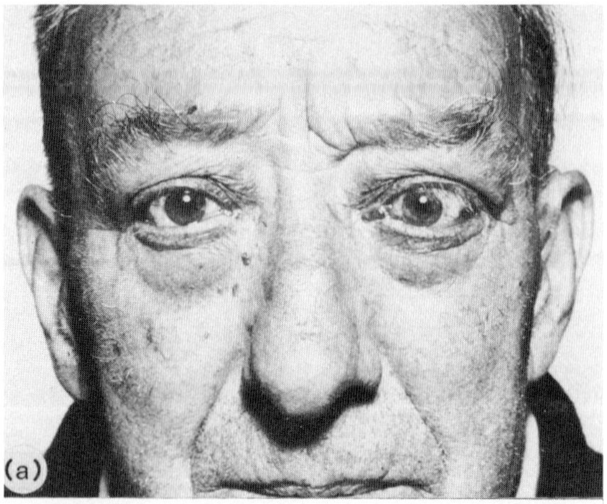

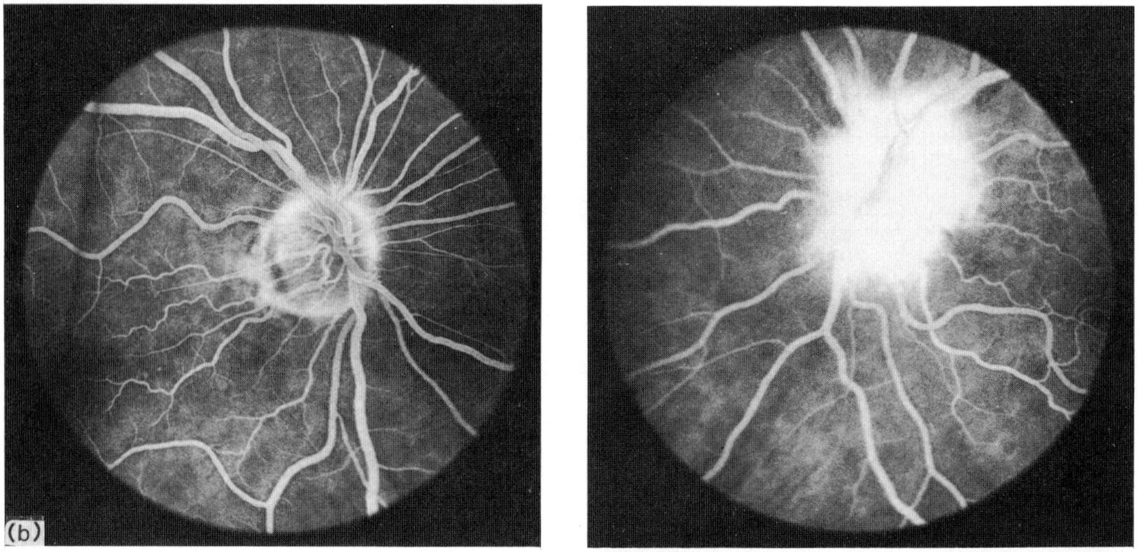

Fig. 3.3 Thyroid ophthalmopathy. A 66-year old man presented with diplopia and orbital discomfort. He had previously been thyrotoxic and become hypothyroid after treatment with radioactive iodine. Recent thyroid tests were normal. The orbits were extremely tense and ocular movements were limited (a). There was visual loss on the left, with disc oedema, confirmed by fluorescein angiography (b). CT showed grossly thickened medial recti, and also an increase in orbital fat (c), especially in the lateral intraconal compartment; the left optic nerve appears displaced medially and may be abnormally thin. This case demonstrates the predominant involvement of the orbital fat in some patients with thyroid ophthalmopathy.

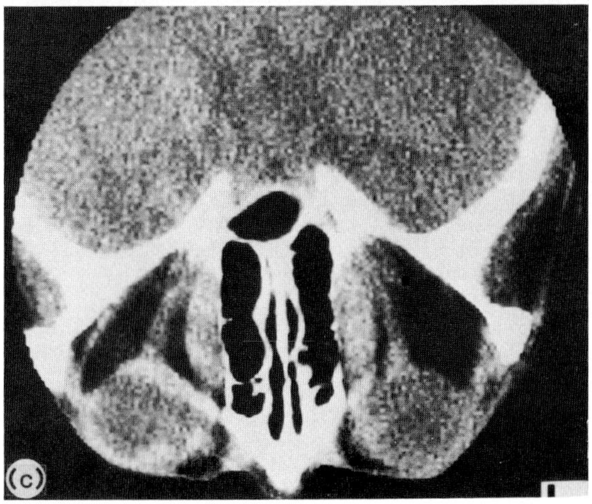

drugs. Some centres use orbital radiotherapy, but the success of medical management has greatly reduced the need for surgical decompression. Serial CT examinations during drug treatment may show reduction in the size of the affected muscles (Fig. 3.1.). Enzmann *et al.* (1979) reported follow-up studies after radiation therapy in 15 patients. Clinical amelioration preceded CT evidence of improvement, and indeed regression of CT changes was discernible only in those with extended follow up.

We have seen one patient with CT changes exactly similar to those of thyroid disease, in whom tests of thyroid function have always been normal (Fig. 3.4).

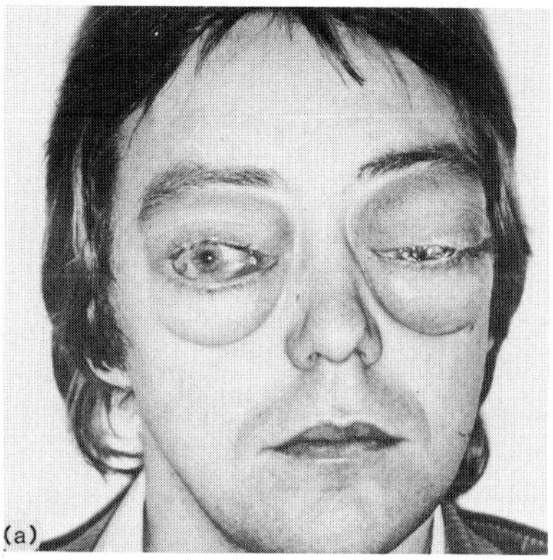

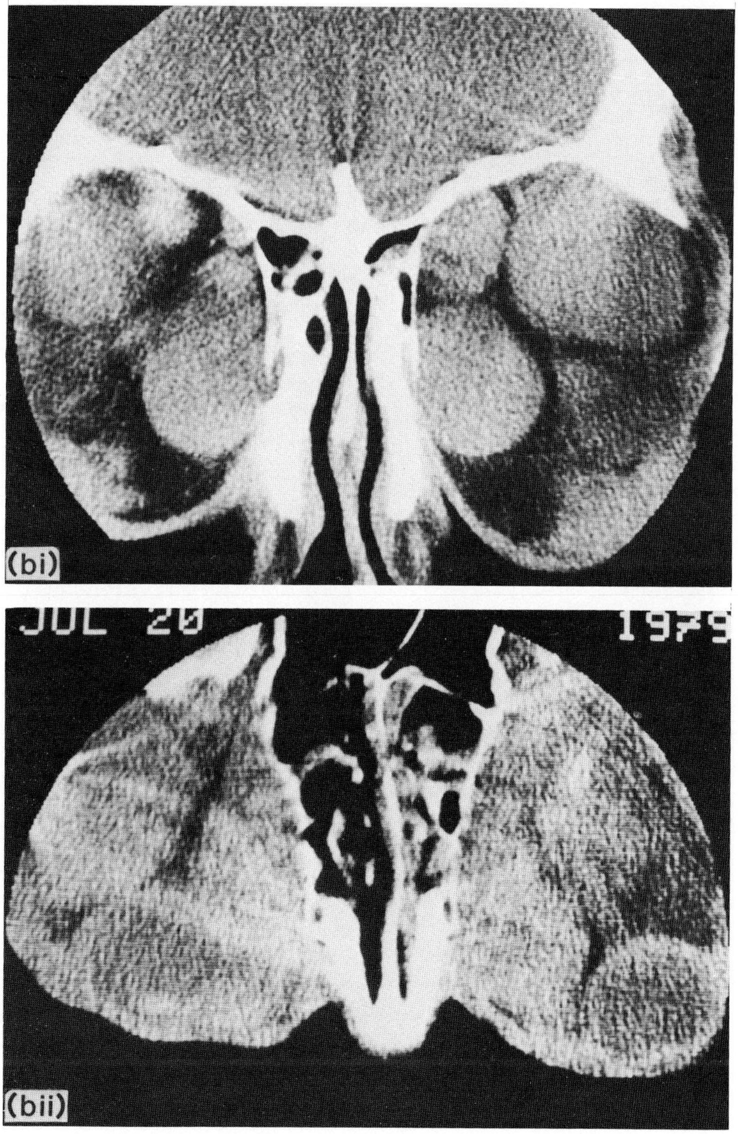

Fig. 3.4 This 23-year old man has had proptosis for 20 years (a); bilateral orbital decompression was carried out during childhood. Extensive investigation has failed to confirm thyroid or any other systemic disease. Vision in the right eye is normal and there is a tarsorrhaphy on the left. (b) CT (1979): gross enlargement of the extraocular muscles; the left superior rectus is about 2.5 cm in diameter. The orbits are markedly expanded, and the left optic nerve appears stretched. (Courtesy of Mr J. Winstanley. Case to be published in detail in the *Br. J. Ophthal.*, 1981).

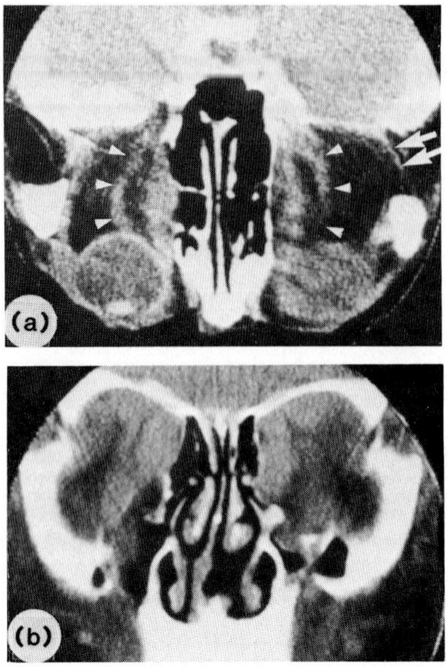

Fig. 3.5 Post-surgical appearances in thyroid ophthalmopathy. (a) After malotemporal decompression; note exuberant orbital fat, predominant enlargement of medial rectus muscles and abnormal course of optic nerves (arrowheads). Double arrows indicate the periorbita. (b) After internal decompression of the left ethmoid and maxillary sinuses.

Surgical decompression may take the form of the classical malotemporal approach (Nafziger's or 'pawnbroker's' operation) or of internal decompression into the ethmoid and maxillary sinuses. The results of these operations can be monitored by CT, and failure of visual improvement can occasionally be demonstrated to result from inadequate decompression of the optic nerve at the orbital apex. When the lateral wall of the orbit has been removed, the periorbita can be seen as a thin line of soft tissue attenuation separating the low-attenuation orbital and extracranial fat (Fig. 3.5). Decompression into the ethmoid and sphenoid sinuses produces maximal relief at the orbital apex and we have experienced gratifying results (Fig. 3.5).

Inflammatory diseases of unknown aetiology

(a) Orbital granuloma (pseudotumour)

The high incidence of granuloma formation within the orbit, as compared with other sites, defies explanation. There is increasing evidence that the granuloma represents a delayed hypersensitivity reaction, a function of T-cell mediated immunity, and diagnostic immunological tests are hopefully to be developed. Orbital involvement may in some cases be associated with other granulomatous lesions, such as retroperitoneal fibrosis, or other systemic diseases such as Wegener's granuloma, polyarteritis nodosa or sarcoidosis. However, the majority of patients with orbital granuloma present, often acutely, with pain, unilateral orbital involvement and ophthalmic signs which are determined by the anatomical site of inflammation. Thus, a spectrum emerges, with anterior involvement (ocular signs, uveitis, scleritis, etc), orbital involvement (painful ophthalmoplegia and proptosis), or with orbital apex problems (ophthalmoplegia and visual loss). The orbital fissure syndrome was first recognized in 1896 by Rochon-Duvigneaud; it is characterized by painful ophthalmoplegia, but visual loss does not occur, as the optic nerve traverses the optic canal, and this serves to differentiate an orbital apex syndrome from a superior orbital fissure syndrome. Painful ophthalmoplegia with paralysis of the III, IV and VI cranial nerves and a reduced corneal response was described in 1954 by Tolosa in a patient with a cavernous sinus syndrome who was shown at necropsy to have granulomatous tissue enveloping the contents of the cavernous sinus. Numerous eponymous titles have been ascribed to lesions of the cavernous sinus, but the clinician may serve his patient with greater clarity by attempting accurate localization based on an understanding of the trigeminal nerve and by pursuing his search for the aetiology. Finally, granulomatous tissue may involve not only the orbital contents, but the orbital fissure, cavernous sinus, intracranial dura and hypophyseal region (Fig. 3.14, p.40).

CT examination shows a spectrum of changes, from those which are scarcely distinguishable from normal to those in which almost none of the normal orbital anatomy can be appreciated.

The extraocular muscles may be involved, with increase in size, and although one muscle is usually affected (Trokel and Hilal, 1979), this is not invariable. However, whereas in thyroid ophthalmopathy, the belly of the muscle is usually the site of maximum expansion, in granulomatous disease the ocular insertion of the muscle is frequently seen to be abnormal. Keane (1977) described one case of 'acute orbital myositis': a 27-year-old woman who presented with a two-week history of acutely painful right proptosis. Examination showed ptosis, decreased ocular movements (especially abduction) and medial conjunctival injection, while CT demonstrated swelling of the right medial rectus, which enhanced with intravenous contrast medium. When the patient returned one month later, complaining of similar symptoms in the other eye, examination showed similar changes, with very limited abduction on the left, while the CT revealed marked swelling of the left medial rectus. We have seen a small number of cases of apparent orbital myositis (Fig. 3.6).

A blurred outline of the extraocular muscles in cases of orbital granuloma is presumably the result of oedema and inflammatory infiltration of the orbital fat and ocular muscles; the same mechanism results in poor definition of the optic nerve. The attenuation coefficients of normal fat are below those of water, so that an increase in water content results in an increase in attenuation coefficients, and not a decrease, as occurs with oedema in highly cellular tissue (Fig. 3.7). The orbital fat may present a slightly spiculated appearance due to abnormal prominence of the fibrous septa. These alterations in the fat, in their mildest form, produce what may be described as a 'dirty orbit', in which the outlines of the major structures are poorly defined, and the contrast between them and the surrounding fat is reduced. When the changes are advanced, however, it may be impossible to distinguish the muscles and optic nerve from the enveloping granulomatous tissue. Orbital granuloma is one of the few conditions in which all anatomical detail within the orbit is lost.

As has been noted above, the optic nerve often appears slightly irregular in outline. The posterior margin of the globe may show thickening which in severe cases also extends more anteriorly. Injection of intravenous contrast medium will produce intense enhancement of this thickened portion of the globe, an observation which may be useful in differential diagnosis (Fig. 3.8).

The lacrimal gland may be enlarged in orbital granuloma, either as a site of primary granulomatous infiltration, or as part of a generalized orbital involvement. The clarity of visualization at CT will depend on the degree of change in the surrounding

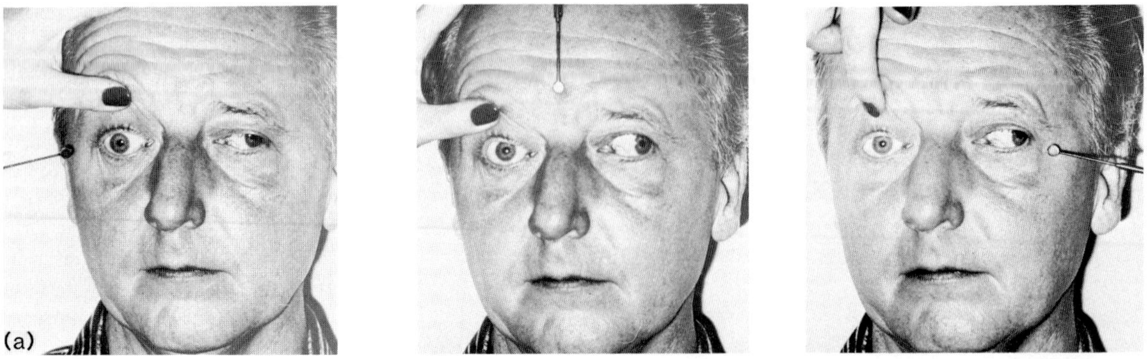

Fig. 3.6 Orbital myositis. This 57-year old man presented with double vision and ptosis, progressing over five years. There was bilateral ptosis, complete on the right, marked divergence of the visual axes and severe limitation of all ocular movements without evidence of tethering (a), gaze to the right (left) up gaze (centre) and to the left (right). Extensive investigations for myasthenia gravis and thyroid disease were negative. A diagnosis of probable orbital myositis was made. CT: The divergent squint is evident (note the position of the lenses and the form of the optic nerves), both medial and possibly lateral recti are thickened (b). On the left, the superior and medial rectus and superior oblique muscles are thickened; there may also be less marked thickening of the rectus muscles on the right (c) coronal cuts.

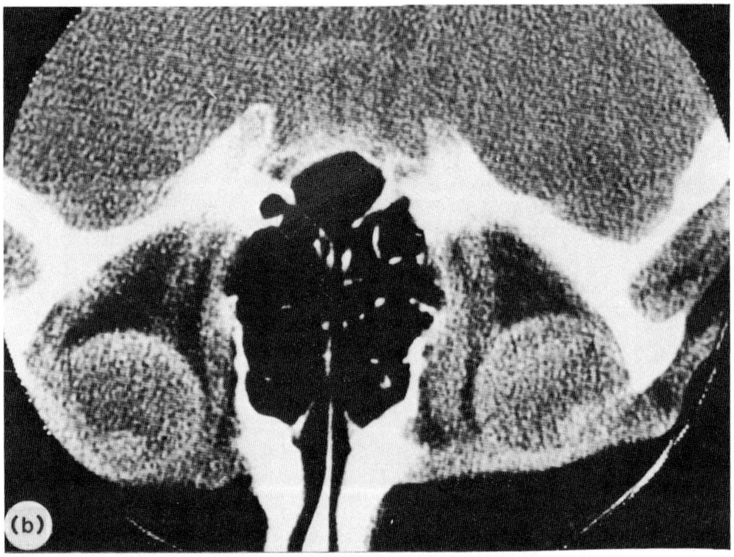

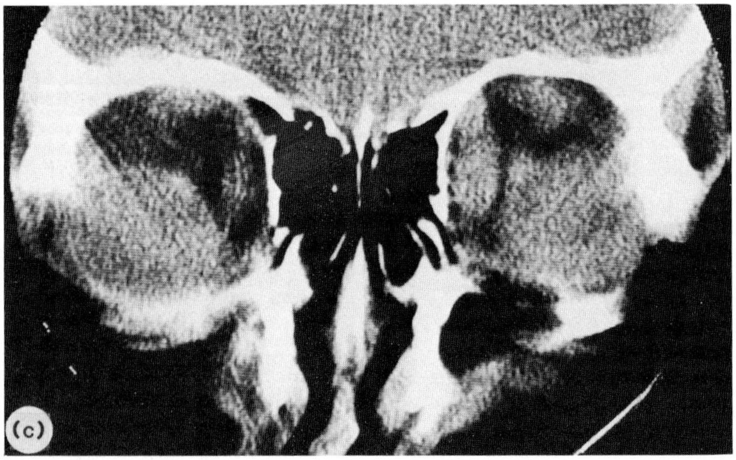

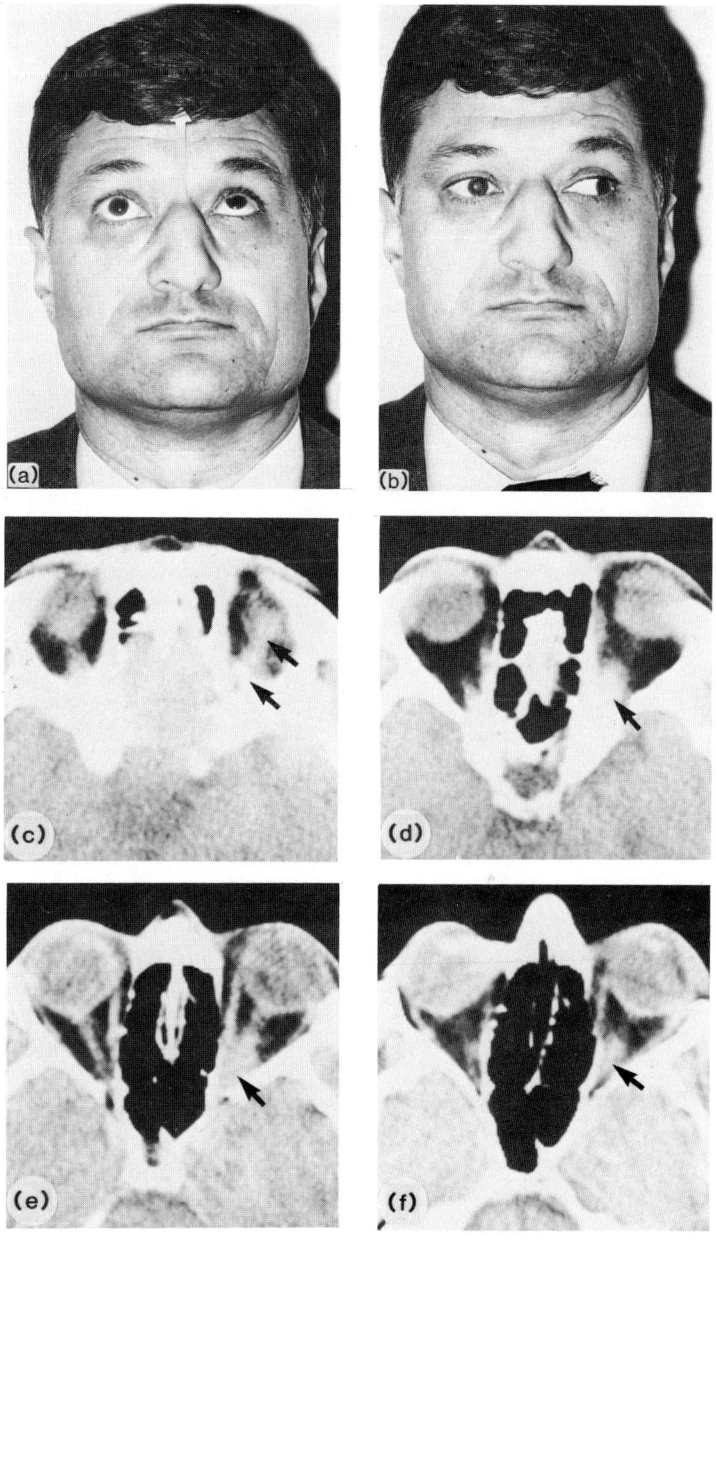

Fig. 3.7 Orbital apex syndrome. A 48-year old man presented with rapid visual loss in the right eye with proptosis and generalized ophthalmoplegia as shown by reduced elevation and left gaze (a, b); corneal sensation was reduced. The diagnosis of an orbital apex lesion was confirmed by CT, demonstrating an amorphous mass (arrows) extending from the level of the superior rectus, which appeared expanded (c) to the inferior rectus (f). The optic nerve is concealed by the lesion (e). Biopsy via the ethmoid sinuses showed non-specific granuloma.

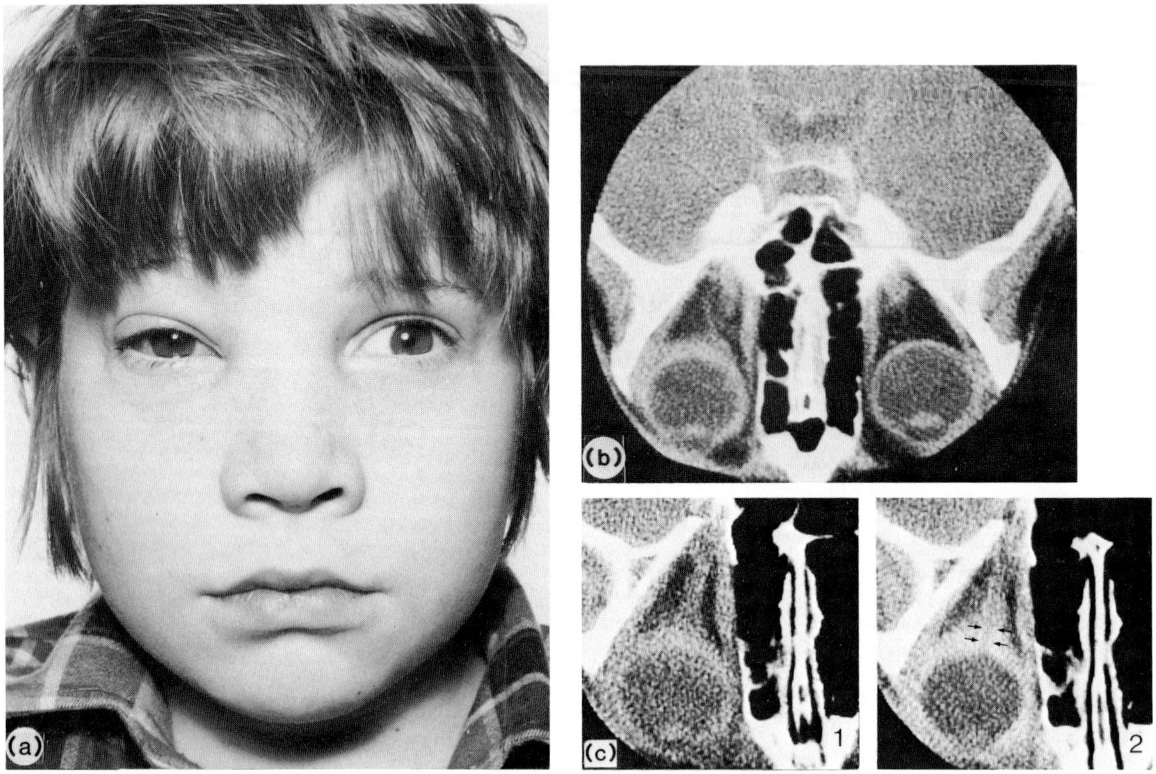

Fig. 3.8 Acute scleritis. A 9-year old boy presented with painful ophthalmoplegia and visual loss. The right orbit was inflamed, tender and the lids were swollen (a). CT (b) showed thickening of the right sclera, most marked posteriorly and some increase in attenuation of the right intraconal fat. The superior ophthalmic vein was prominent (c). There was marked enhancement with intravenous contrast medium (1: before; 2: after injection) involving the globe and the surrounding tissues, including the optic nerve sheath, within which the optic nerve can be seen (arrows).

tissues and enhancement of the lesion may occur after intravenous contrast medium (Fig. 3.9).

As in thyroid eye disease, proptosis and, less commonly, orbital expansion are sometimes present (Fig. 3.10). Thickening of the lid and adjacent tissues may be seen, indicating forward extension of the inflammatory changes.

A classification of orbital granuloma based on CT findings was suggested by Hilal and Trokel (1977):

Group I: swelling of one or more extraocular muscles, with preservation of their normally sharp outlines (25% of their cases) (Fig. 3.11).

Group II: no positive findings other than proptosis and sometimes increased prominence of the sclera (50%).

Group III: diffusely increased attenuation of the retrobulbar fat, which tends to blend with the extraocular muscles (25%).

It is somewhat surprising that these workers did not recognize a true 'pseudotumour' group: the large proportion of essentially negative scans must be considered in relation to the clinical and laboratory criteria for the diagnosis of orbital pseudotumours.

Alper (1979) compared a small series of patients having suspected or proven granuloma with a similar group of patients with Graves' disease. He made the following differential points:

1. The insertions of the extraocular muscles are normal in Graves' disease, but are thickened and show contrast enhancement in granuloma. Conversely, the apex of the muscle cone is less commonly affected in the latter.
2. Increased volume and forward prolapse of the orbital fat are not seen in orbital granuloma, whereas increased attenuation and contrast enhancement are typical.

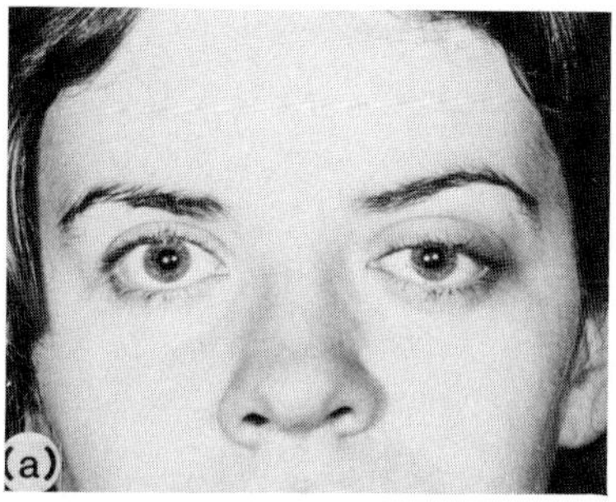

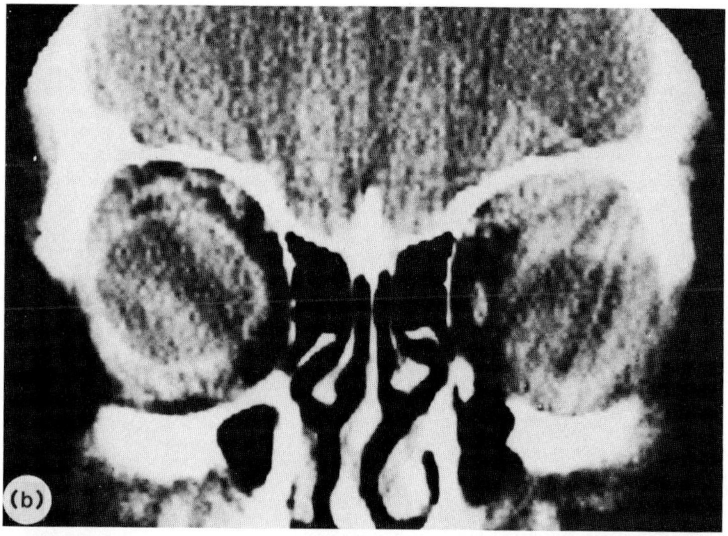

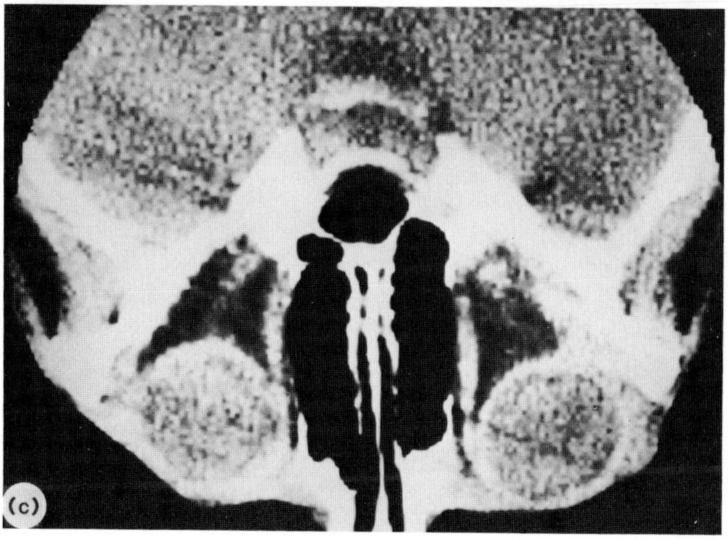

Fig. 3.9 Orbital granuloma involving the lacrimal gland. This 28-year old woman complained of pain in the upper, outer part of the left eye, with redness and watering, for six weeks. There was left-sided ptosis, with depression of the globe (a), and a tender mass in the region of the lacrimal gland. CT (b,c) demonstrated a poorly-defined extraconal mass extending along the roof and lateral wall of the orbit, shown by biopsy to be a granuloma.

Fig. 3.10 Orbital granuloma. At the age of 20, this woman had an episode of acute, painful left proptosis with ophthalmoplegia. Systemic steroid therapy led to rapid resolution, but as this was only partial, biopsy was carried out, showing a granuloma. Clinical and CT follow-up showed little change over three years: she now has slight left proptosis and congestion of the medial conjunctiva (a). CT (b,c) There is a nodular mass of slightly higher attentuation than brain, extending along the medial side of the orbit from the apex to the conjunctiva (arrow) where it corresponds to the congested area seen in (a). It is both intra- and extraconal. The rectus muscles are largely affected by the mass which displaces the superior ophthalmic vein (small arrows). The left orbit is slightly expanded.

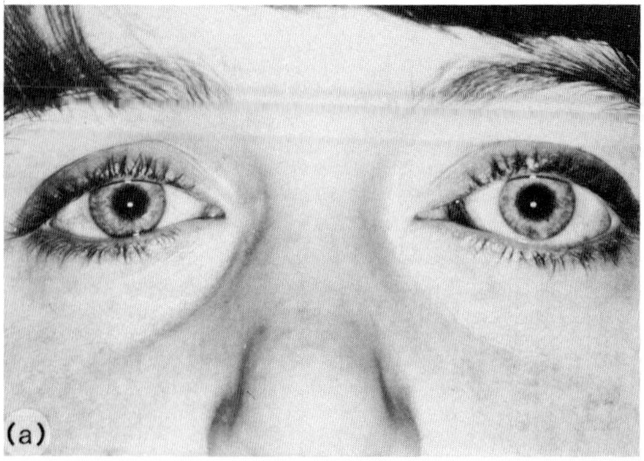

(a)

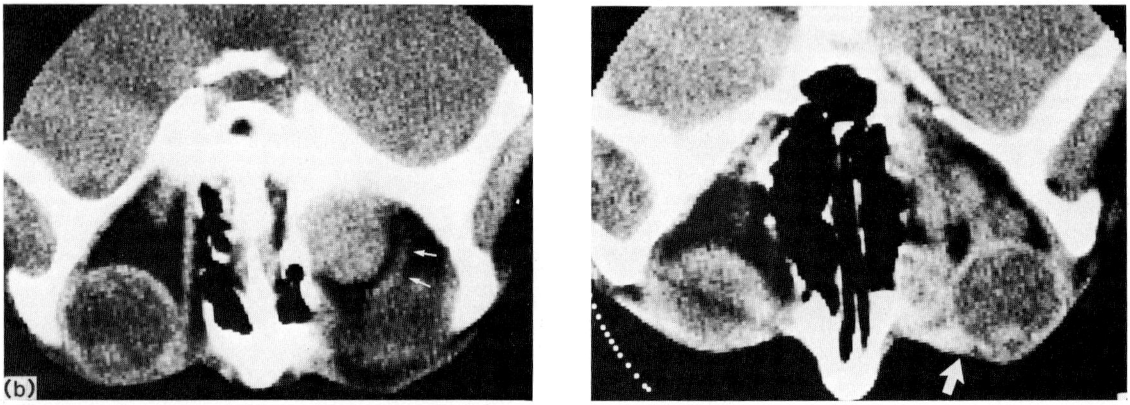

(b)

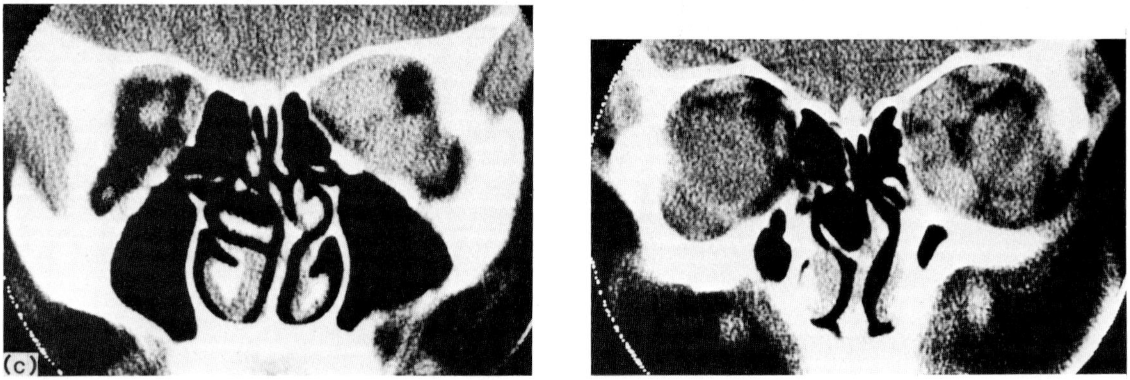

(c)

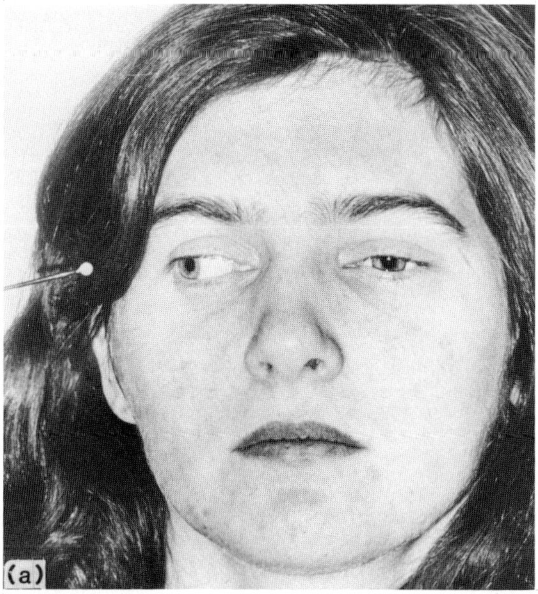

Fig. 3.11 *Orbital granuloma involving muscles.* A 19-year old nurse presented with horizontal diplopia. She had impaired adduction of the left eye with a slightly enlarged left pupil (a) suggesting a left partial IIIrd nerve palsy. However, CT (b) demonstrated thickening of the left medial rectus (arrows), facilitating biopsy, which showed granulomatous changes. The condition responded to steroids.

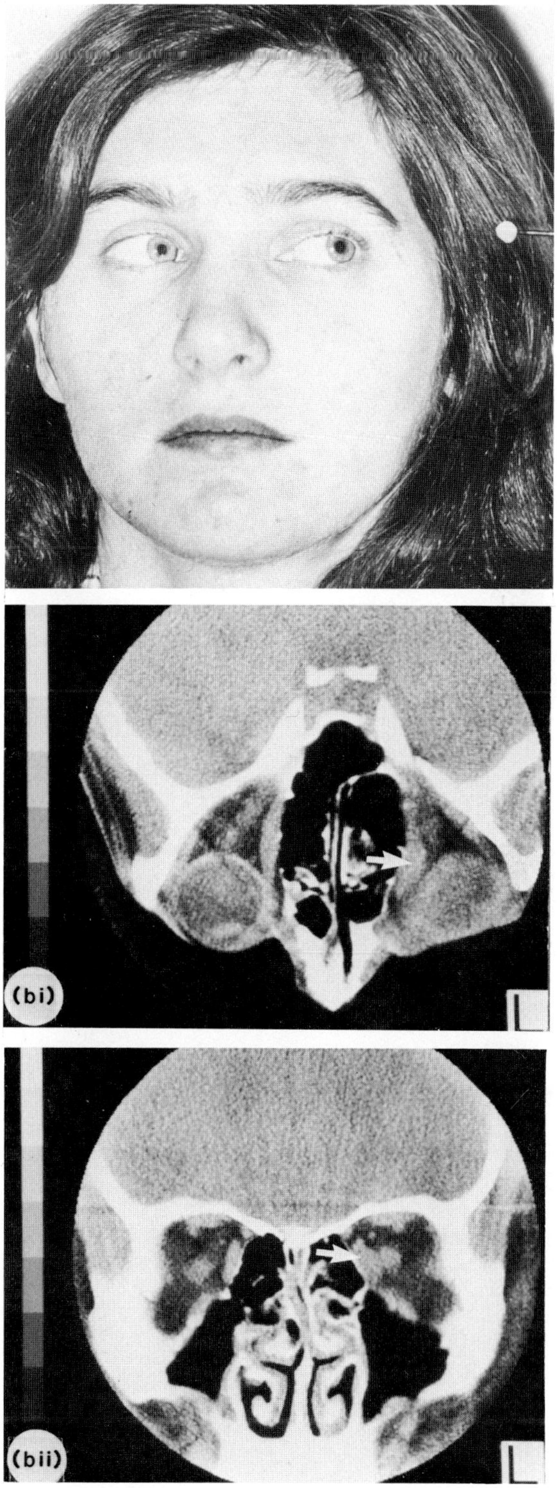

3. Thickening and enhancement of the uveoscleral rim of the globe may be marked in granuloma; the optic nerve may also be thickened, although stretching and thinning of the nerve is more common in both conditions.

4. Bilateral CT evidence of disease in patients with unilateral clinical involvement is much more common in thyroid ophthalmopathy than in granuloma.

As Alper noted, the observation of bilateral orbital disease in patients suspected of having orbital granuloma does not necessarily render the diagnosis less likely. It might be expected that CT would show evidence of subclinical disease in a number of patients with clinically unilateral involvement, and indeed Enzmann *et al.* (1976b) showed bilateral involvement in one third of a small series.

Orbital phlebography was previously used to confirm the clinical suspicion of orbital granuloma. It was not infrequently noted that the superior ophthalmic vein on the affected side was very narrow or occluded in its posterior intracranial portion, and that the contralateral vein was larger than usual. This observation may also be made at CT. Moseley *et al.* (1978) found that the extraocular muscles and superior ophthalmic vein were clearly visible in a considerably higher percentage of patients with clinical evidence of proptosis but no specific radiological abnormality than in a control group. It is possible that such patients have a minor degree of orbital inflammatory change.

Rapid onset, a characteristic clinical picture and an immediate response to systemic steroids in a patient in the second, third or fourth decade suggest a diagnosis of orbital or cavernous sinus granuloma, but without biopsy this diagnosis is conjectural. Histologically 'proven' cases of orbital pseudotumour have turned out at a later date to be inflammatory changes in association with meningiomas, sinus carcinomas, other tumours or aneurysms (Jakobiec and Jones, 1979). If after steroid treatment, symptoms recur, CT is of value in localizing the lesion and facilitating biopsy by the simplest route (Fig. 3.12).

(b) Specific granulomatous diseases

The commonest of these are: 1. Wegener's granuloma, 2. sarcoidosis and 3. histiocytosis X.

Wegener's granulomatosis. Orbital involvement is commonly unilateral (being more frequent on the right side, for reasons which are not clear). CT may, however, show evidence of bilateral orbital involvement and disease in other sites, such as the brain. The latter changes are non-specific (Fig. 13.3).

The ophthalmological manifestations of Wegener's granuloma were reviewed by Haynes *et al.* (1977); they are seen in 40–50% of cases and represent the mode of presentation in

Fig. 3.12 Disc oedema in orbital granuloma. Biopsy of a gastric tumour carried out one year previously in this 77-year old man had shown a moderately differentiated adenocarcinoma. He subsequently complained of progressive blurred vision and pain in the right orbit exacerbated by abduction. There was mild proptosis, and eye movements were limited in all directions but particularly on adduction, with evidence of tethering (a). The right optic disc was swollen, whereas the left was normal (b). CT (c) showed a mass lying between the medial wall of the orbit and the optic nerve. Biopsy, performed through a medial orbital approach was reported as granulomatous vasculitis, without evidence of tumour. Two and a half years later, there had been no change in his visual status.

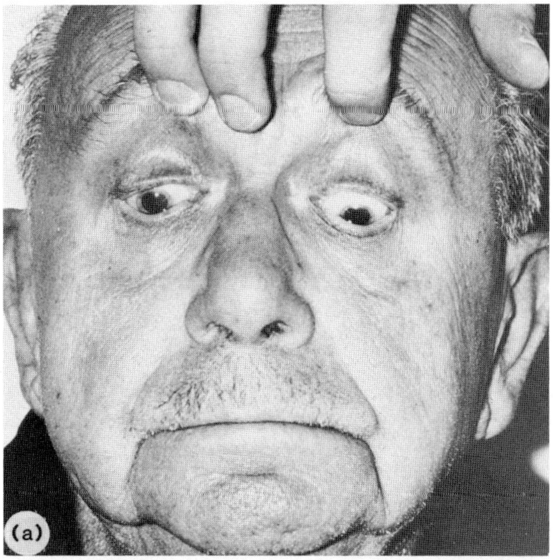

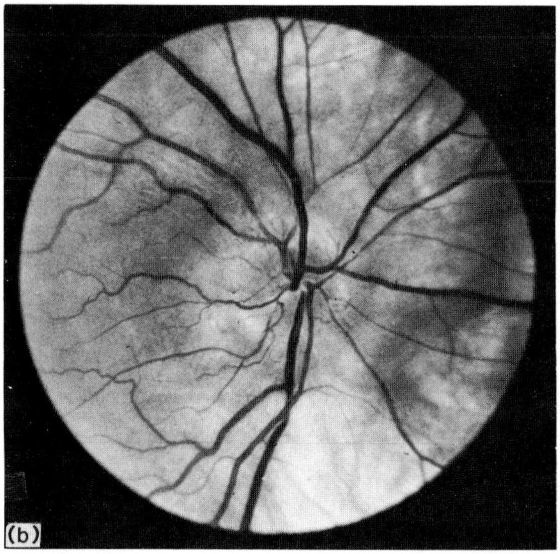

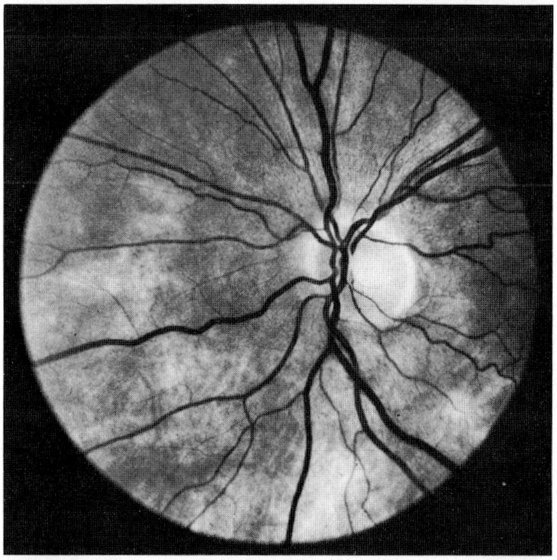

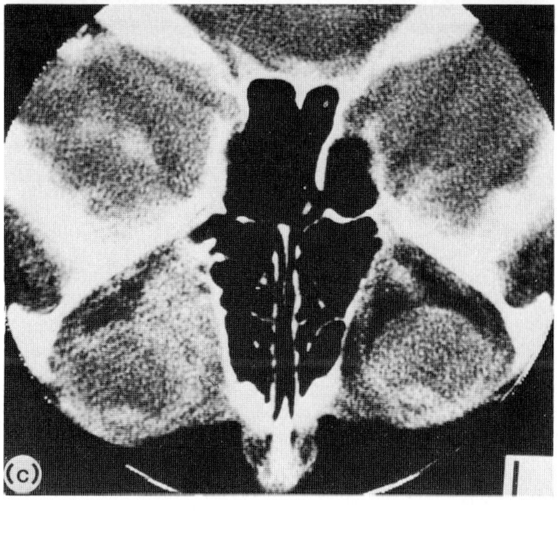

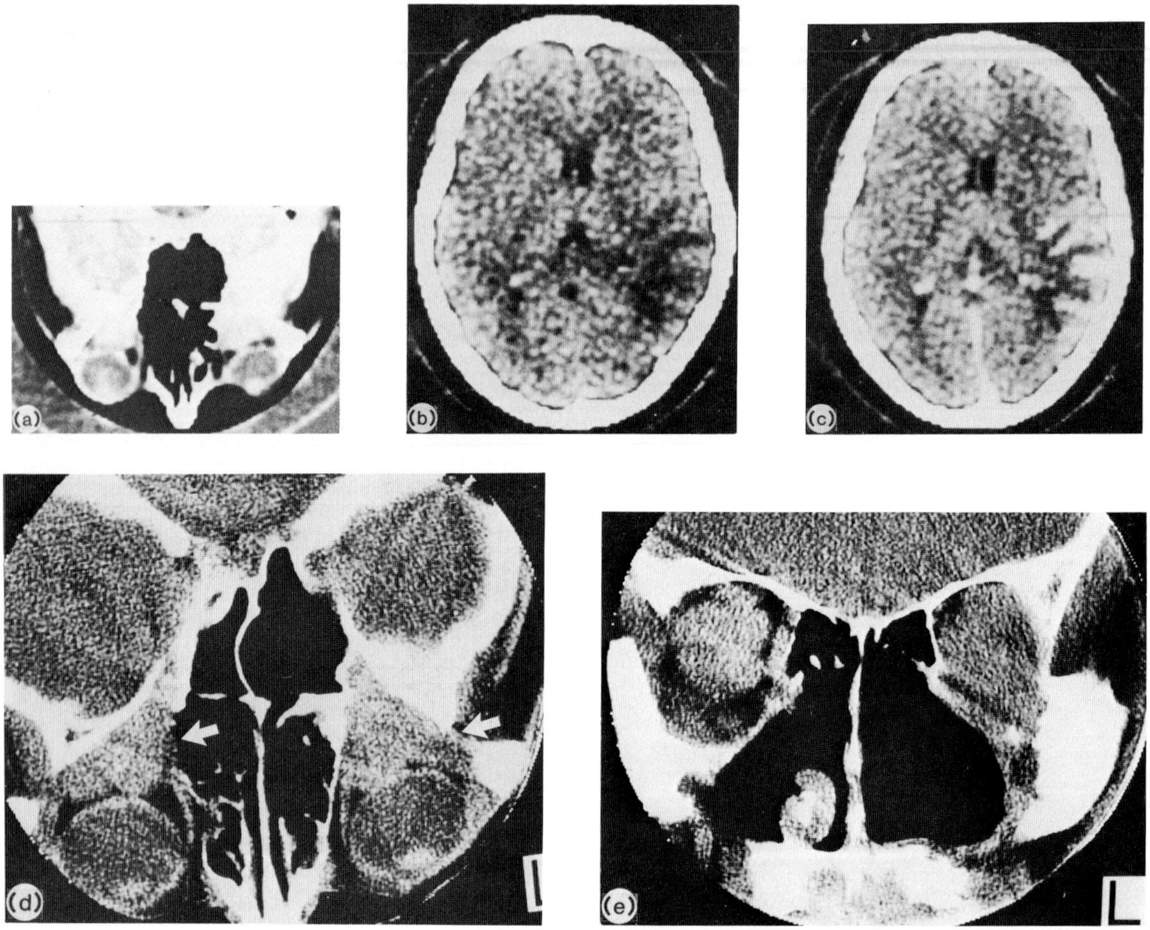

Fig. 3.13 Wegener's granuloma. Extensive nasal surgery had been carried out on this 35-year old man, for Wegener's granuloma. When seen in 1976, he had bilateral proptosis due to masses which appeared intraconal (a) and signs of a recent right parietal infarct (b, before; c, after intravenous contrast medium). High resolution orbital CT carried out two years later (d–f) showed the extent of the bone destruction (only the nasal septum and right inferior turbinate remaining (e)), and the nodular nature of the bilateral intraconal masses. The orbital walls were also deficient (arrows), but this may be largely iatrogenic.

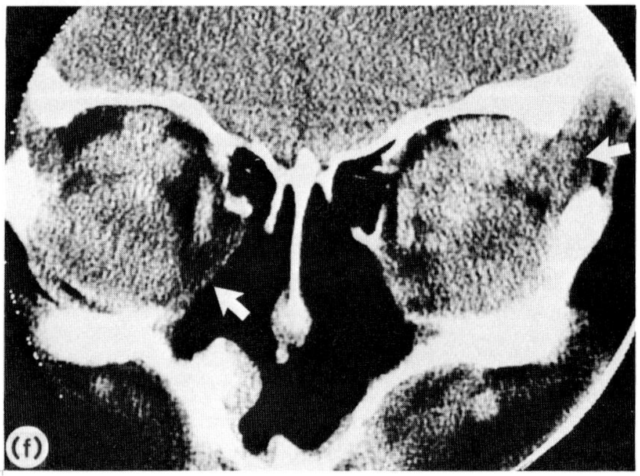

about one quarter of those affected. Proptosis, the most common single manifestation, is seen in about 20% of patients. Conjunctivitis and scleritis are not uncommon, occurring in 15% of cases, though uveitis is much less frequent. Optic nerve involvement, either on a vascular basis or as the result of granulomatous infiltration, also occurs in about 15% of cases. Clinically disseminated or limited forms of Wegener's can be seen and the pathological picture is extremely varied, though fibrinoid necrosis in arteries or arterioles with perivascular granuloma formation is a characteristic feature.

Diseases closely related to Wegener's granuloma but apparently distinct are lymphomatoid granulomatosis, in which orbital involvement is rare, and idiopathic or lethal midline granuloma, in which the systemic disturbance is lacking.

In all these related conditions, the orbit may be involved by direct extension from the paranasal sinuses, particularly the maxillary antra and ethmoid cells, or, much less frequently, by apparently discrete orbital granuloma. The only patient in the series of Haynes *et al*. (1977) who was shown to have orbital involvement without contiguous sinus disease, had lymphomatoid granulomatosis. CT shows the classical changes of homogeneous soft tissue masses with extensive expansion and erosion of the bony walls of the nasal cavity and/or paranasal sinuses, with extension of the granulomatous tissue to the orbit, usually the retrobulbar space. When the granuloma is confined to the orbit, the appearances are similar to those seen in non-specific orbital granuloma, with involvement of the muscles, the surrounding fat, and the formation of soft tissue masses. Wegener's granuloma is one of the conditions in which all detail in the retrobulbar space may be effaced. (Fig. 3.14).

Haynes and his co-workers (Verness *et al*., 1978) also described the CT appearances in Wegener's granuloma. Two patients with a previous history of proptosis, but without active disease, had normal CT scans. In four other patients, the salient findings were proptosis, large retrobulbar masses of soft tissue attenuation, unilateral, often filling the entire retrobulbar space, thickening of the sclera, and destruction of the ethmoid cells and the medial and inferior walls of the orbit. The effects of intravenous contrast medium were variable: one very 'active' case showed massive enhancement, while in another there was no change. The authors suggested that where visual loss in patients with Wegener's granuloma was not associated with a retrobulbar mass, it was probably due to vasculitis of the optic nerve. They also stressed that early radiological detection of orbital involvement might be instrumental in the decision to use immunosuppressive drugs or decompressive surgery, and could thereby prevent loss of vision.

Sarcoidosis. This chronic granulomatous multisystem disease

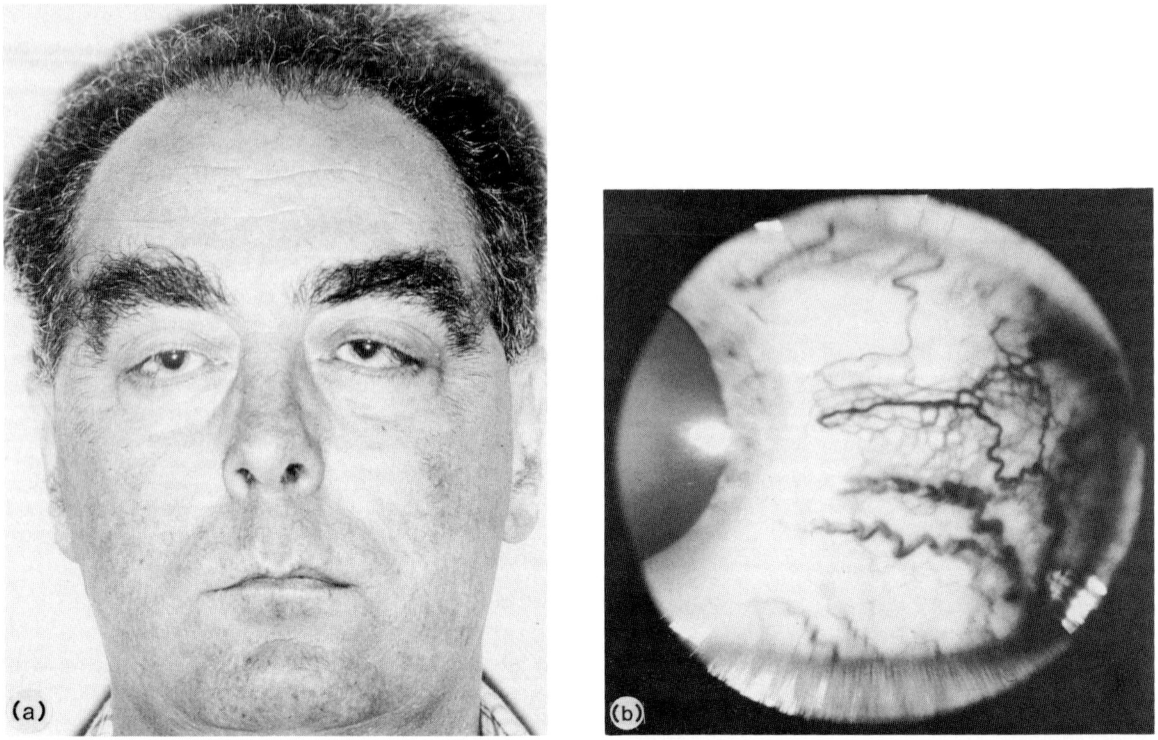

Fig. 3.14 Diffuse orbital and intracranial granulomatosis. A 55-year old man was referred with bilateral proptosis, and ophthalmoplegia (a). Examination showed normal vision, tense orbits, generalized ophthalmoplegia, dilated episcleral vessels (b) and bilateral papilloedema. There was disc swelling with retinal striae (c) and fluorescein angiograms (d) confirmed disc leakage, with numerous choroidal striae in each eye. Lumbar puncture showed an elevated CSF presence of 350mm of water. CT in 1976 (e) showed an irregular intraconal mass on the left side. Two years later (f) after a left lateral orbital decompression, at which diffuse inflammation of the dura mater, cavernous sinus and orbits was found, granulomatous tissue was visible in both orbits and the left temporal fossa. By 1978 (g, h) both orbits were packed with masses of soft-tissue attenuation, obliterating the normal anatomy.

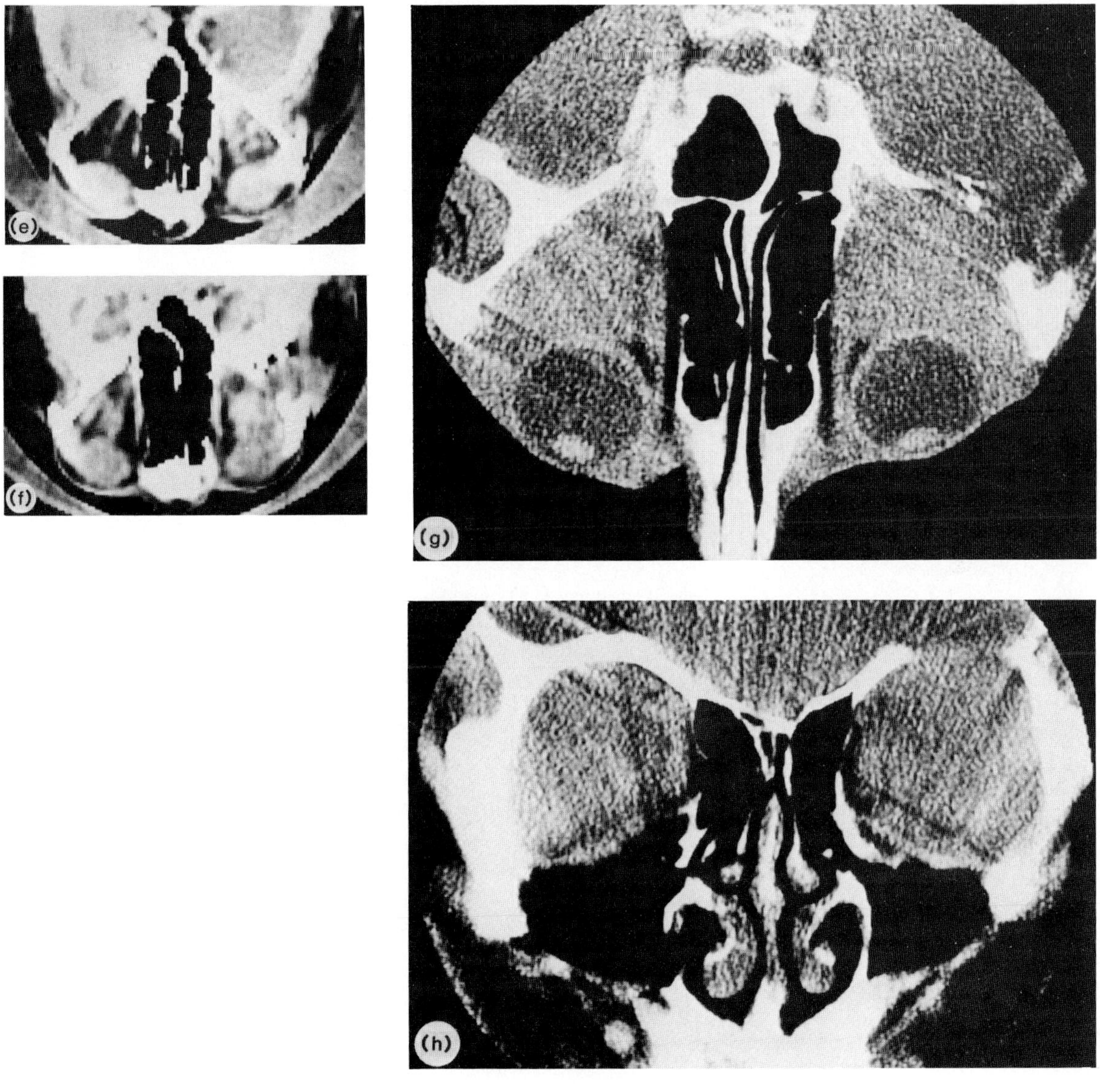
(e)
(f)
(g)
(h)

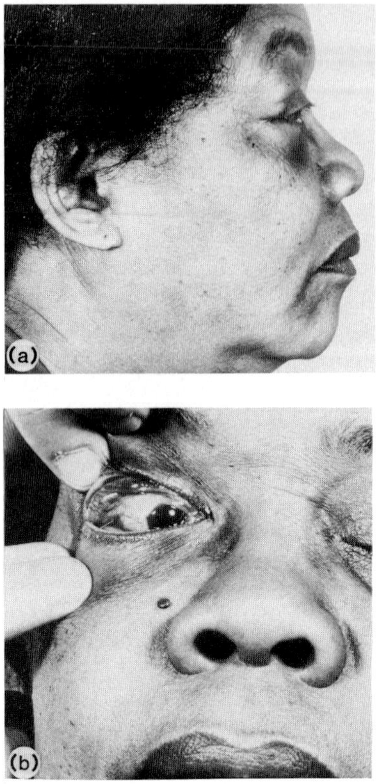

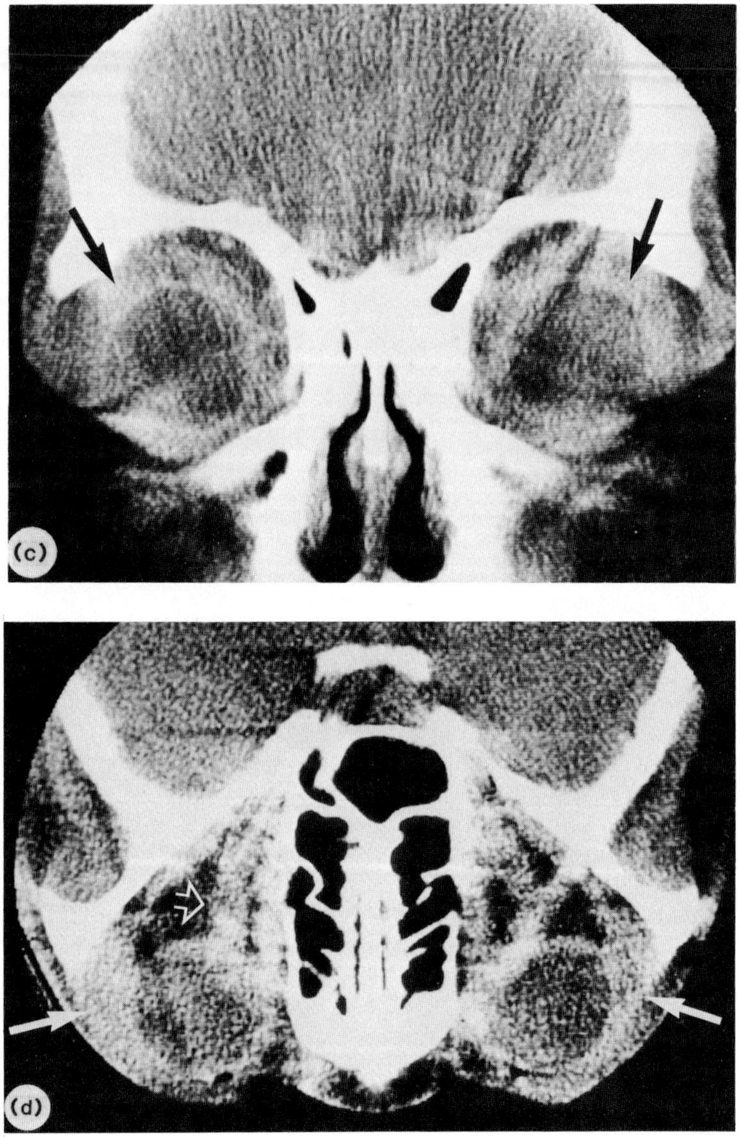

Fig. 3.15 Mikulicz's syndrome. Enlargement of lacrimal and parotid glands was seen in this 50-year old black West Indian woman with known sarcoidosis (a,b). CT (c,d) showed enlargement of lacrimal glands (arrows) more marked on the right side where the optic nerve appeared to be displaced medially (open arrow).

affects the lungs, lymph nodes, skin and skeleton and produces inflammatory ocular and orbital changes. Ocular involvement is seen in 20% to 30% of patients. Anterior uveitis is the most common ocular finding, but posterior segment disease is not rare (Spalton and Sanders, 1981). About 7% show orbital changes and the lacrimal gland is the principal site for granuloma formation. CT shows enlargement of the lacrimal gland, sarcoidosis accounting for about 5% of cases of tumefaction of the gland (Fig. 3.15). The rare orbital granulomata has been reported, though we are not aware of a report of the CT findings, and optic nerve involvement may be manifest by swelling of the nerve. CT may also demonstrate evidence of intracranial sarcoidosis with granulomas, basal meningitis and hydrocephalus (Fig. 4.9b).

Histiocytosis X has a number of forms. In the most severe, juvenile form (Letterer-Siwe disease) bilateral proptosis is associated with characteristic skin lesions and systemic changes. Hand-Schuller-Christian disease also affects children, is more benign and referred to as subacute or chronic. Exophthalmos occurred in 15 of 117 patients in one series (Enriquez *et al*., 1967); it may be bilateral, and is occasionally pulsatile when extensive erosion of the bony walls of the orbit has occurred. Ophthalmoplegia is uncommon. Xanthomatous deposits may be seen in the eyelids or exceptionally in the posterior choroid in Letterer-Siwe disease. Disc oedema with haemorrhages and exudates, which may progress to optic atrophy, can result from intraorbital deposits or from raised intracranial pressure.

At CT the hallmark of these conditions is the combination of bone destruction and soft-tissue infiltration, giving rise to mass lesions, especially in the sinuses and orbits (Fig. 3.16). Affection of the sellar and hypothalamic region may give rise to the classical symptoms of polyuria and polydipsia in Hand-Schuller-Christian disease (Fig. 3.17).

Polyarteritis nodosa. The main ocular presentation is with bilateral episcleritis, but occasionally polyarteritis nodosa may present as an orbital pseudotumour. Thus any patient with biopsy

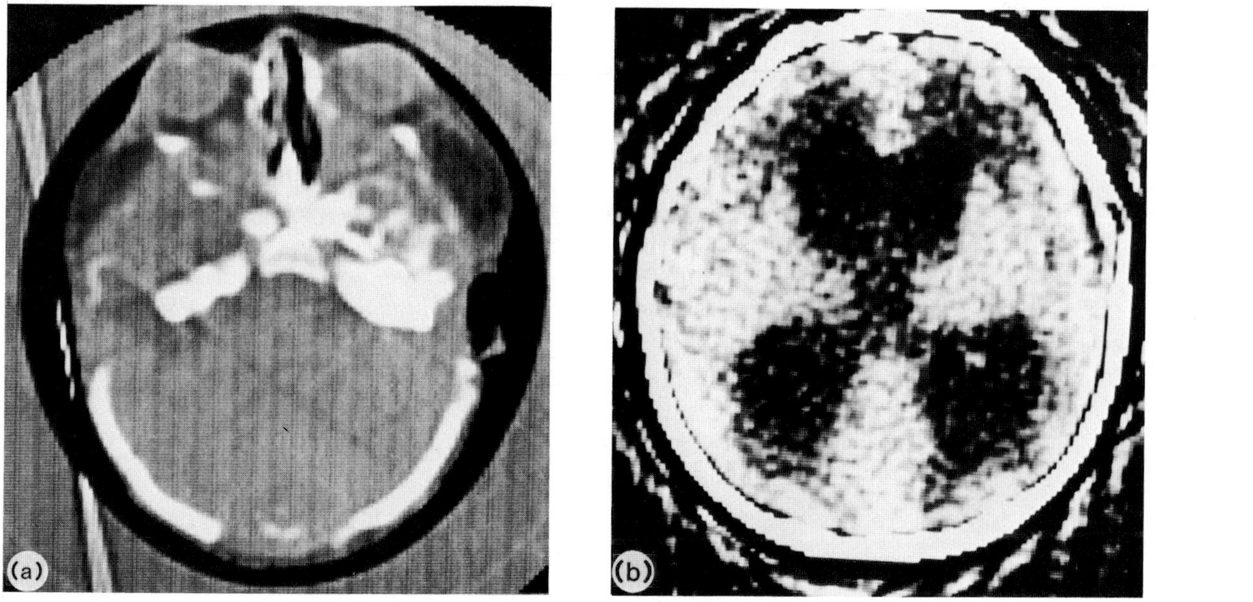

Fig. 3.16 Histiocytosis X (Letterer-Siwe disease). A 2.5-year old child with systemic disease, and the typical skin rash. CT: (a) there is extensive destruction of the skull base, orbital walls, temporal and occipital bones. Soft tissue masses fill the retrobulbar spaces (b) Marked hydrocephalus is present, with periventricular lucencies (see Chapter 5).

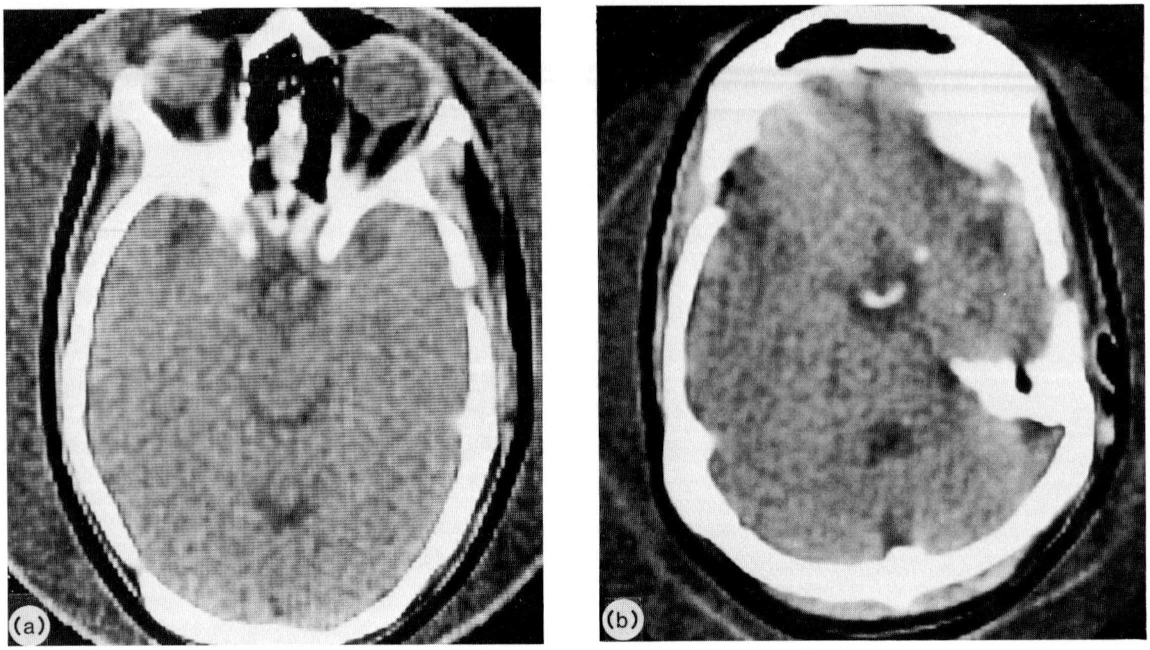

Fig. 3.17 Histiocytosis X (Hand-Schuller-Christian disease). This 29-year old man presented with diabetes insipidus. There was no clinical evidence of orbital involvement. CT: bilateral temporal osteolytic lesions are present. There is probably also bone destruction in the region of the tuberculum sellae and soft tissue is seen within the chiasmatic cistern.

confirmed orbital pseudotumour who develops renal, cutaneous or peripheral neuropathy merits consideration of the diagnosis of polyarteritis nodosa. The small and medium sized arteries are involved.

Amyloidosis may be localized or part of a systemic process and because of its relationship to the plasma cell can be considered here. The localized form may be restricted to the orbit and systemic tests for amyloid may be negative (Fig. 3.18). We have seen one patient with systemic amyloid who showed thickening of the extraocular muscles (Fig. 6.42); this may lead to complete ophthalmoplegia (Howard, 1966).

Chronic nasal polyposis. In this condition, which may have an allergic basis, there is recurrent massive polyp formation by the mucosa of the nose and paranasal sinuses. These cavities become expanded, but in contradistinction to Wegener's granuloma, it is uncommon for destructive bone lesions to occur. The orbit may, however, be compressed as a result of the grossly exuberant hypertrophy of the mucosae.

Infective conditions

Orbital cellulitis is usually the result of spread of infection from the paranasal sinuses and lids, and may be due to a variety of organisms, of which staphylococci or streptococci are the most frequent. Rarely, haematogenous spread to the orbit may occur.

Fig. 3.18 Advanced orbital amyloid. This elderly man had been diagnosed clinically as suffering from thyroid ophthalmopathy many years previously. He showed proptosis, most marked on the right, where there was a large mass in the region of the upper lid depressing the globe (a), and restricted eye movements. There was also hepatosplenomegaly, although liver biopsy gave a normal result. CT (b, December, 1978): There is a soft tissue mass above and lateral to the right eye, from which the rectus muscles cannot be separated. The optic nerve cannot be identified with certainty. The orbit is expanded. Similar, less marked changes are present on the left, where the superior rectus muscle is thickened. There is widespread inflammatory change in the ethmoid sinuses, whose lateral walls appear defective. Orbital biopsy on the right showed tissue characteristic of amyloidosis; there was no evidence of systemic amyloidosis. (c, August, 1979): progression of the changes described above.

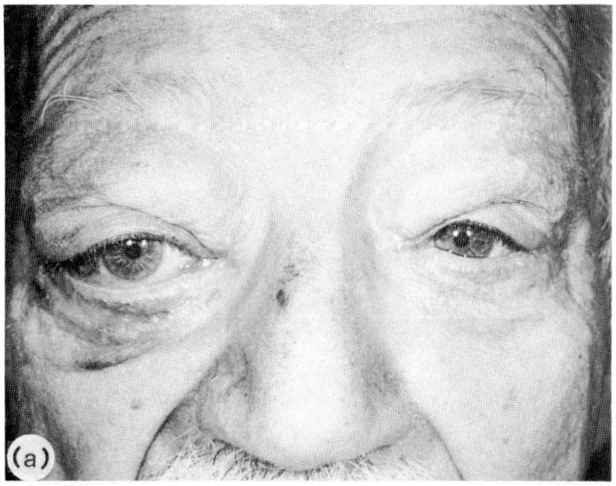

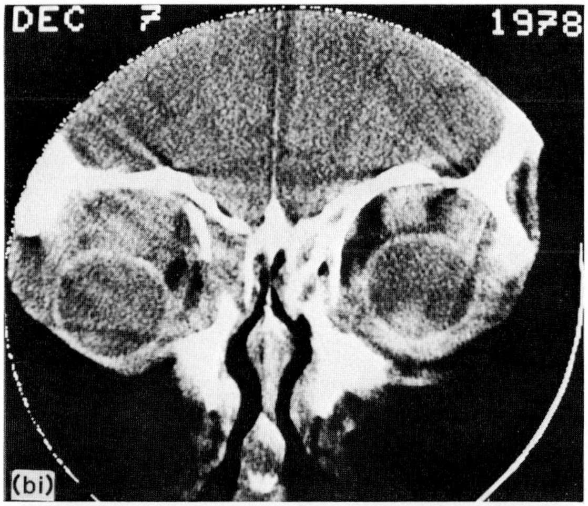

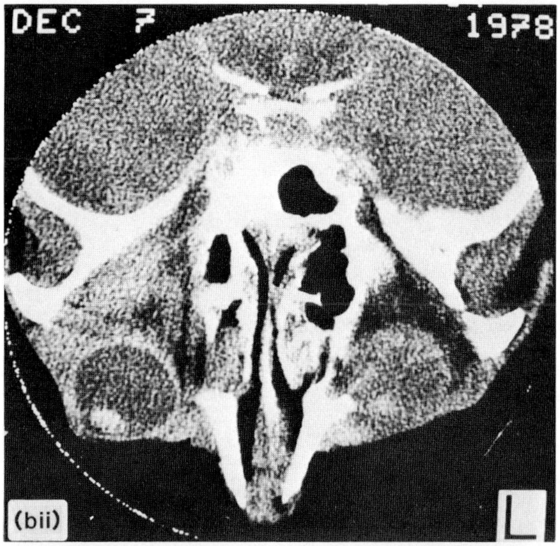

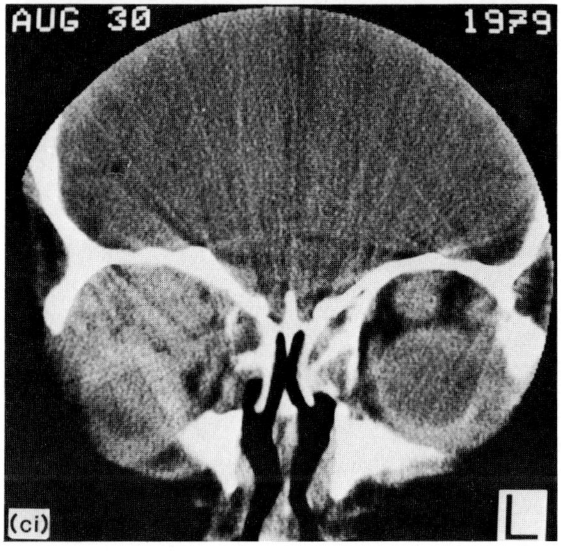

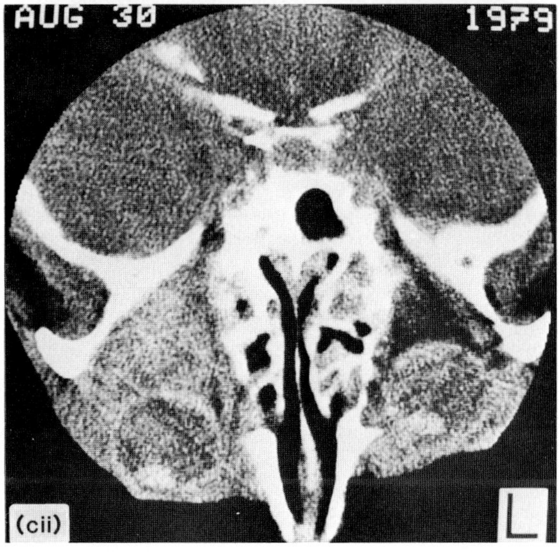

The CT changes of cellulitis are similar to those of orbital granuloma: swelling and poor definition of the retrobulbar structures, especially the extraocular muscles, and irregularly increased attentuation in the orbital fat (Fig. 3.8 p.32). In rare cases, gas may be seen in the retrobulbar space, usually as the result of a breach of the bone between the orbit and the adjacent sinus, rather than of infection with gas-forming organisms. Foreign bodies may be present, including the results of ophthalmic surgery (e.g. encircling bands) and injuries may be a cause of infection.

Goldberg *et al.* (1978) described five cases of cellulitis, two post-traumatic and the others associated with sinus disease. These workers indicated the value of CT in distinguishing cellulitis limited to the preseptal tissues, i.e. essentially extraorbital and not requiring surgical exploration, from true orbital cel-

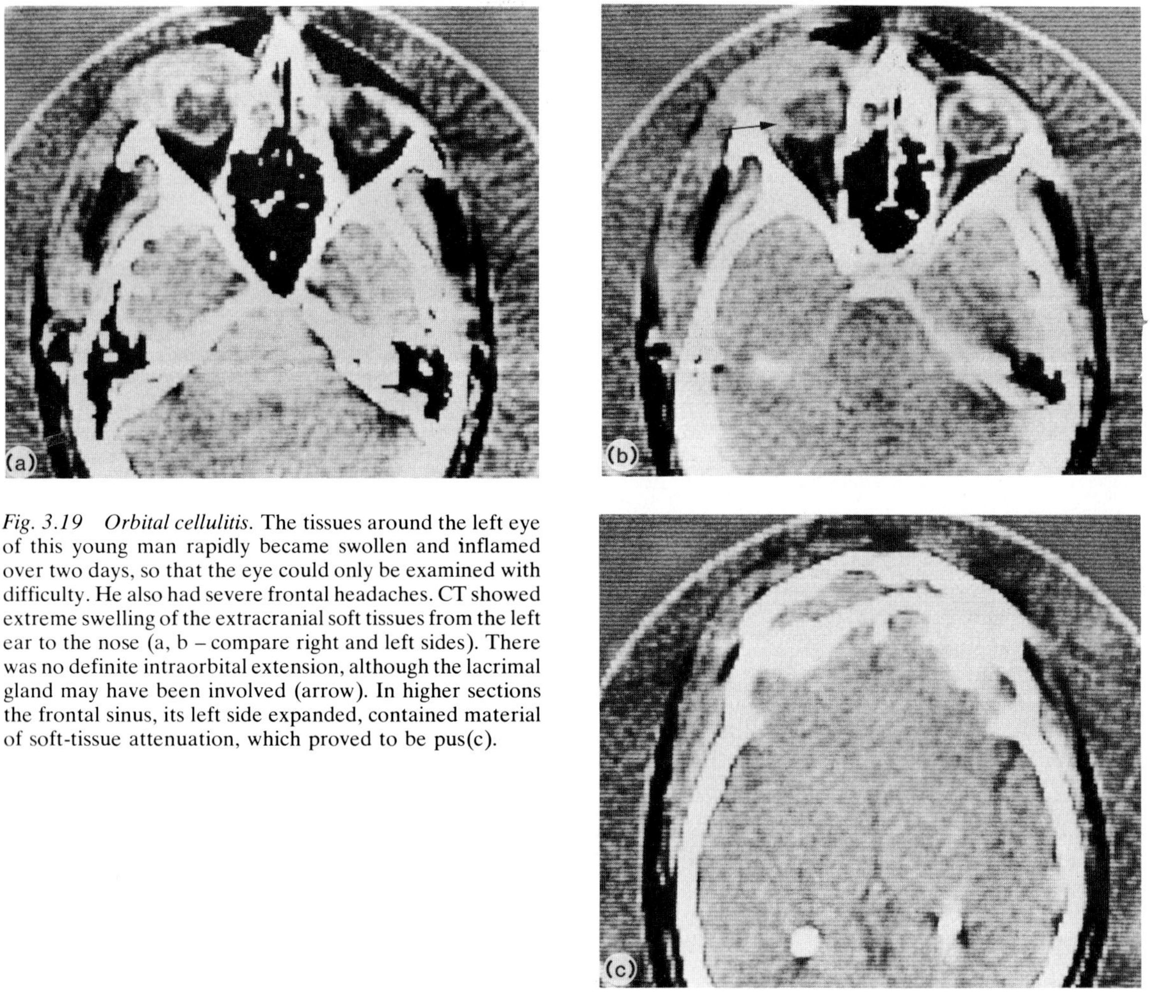

Fig. 3.19 Orbital cellulitis. The tissues around the left eye of this young man rapidly became swollen and inflamed over two days, so that the eye could only be examined with difficulty. He also had severe frontal headaches. CT showed extreme swelling of the extracranial soft tissues from the left ear to the nose (a, b – compare right and left sides). There was no definite intraorbital extension, although the lacrimal gland may have been involved (arrow). In higher sections the frontal sinus, its left side expanded, contained material of soft-tissue attenuation, which proved to be pus(c).

lulitis. This distinction may be very difficult on clinical grounds when there is marked swelling of the overlying soft tissues (Fig 3.19). They also suggested that in the appropriate clinical context, a well-defined intraorbital mass at CT was probably an abscess contained by the periosteum, whilst preservation of the outline of the optic nerve indicated that the infection was still extraconal.

Abnormalities indicating the site of the infection may be present, in the form of soft-tissue masses (Fig. 3.19), fluid levels in the paranasal sinuses, or oedema and swelling of the overlying soft tissues; there may be evidence of surgery. In such cases, a search for spread to the intracranial structures with formation of an extracerebral empyema or cerebral abscess should also be made (Fig. 3.20).

Infection in the paranasal sinuses can result in loculation of all or part of a sinus, into which the mucosa continues to secrete. The result is a mucocoele, which by its slow expansion may compress and finally break through the bone, into the orbit. The CT picture of expansion of a loculus or an entire sinus, containing material of soft-tissue or water attenuation, over which the bone is markedly thinned, is characteristic, but its detection may need considerable manipulation of the window level and width controls (Fig. 3.21).

The fungus phycomycetes can produce a chronic form of orbital inflammation, also spreading from the adjacent sinuses, usually the ethmoid cells. The infection may be virulent, with rapid spread to the cranial cavity.

3.2 ORBITAL TUMOURS

Tumours of the eye

The majority of ocular tumours are adequately assessed by fundoscopy with further evaluation by ultrasound. CT may, however, also be of assistance when:

1. Corneal, lenticular or vitreous opacity renders fundoscopy impossible.
2. Retinal detachment is, or is thought to be, the result of a subjacent tumour.
3. In cases of known tumour, it is desirable to assess spread of the tumour to the optic nerve and retrobulbar tissues.

The two common primary tumours of the eye are malignant melanoma and retinoblastoma.

Malignant melanoma

Malignant melanoma is the commonest primary ocular neoplasm occurring in adult life, with a peak in the sixth decade (Fig. 3.22). The tumour, which arises in the choroid, is seen at CT as an

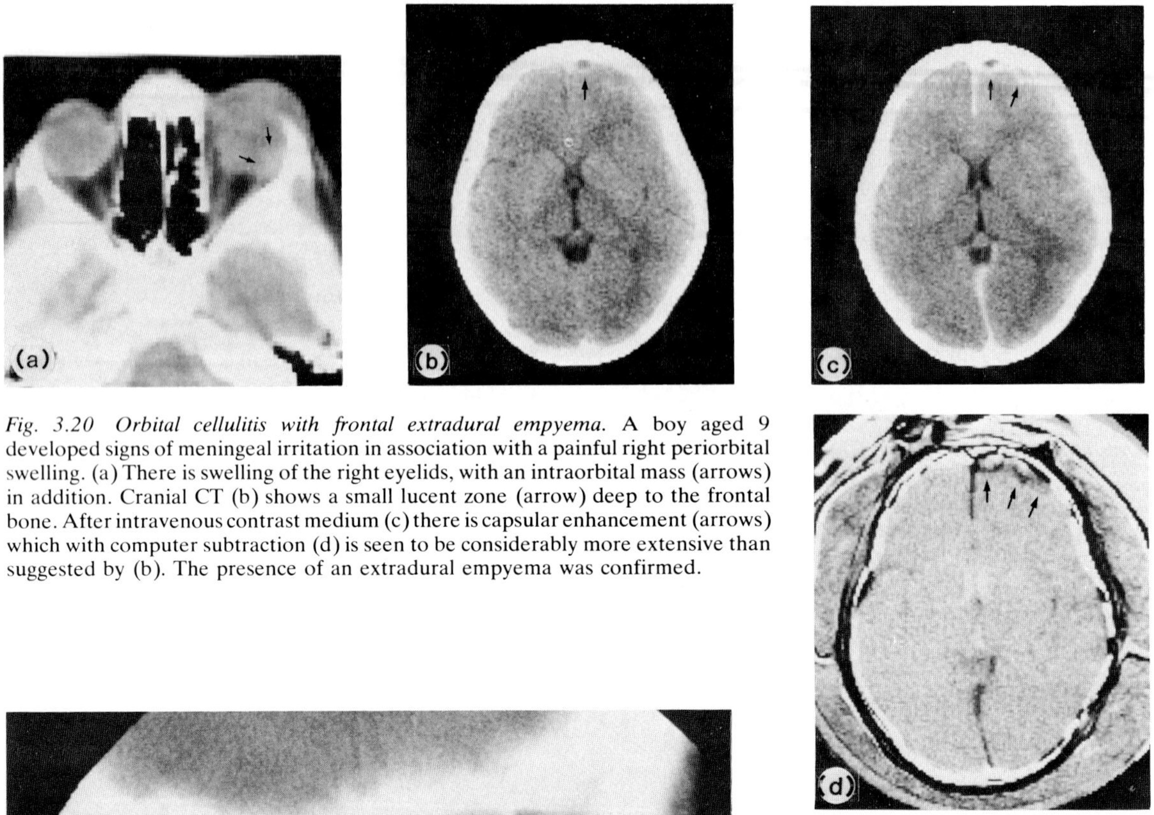

Fig. 3.20 Orbital cellulitis with frontal extradural empyema. A boy aged 9 developed signs of meningeal irritation in association with a painful right periorbital swelling. (a) There is swelling of the right eyelids, with an intraorbital mass (arrows) in addition. Cranial CT (b) shows a small lucent zone (arrow) deep to the frontal bone. After intravenous contrast medium (c) there is capsular enhancement (arrows) which with computer subtraction (d) is seen to be considerably more extensive than suggested by (b). The presence of an extradural empyema was confirmed.

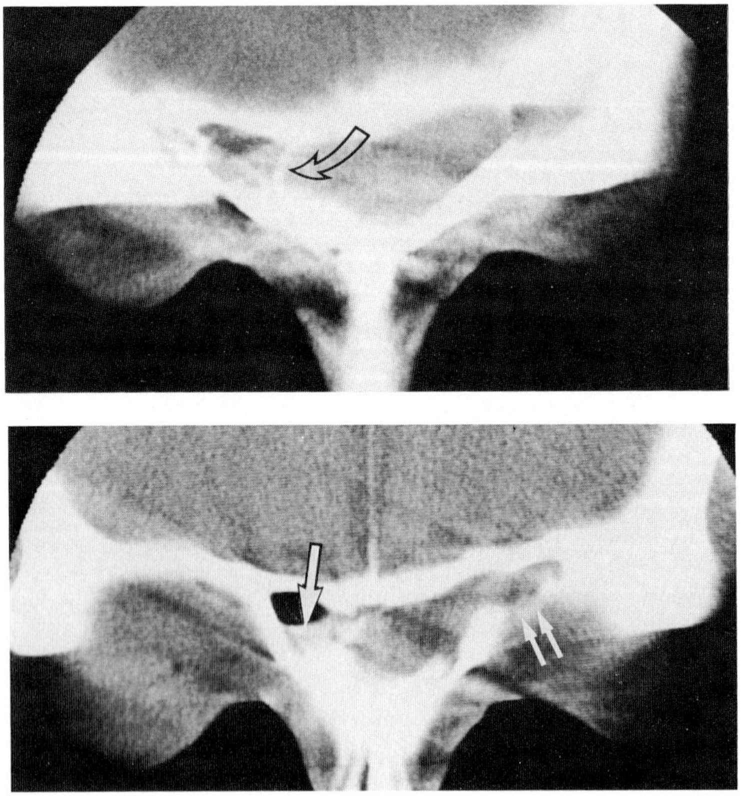

Fig. 3.21 Frontal sinus mucocoele. Two coronal CT sections of a typical mucocoele, showing an expanded sinus filled with material of soft tissue attenuation. The septum is bulged to the right (open arrow), where there is a fluid level (arrow) and the floor of the sinus is eroded (double arrows).

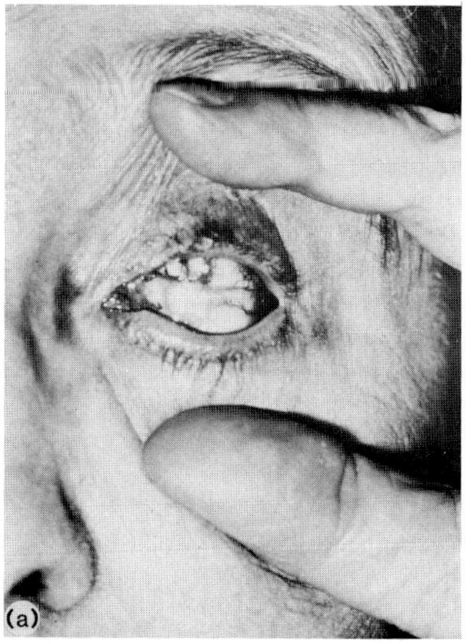

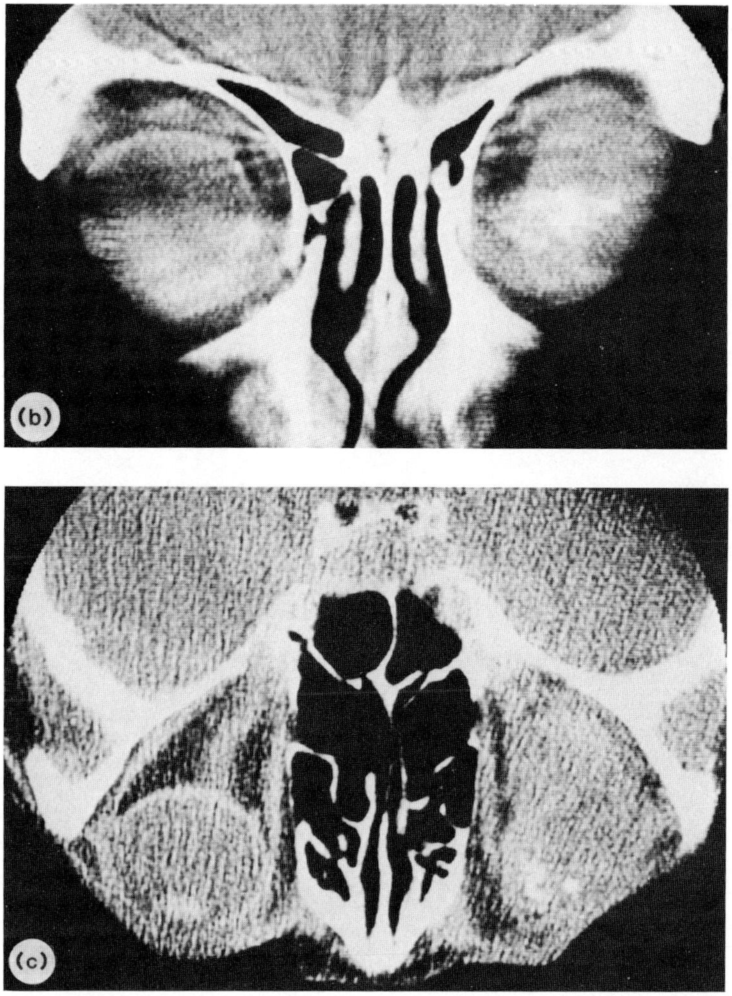

Fig. 3.22 Advanced malignant melanoma. This 68-year old woman presented with a phthisical left globe (a) having deferred consultation for many years. CT: (b) coronal and (c) axial scans. A partially calcified mass, inseparable anteriorly from the globe, almost fills the muscle cone. The patient died within six months, with evidence of metastases.

irregular expansion of the dense outer layer of the globe, bulging towards the vitreous. Retinal detachment may be visible. The attenuation coefficients of the lesion are in the same range as the adjacent normal portion of the globe and higher than those of the vitreous; there is definite enhancement with intravenous contrast medium. Spread of these peripapillary tumours occurs directly to the retrobulbar space and to the optic nerve, which becomes widened, with increased attenuation and enhancement. Haematogenous dissemination may also occur, possibly facilitated by surgery. Extraocular extension occurs in 15% of cases and the nerve is infiltrated in up to 80% of peripapillary lesions. Melanoma metastases in the brain are characteristically of increased attenuation, suggesting the presence of haemorrhage within them, with homogeneous enhancement (Fig. 3.23). There is usually surrounding oedema. Evidence of intracranial haemor-

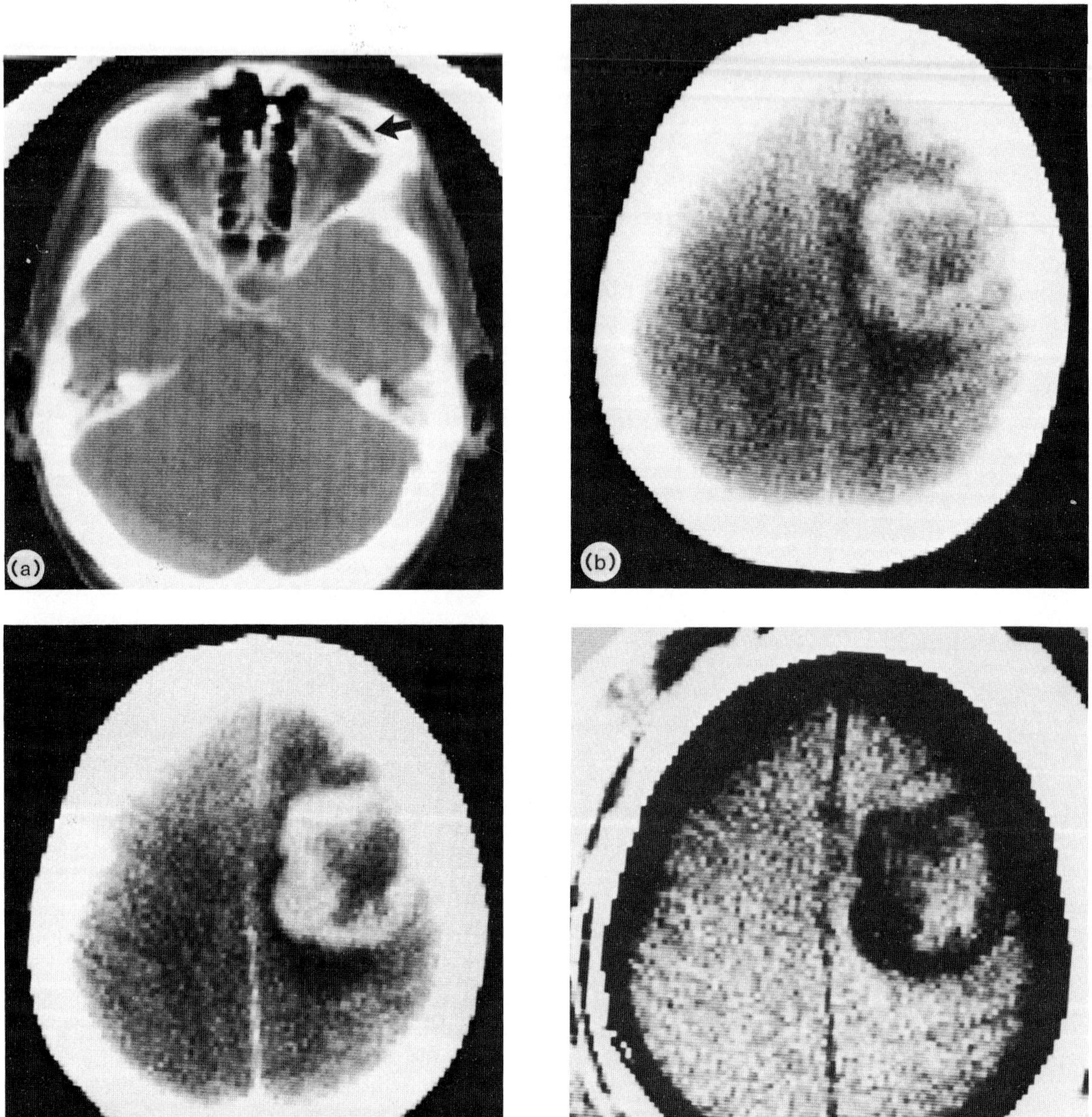

Fig. 3.23 Metastatic malignant melanoma. This 47-year old man had a right enucleation for malignant melanoma and subsequently presented with a rapidly progressive left hemiparesis. (a) Prosthesis in right orbit (arrow). (b) Irregular right frontoparietal lesion of mixed attentuation, suggesting some haemorrhage, with surrounding oedema. (c) After intravenous contrast medium, there is intense enhancement of the lesion, apart from its centre, which is possibly necrotic. (d) Computer subtraction of (b) from (c), showing extent of enhancement.

rhage may be present and indeed subarachnoid bleeding is the mode of presentation in up to 20% of cases (Enzmann *et al.*, 1978).

Retinoblastoma

Retinoblastoma occurs in children; the mortality rate has decreased from 95% to 9% over the past century, due to early diagnosis and improved therapy. The tumour originates in the retina, but has the potential to invade tissues locally and disseminate widely. In particular, if the tumour gains access to the CSF pathways multiple seedlings can arise throughout the central nervous system, as with medulloblastomas and pineoblastomas. Optic nerve extension was seen in 12.7% of cases and orbital spread was seen in 8% of the Harkness Eye Institute cases. Distant spread via the blood stream rarely occurs to produce the picture of fulminating malignancy. Early detection by ophthalmoscopic means is therefore essential, and CT is of value in defining the extent of the lesion. The CT appearances are similar to those seen in malignant melanoma (Fig. 3.24). In the early stages the tumour appears as a high attenuation mass, without enhancement following intravenous contrast medium. Calcification is a useful diagnostic finding, and when found in both eyes is almost pathognomic. Bilateral disc calcification may also be seen with drusen of the disc (Chapter 5), but clinically this causes no diagnostic confusion. The occurrence of calcification after radiotherapy presents a difficult diagnostic problem which either indicates orbital recurrence of the tumour or a postirradiation osteogenic sarcoma, to which these patients are vulnerable. Goldberg and Danziger (1977) divided patients with retinoblastoma into three therapeutic groups: ocular – treated by enucleation; orbital – treated by exenteration, radiotherapy and systemic cytotoxics; metastatic – in which only palliative measures

Fig. 3.24 Retinoblastoma. An 11-year old boy presented with right visual loss and the typical amaurotic 'cat's-eye' (a) (courtesy of Mr D.S.I. Taylor). There was a large intraocular tumour. CT examination of a similar case shows extensive ocular calcification (b), but no evidence of spread to the optic nerve (c). Retinoblastoma was confirmed on enucleation (courtesy of Mr A.I. Friedmann).

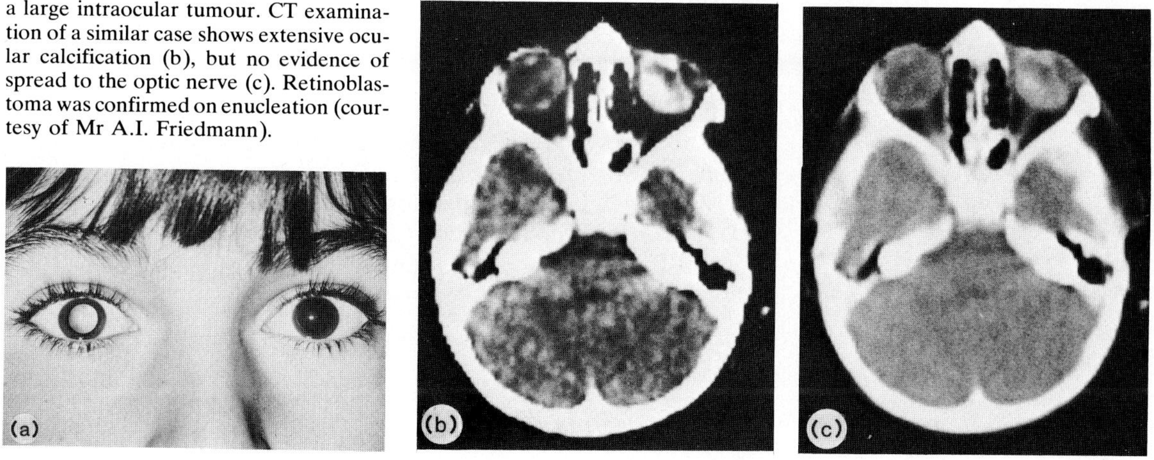

are employed. They noted that mortality was greatly increased in children with orbital recurrence of tumour following enucleation and contended that CT was invaluable as an adjunct to clinical staging.

Calcification within the eye or orbit has a number of other causes. It can be *metastatic*, i.e. the result of hypercalcaemia in parathyroid disturbances, vitamin D intoxication, sarcoidosis or myelomatosis. *Dystrophic* calcification may be seen in cataract (by far the commonest cause of orbital calcification) or in phthisis bulbi, usually of traumatic of infective origin. A lesion commonly associated with calcification is the orbital varix. Relatively rare causes include drusen, choroidal haemangioma, optic nerve meningioma, lacrimal gland tumour and dermoid tumours. Emphasis has recently been focused on the choroidal osteoma, but whether this is a primary or secondary phenomenon remains conjectural.

Metastatic tumours

Metastatic tumours to the eye are more common than previously appreciated (Ferry and Font, 1974) and the CT appearances are non-specific.

Retrobulbar and other tumours

In the often quoted series of Reese (1956), about 90% of patients with proptosis in whom the final diagnosis was of neoplastic disease were suffering from one of seven types of tumour:

Haemangioma	25%
Lymphoma	20%
Lacrimal gland epitheliomas	16%
Lymphangioma	each 7–9%
Metastases	each 7–9%
Peripheral nerve tumour	each 7–9%
Dermoid	each 7–9%

The majority of the remaining patients had rare malignant sarcomas.

The detection of intraorbital mass lesions other than those described previosly is not difficult providing a full series of axial scans, i.e. from the maxillary antra below to the orbital roof above, supplemented if necessary by coronal sections and sagittal sections or reconstructions, is obtained. However, differential diagnosis may present considerable problems. In addition to the clinical features, it will depend on:

1. The situation of the mass.
2. Its form.
3. Specific characteristics of its attenuation coefficients.
4. Additional more or less distinctive observations.

Some tumours will show a typical site and form, and have attenuation coefficients which clearly indicate the diagnosis. Many, unfortunately, will not.

Orbital haemangiomas

These can be regarded as tumours rather than vascular malformations, on the basis of their clinical, radiological and pathological characteristics. The cavernous type, with its well-defined limiting capsule, is the most common, representing between 13 and 23% in different series of primary orbital neoplasms. There is a female sex preponderance (70%), and the incidence is highest in middle age.

The orbital cavernous haemangioma is a gratifying tumour to deal with because diagnosis is possible on clinical grounds, with confirmation by CT and surgical excision is extremely satisfactory. The development of these tumours within the muscle cone produces axial proptosis, which evolves gradually (Harris and Jakobiec, 1979). Diplopia is not a common complaint; it may be produced when the ocular motor nerves are compressed or the normal range of movements of the globe or optic nerve is limited by the tumour. In some instances proptosis is minimal, leading the clinician to suspect an intracranial cause for the optic nerve compression. This may be accounted for by atrophy of orbital fat which allows the orbit to contain a moderate sized mass without protrusion of the eye. *An orbital CT scan is therefore recommended in all cases of visual failure*. Mild disc oedema is a common finding.

At CT the cavernous haemangioma is one of the few characteristic lesions (Fig. 3.25). The large majority are solitary lesions, situated within the muscle cone, inferolateral to the optic nerve, which is frequently considerably displaced, although this fact may be apparent only on coronal sections. Hoyt (1979 personal communication) has suggested that the preferred site of the tumour may be explained by the fact that the inferotemporal quadrant of the intraconal space is not entered by the optic nerve during normal eye movements, a fact clearly demonstrable at CT (Fig. 2.2). The tumour is rounded, smooth (the minor lobulations characteristic of pathological specimens are not usually evident) and clearly defined. Some of the larger tumours may become pear-shaped as they tend to fill the orbital apex. In such cases demonstration that the tumour is separate from the optic nerve is greatly facilitated by coronal and/or oblique sections; sagittal reconstructions may also be helpful.

Attenuation values of cavernous haemangiomas are slightly higher than the adjacent soft tissue structures, and intravenous contrast medium produces a dense, homogeneous increase. Calcification is well recognized as occurring in cavernous haemangiomas, but in our experience is rare at CT. The orbit is enlarged in about 50% of cases.

Failure to confirm the presence of a cavernous haemangioma by angiography or phlebography should not sway the diagnosis, since it is axiomatic that the slowly flowing vascular pools may not fill with contrast medium.

Other vascular tumours
Other vascular tumours are less common; the classification by Reese indicates their structural origin:

Polymorphous origin	*Monomorphous origin*
Angioblastic	Haemangioendothelioma
Capillary	Haemangiopericytoma
Cavernous	Leiomyoma, leiomyosarcoma
Racemose	
Telangiectatic	

Lymphangiomas. In children, lymphangiomas produce a distinct clinical picture with episodes of proptosis attributed to haemorrhage within the tumour. The tumours are usually benign and recurrent haemorrhage may play a part in the production of orbital blood cysts. Proptosis may be exacerbated by upper respiratory tract infections (Fig. 3.26).

Treatment is often troublesome because the diffuse nature of the tumour, without a clear capsule, makes surgical excision difficult. It is of interest that electron microscopy shows that while the cavernous haemangioma is composed of endothelial cells surrounded by one or two layers of muscle cells, enclosed by basement membrane material, lymphangiomas are composed of flattened endothelial cells, with unstable junctions and surrounded by a discontinuous basement membrane (Jakobiec and Tannenbaum, 1975). These findings may contribute to an understanding of the clinical behaviour and CT features of these tumours.

Haemangiopericytomas usually occur outside the muscle cone, but resemble cavernous haemangiomas both clinically and radiologically although Hilal and Trokel (1977) noted that the lesion tends to lie on the nasal side of the optic nerve. Surgical excision requires dexterity and gentle handling, for these tumours are fragile and have a thin capsule. They may recur after removal, particularly when excision is incomplete, and have the potential to metastasize.

Lacrimal gland tumours
These are of three main types: mixed tumours analogous to parotid gland lesions, carcinomas, and malignant lymphomas. Dermoid cysts and simple adenomas are rare; in the remaining cases, it usually transpires that the 'tumour' is inflammatory.

A study of 115 cases of expanding lesions of the lacrimal gland by Reese showed the following distribution:

Dacroadenitis	26
Sarcoidosis	5
Malignant lymphoma	28
Carcinoma	27
Mixed tumour	25
Dermoid cyst	2
Adenoma	2

The common tumours therefore are equally distributed between malignant lymphomas, mixed tumours and carcinomas.

Clinical features. Lacrimal gland tumours usually present with a

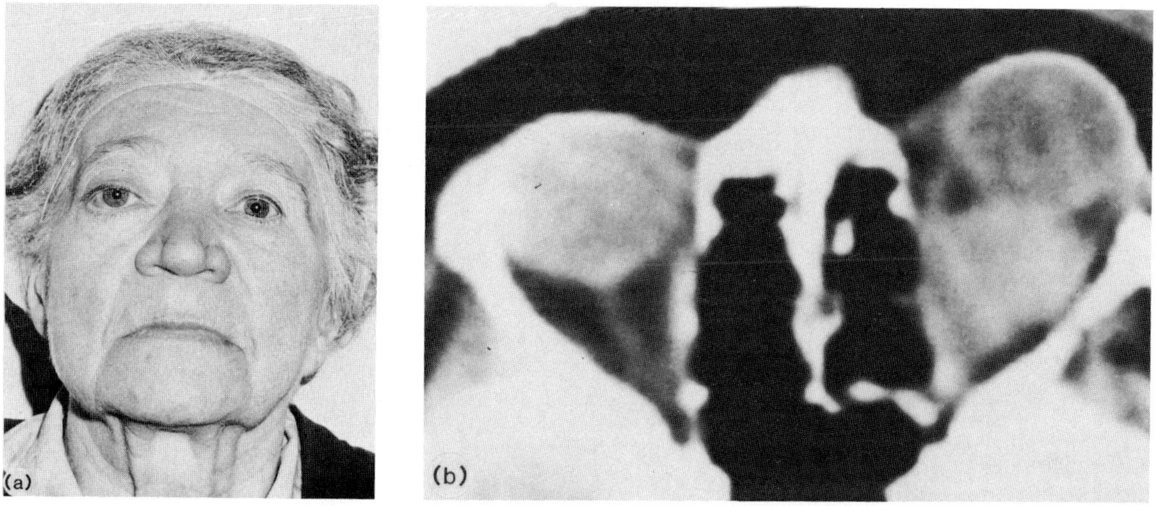

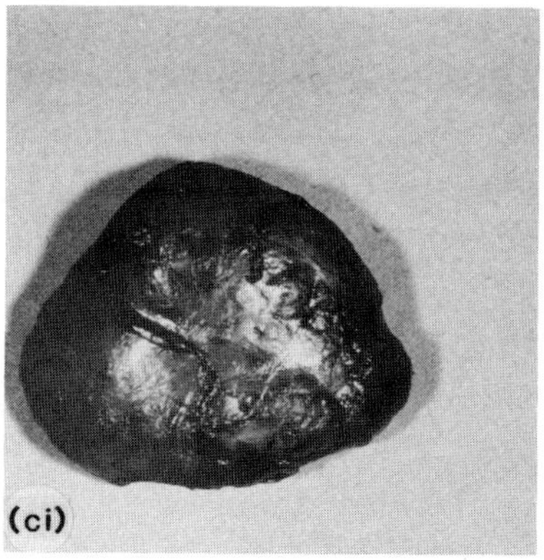

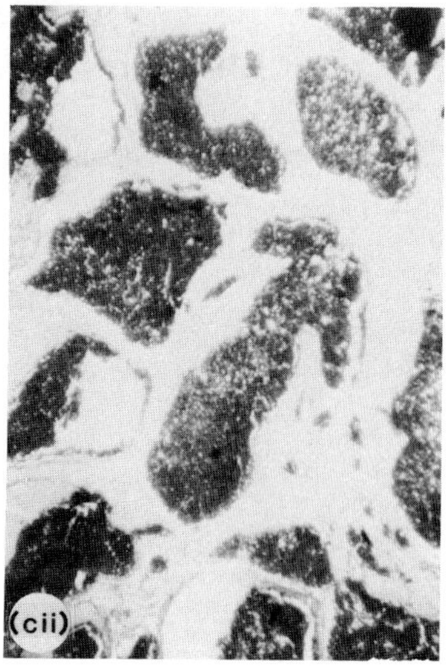

Fig. 3.25 Cavernous haemangioma. An elderly lady gave a history of painless proptosis for 12 years, with some distortion of central vision. There was axial proptosis of 7 mm on the right with resistance to retropulsion (a). Fundus examination showed choroidal striae. CT (b) revealed a rounded, slightly pear-shaped intraconal mass of higher attenuation than the globe. The lamina papyracea was concave. A typical cavernous haemangioma (c) was removed.

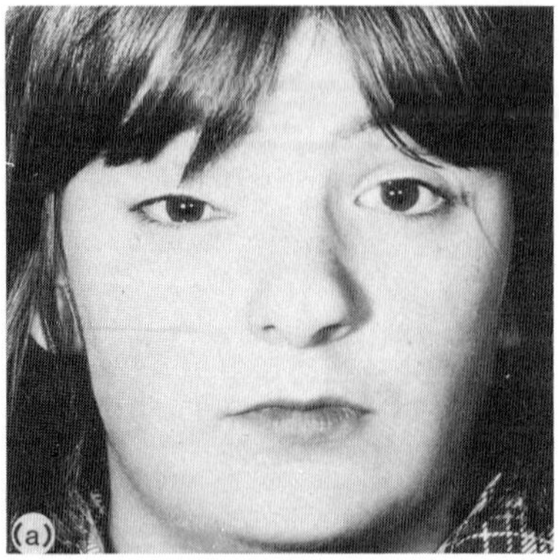

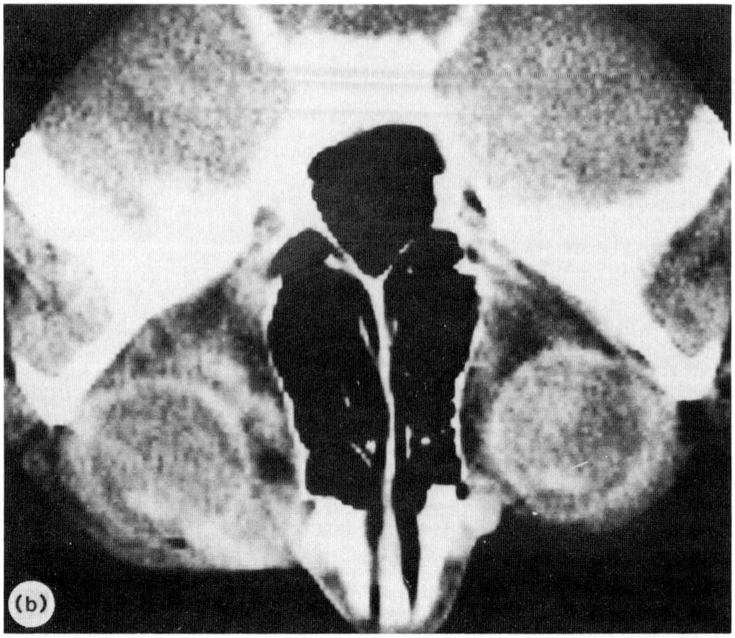

Fig. 3.26 Lymphangioma. A 9-year old boy was referred with a history of intermittent right proptosis, often associated with respiratory infections. Examination showed ptosis, and a palpable mass superomedial to the right orbit (a). He had previously suffered nose bleeds and a partial excision of a lesion on the nose confirmed the diagnosis of lymphangioma. CT showed an irregular area of increased density within the muscle cone (b) and a mass medial to the right globe, displacing it laterally (c).

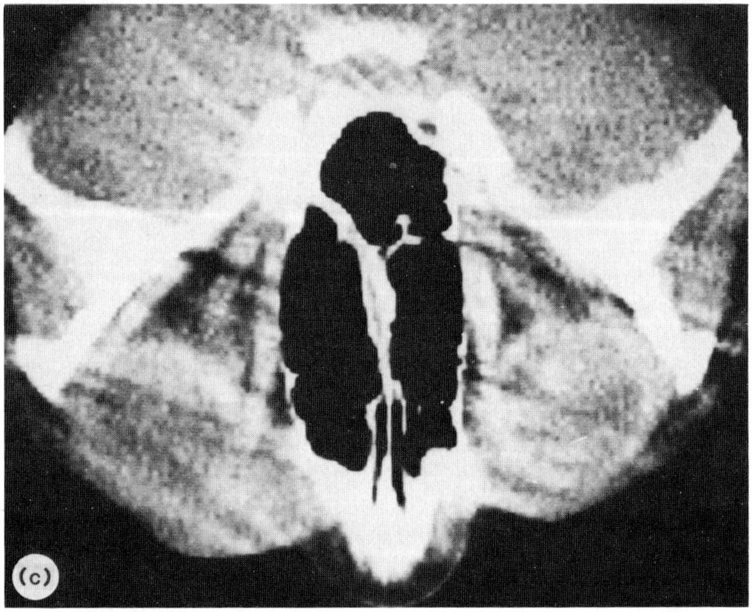

laterally placed mass in the upper lid. Increased watering of the eye may be noted. Pain and rapid progression often suggest a carcinoma. Other features depend on the extent of the lesion, and may include proptosis, diplopia, or visual symptoms produced by distortion of the globe. Granuloma of the lacrimal gland may also simulate a carcinoma.

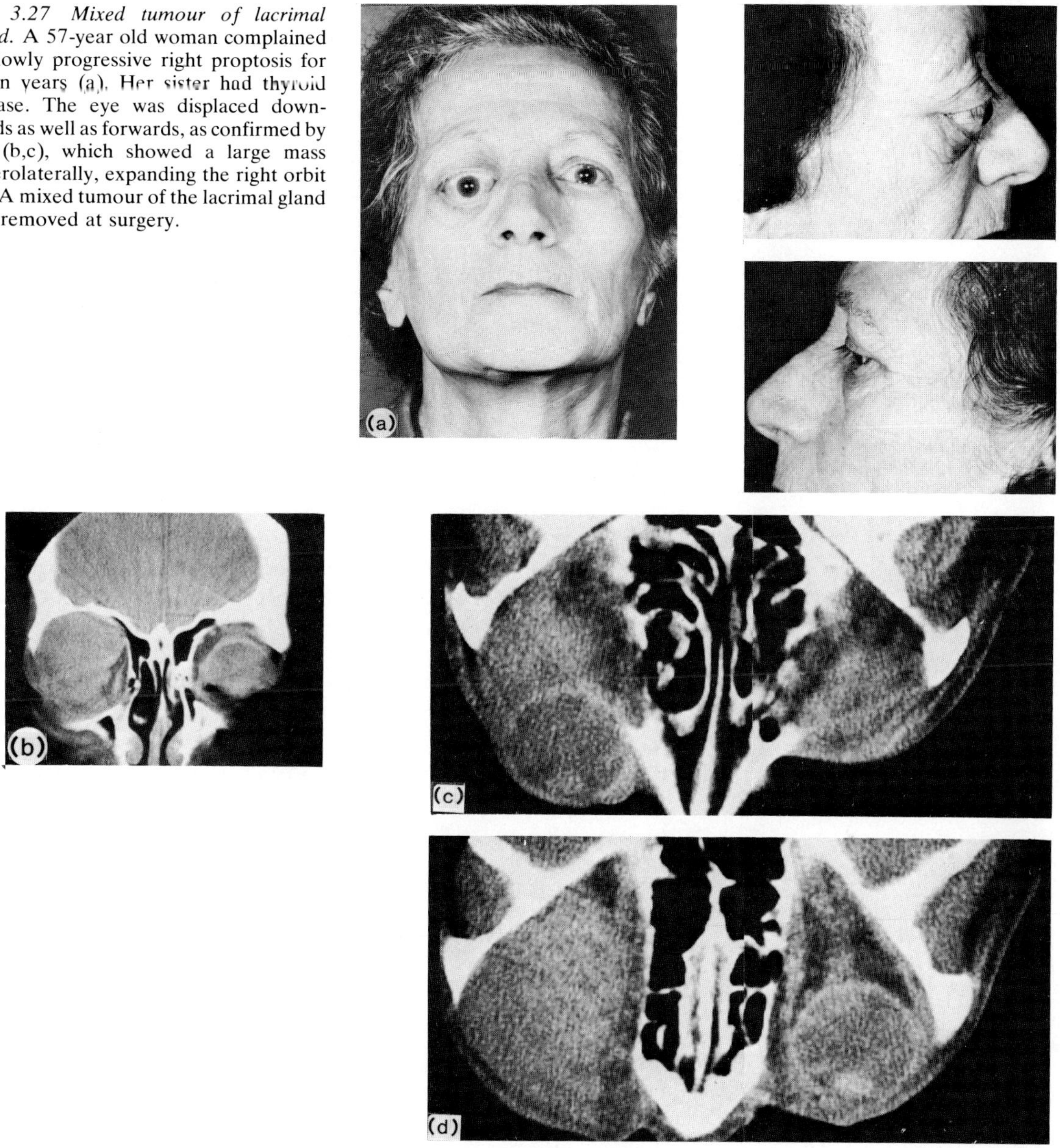

Fig. 3.27 Mixed tumour of lacrimal gland. A 57-year old woman complained of slowly progressive right proptosis for seven years (a). Her sister had thyroid disease. The eye was displaced downwards as well as forwards, as confirmed by CT (b,c), which showed a large mass superolaterally, expanding the right orbit (d). A mixed tumour of the lacrimal gland was removed at surgery.

Mixed tumours (Fig. 3.27). Wright *et al.* (1979) have pointed out that successful management of so-called benign mixed cell lacrimal gland tumours depends on excisional biopsy *en bloc*, since seeding of tumour at the time of operation inevitably leads to recurrence, with possible malignant transformation.

Pathologically, these tumours exhibit marked pleomorphism, both from case to case and in different portions of the same tumour. They are usually contained within a capsule, although this may be closely attached to the periosteum and may have small nodular extensions, two factors which contribute to incomplete removal and local recurrence.

Carcinomas. These are usually adenocystic carcinomas with histological features of numerous small cells with hyperchromatic nuclei. They have a highly malignant course so that early recognition may be important. Frozen section examination at surgery is recommended, and if the diagnosis of carcinoma is confirmed exenteration is indicated. However, despite the aggressive approach the mortality rates remain high.

With the exception of dermoid tumours, which are discussed below, the various types of lacrimal gland tumour show no major indication of their origin: the lesion lies outside the muscle cone, superolaterally in the anterior part of the orbit, displacing the globe inferomedially and frequently extending towards the upper lid, where it is often palpable. Its form is extremely variable, ranging from a small, well-defined lesion to a large, amorphous mass filling the whole orbit; when the latter appearance is associated with a short history, lacrimal gland carcinoma can perhaps be suggested, but the clue to the site of origin may then be lacking. Attenuation coefficients are characteristically in the soft tissue range, and increase non-specifically after intravenous contrast medium; the lacrimal gland has, of course, no blood–tissue barrier. In one case of lymphoma we examined, the attenuation coefficients suggested haemorrhage within the tumour; calcification is well recognized histologically, in both mixed tumours or carcinomas, but is rarely seen at CT (Fig. 3.28).

Associated abnormalities aid in diagnosis; localized pressure erosion of the anterolateral portion of the orbital roof above the lacrimal fossa supports the suggestion that the tumour arose from the lacrimal gland; such erosion may become extensive (Fig. 3.29). At the time of presentation, up to 90% of *mixed tumours* will show this type of pressure erosion, which may even create a small defect in the floor of the anterior cranial fossa; bony sclerosis is also infrequently present. Similar pressure erosion is seen in more than half of lacrimal gland *carcinomas*, but up to 25% of these latter tumours will show irregular bony destruction. This important differential diagnostic feature may require both axial and coronal CT scans for adequate demonstration, and should always be sought when the lacrimal gland appears enlarged. Similar destructive changes are rarely seen with lacrimal gland suppuration. Infiltration of the lateral rectus muscle is not uncommon, but is non-specific. Bilateral enlargement of the lacrimal glands should suggest some other disease process, e.g. Mikulicz's syndrome (Fig. 3.15 p.42).

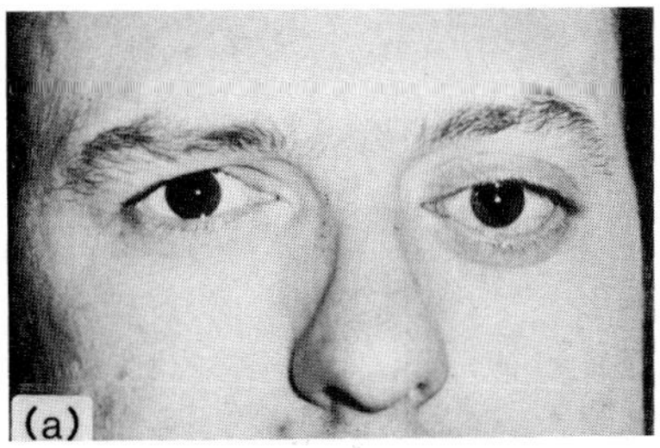

Fig. 3.28 Carcinoma of the lacrimal gland. This 37-year old man presented with a six-month history of slowly progressive left proptosis, which had recently become painful. Abduction was limited and painful. The globe was depressed and there was conjunctival hyperaemia (a). A mass was palpable near the lateral canthus. CT showed the mass to extend from the lateral canthus to the orbital apex, displacing the optic nerve medially (b). There was bone erosion (c,d) and calcification within the mass (c, arrow). Contrast medium produced marked enhancement (shown in (e), a computer subtraction). An adenoid cystic carcinoma of the lacrimal gland was radically excised, but unfortunately the patient returned two years later with a massive intracranial recurrence which proved lethal (f: before; g: after intravenous contrast medium).

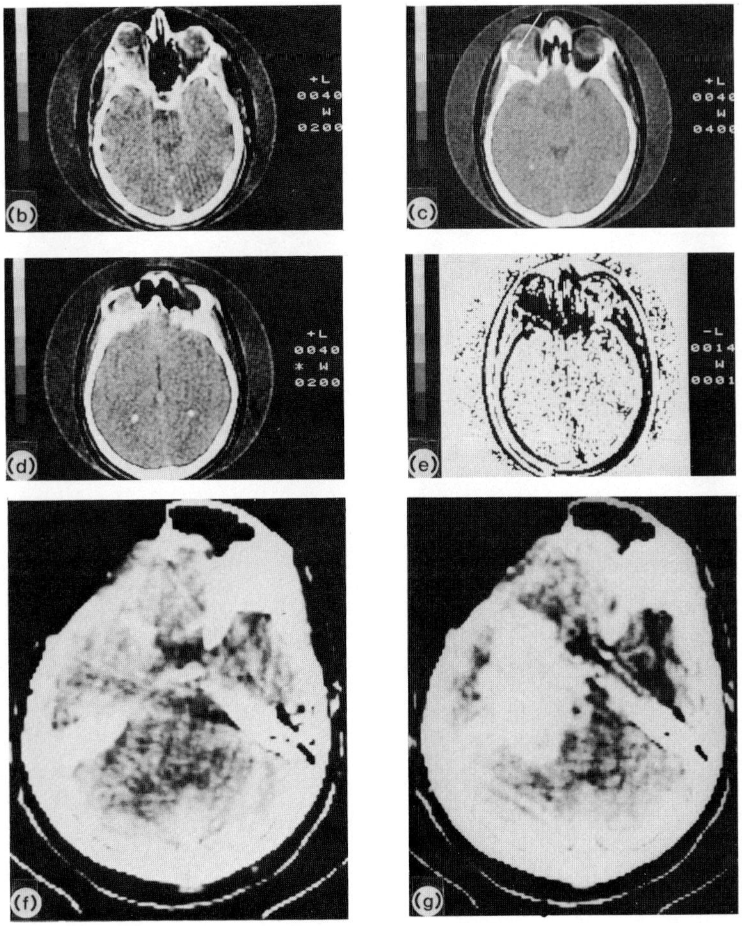

Dermoid cysts

Many of the foregoing remarks on lacrimal gland tumours apply also to dermoid cysts. Useful diagnostic observations in these generally well-encapsulated extraconal lesions are that their attenuation coefficients are frequently lower than those of other intraorbital masses, as a result of their fat content, and that pressure erosion of bone is usually very localized. It should be noted, however, that:

1. Not all dermoids contain enough fat to render the attenuation coefficients visibly low.
2. 'Low' in this context does not necessarily imply less than the attenuation of water (0 EMI units).
3. Even a fat-containing tumour may appear denser than the normal orbital fat, so that examination of the attenuation coefficients directly, by printout or by interrogating the data, may be necessary.

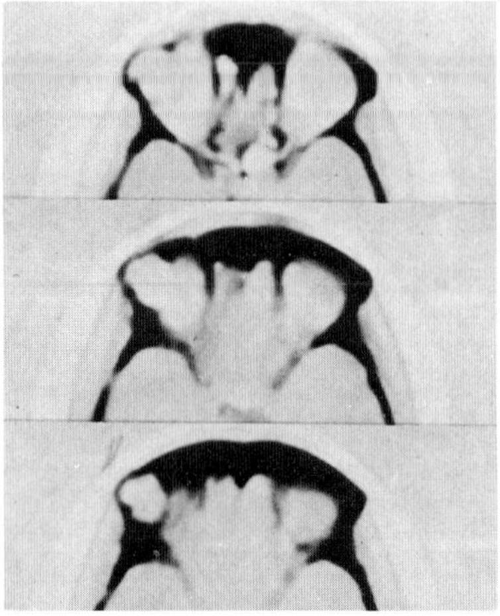

Fig. 3.29 Typical erosion of left orbital roof by lacrimal gland tumour.

4. These features may be obscured if inflammatory changes are present.

Given these caveats, the observation that a tumour in the anterior part of the orbit contains material of less than soft-tissue attenuation, particularly if there is a fluid level between sebaceous and lipid material, should raise the suspicion of a dermoid cyst (Fig. 3.30). These cysts may occur more posteriorly in the orbit, where some of the characteristic features may be absent.

Pressure erosion of the orbital margin by dermoid cysts is from within; this may be helpful in differentiating such a tumour from a mucocoele of the frontal sinus, which may also contain material of around water attenuation, but which expands towards the orbit. Plain radiography should assist in differential diagnosis, but clearly gives less information as to the intraorbital extent of the lesion.

Peripheral nerve tumours

Schwannoma (neurilemoma). This rare orbital tumour can occur anywhere in the orbit, but most commonly occupies the muscle cone to produce axial proptosis (Fig. 3.31). The tumour is benign and slowly progressive and histologically is composed of a proliferation of Schwann cells. It is found in 1.5% of cases of neurofibromatosis (Jakobiec and Jones 1979). CT shows a well-defined mass radiologically indistinguishable from a cavernous haemangioma.

Neurofibroma. This tumour may occur anywhere in the orbit, may be associated with neurofibromatosis, and results from a proliferation of Schwann cells, endoneural cells and axons. It is rarely encountered.

Plexiform neurofibroma. This tumour occurs as part of neurofibromatosis and is usually associated with ocular changes, sphenoid dysplasia and locally related pigmentation. The lesion is usually benign and presents a difficult problem in cosmetic surgery. However, in about 10% of cases a more malignant course follows, and we have seen one patient in whom orbital exenteration was necessary.

Other orbital tumours

Sarcomas of the orbit

Rhabdomyosarcoma is the commonest primary malignant orbital tumour in childhood; it is rare over the age of 20 years. Embryonal, alveolar and differentiated types are recognized, in descending order of frequency. Growth is generally rapid, and prognosis poor; metastases are common, and cerebral lesions

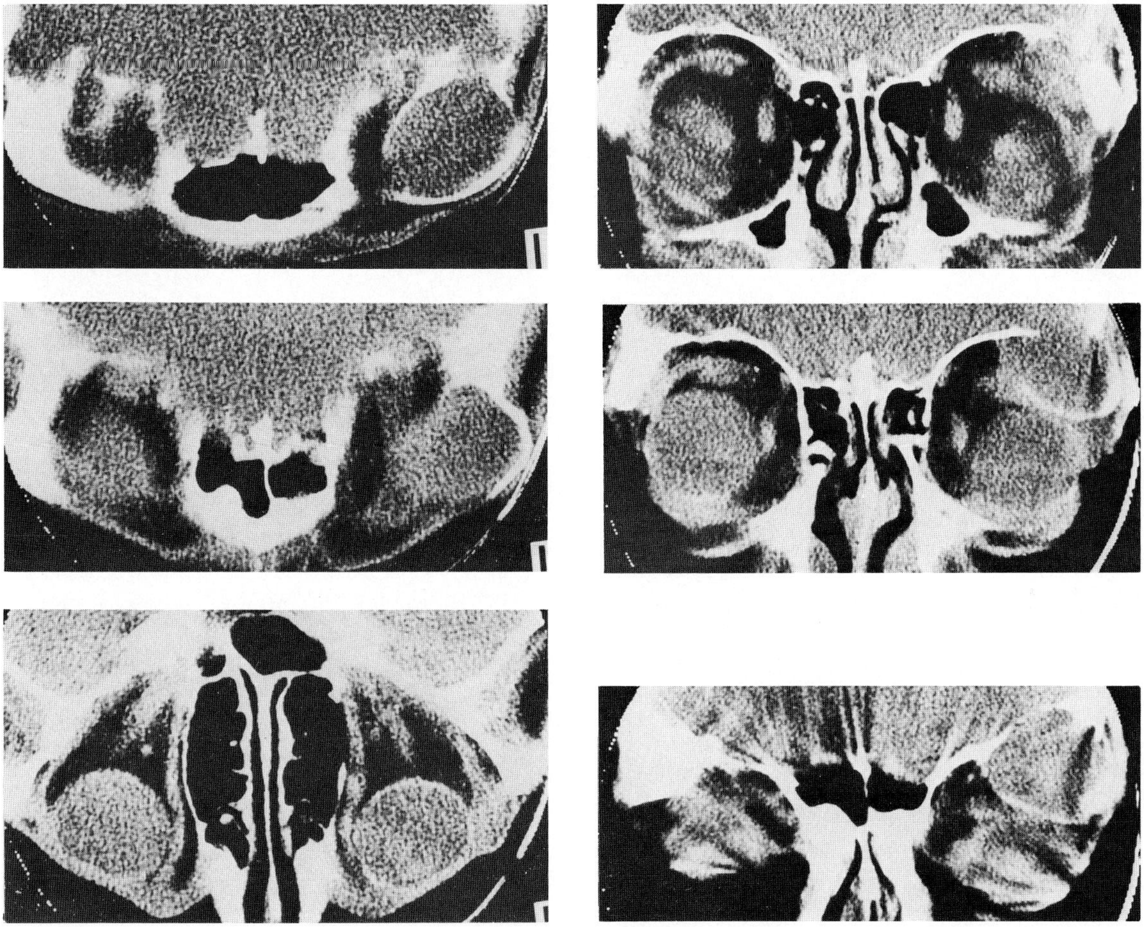

Fig. 3.30 Orbital dermoid. A 39-year old man presented with slowly progressive proptosis and depression of the left eye; vision was normal. CT: (left) axial cuts, descending; (right) coronal cuts, coming forwards. A homogeneous mass of slightly less than brain attenuation has expanded the bone of the orbital roof in the region of the lacrimal gland. The bone appears defective and intracranial extension is possible. The eye is displaced downwards. The orbital extension remains extraconal; it is well defined and probably encapsulated. Surgery: dermoid cyst.

may be observed at CT; the brain should therefore be examined routinely in children with these tumours.

CT shows a bulky or infiltrating intra- and extraconal tumour, often invading the orbital walls. It is usually evident that the mass is distinct from the globe and optic nerve. Marked enhancement after intravenous contrast medium has been described. The appearances are thus not specific, but the value of CT in assessing the extent and spread of the lesion, as well as the response to treatment, is evident (Fig. 3.32).

Other tumours derived from the mesenchymal tissue of the orbit, whose rarity is indicated by the fact that Reese's series of 230 cases contained only six examples of sarcomas, include

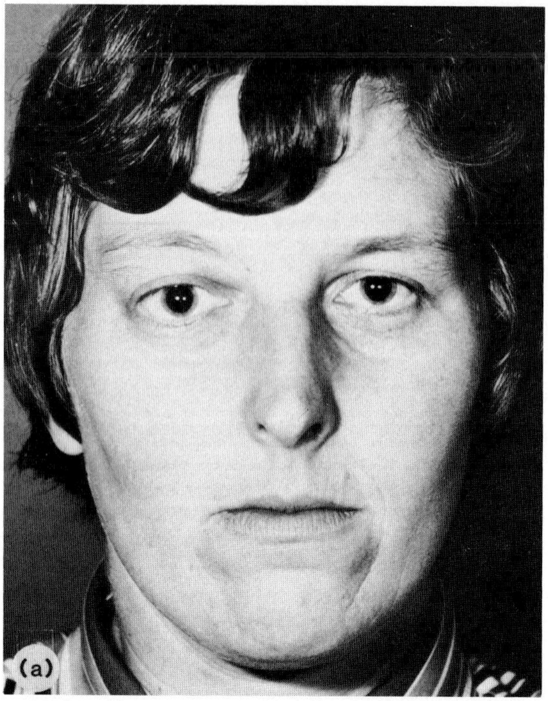

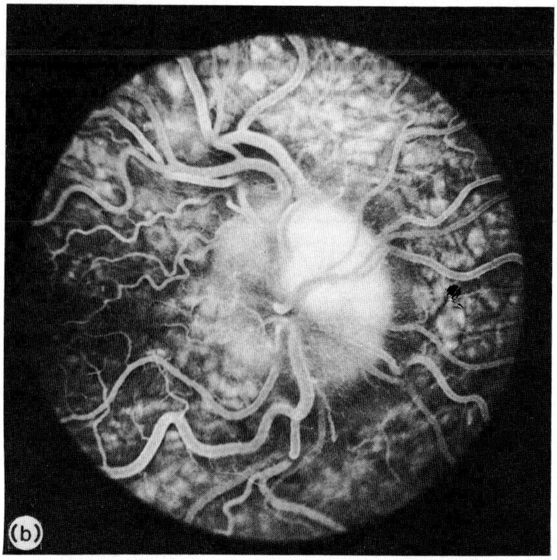

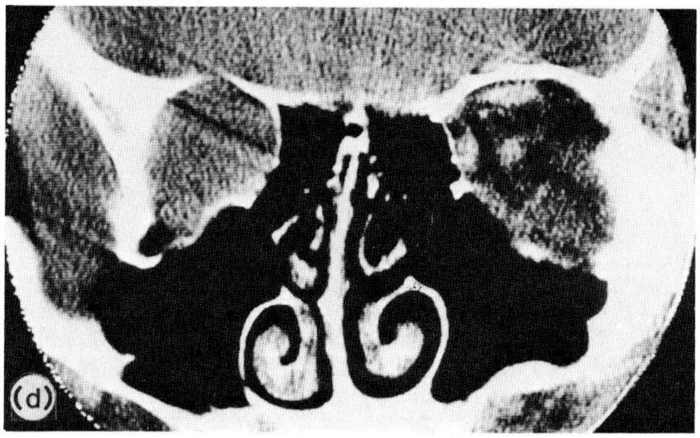

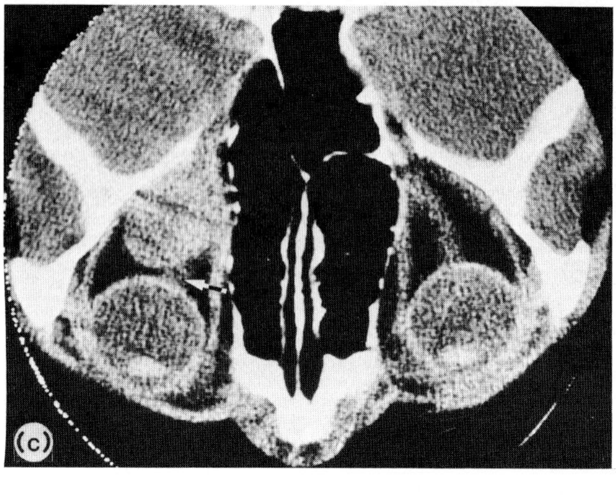

Fig. 3.31 *Schwannoma.* A 36-year old woman complained of right proptosis and blurred vision. There was irreducible axial proptosis (a) and visual acuity was reduced to 6/36; the optic disc was swollen (b). Axial (c) and coronal (d) CT sections showed a rounded intraconal tumour at the orbital apex, closely related to the optic nerve (arrow). The orbit was expanded. At surgery, the lesion was found to be a Schwannoma.

osteosarcoma, chondrosarcoma, myxosarcoma, fibrosarcoma and leiomyosarcoma (Reese, 1956).

Malignant granular cell myoblastoma is a further rare tumour presenting at any age and with a fairly benign prognosis.

Lymphomatous tumours of the orbit
The spectrum of lymphomatous infiltration of the orbit is wide, and recent immunopathological tests have facilitated the specif-

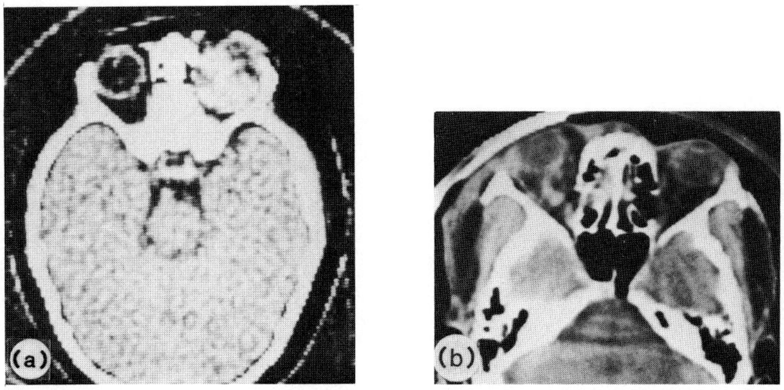

Fig. 3.32 Rhabdomyosarcoma. (a) A child of 4 years, with rapidly progressive right proptosis. CT showed an amorphous mass filling the retrobulbar space and enlarging the orbit. (b) A child of 7 years, who was noted to have orbital swelling after a blow to the face (note superficial soft tissue swelling). An amorphous intraconal retrobulbar mass seen at CT was originally thought to be a haematoma, but exploration revealed a rhabdomyosarcoma.

icity of diagnosis. Thus most orbital lymphomas are due to abnormalities of the B cell system, whereas the T cell disturbances (e.g. Hodgkin's disease) rarely involve the orbit. Aggregation of mature lymphocytes to form reactive lymphocytic hyperplasia is regarded as a form of pseudotumour rather than a lymphoma.

Classification of the non-Hodgkin's lymphomas has led to the following subdivision:

1. Undifferentiated lymphoma
2. Histiocytic lymphoma (reticulum cell sarcoma)
3. Mixed lymphoma
4. Malignant lymphoma – poorly differentiated
5. Malignant lymphoma – well differentiated

It is extremely rare for a patient with systemic lymphoma to *present* to an ophthalmologist; only three of 1269 patients in Rosenberg's series did so, although another 13 patients developed proptosis during the course of their disease (Rosenberg *et al.* 1965).

Patients may have had proptosis for variable periods ranging from days to years. The lymphoma may arise anywhere within the orbit, though the lacrimal gland and anterior orbit are preferential sites. Subconjunctival lymphomas are sometimes visible as salmon pink swellings, though some of these may represent lymphocytic hyperplasia.

Orbital reticulum cell sarcoma is of interest to ophthalmologists. It is always part of a systemic disease, which occurs in the fifth, sixth and seventh decades and carries a poor prognosis. Brain involvement may occur, but is seen more frequently in the absence of systemic disease, as reticulum cell sarcoma (microglioma) of the brain. In this condition the orbit is not usually involved, but there is neoplastic seeding in the vitreous and anterior chamber so that these patients present with uveitis. Diagnosis can be difficult initially, with normal haematological, bone marrow, and CSF examination, so that when vision is reduced it may be necessary to resort to vitreous biopsy. In two recent patients with bilateral uveitis an abnormal monoclonal band was present on electrophoresis as the only abnormality, and death followed within two years.

CT scanning shows a poorly defined mass, or in some cases diffuse infiltration of the whole orbit (Fig. 3.33). Lymphoid tumours may be extraconal and anterior to the orbital septum (Hilal and Trokel, 1977). In microgliomatosis a cerebral scan may show multiple well-defined high density lesions in the cerebral hemispheres or less obvious infiltrating lesions.

Metastases to the orbit

Metastatic disease should be considered in any patient presenting with orbital signs, particularly in the sixth and seventh decades. The clinician may be aided by a past history of carcinoma of some other site and such information should always be actively sought. The presence of orbital apex or orbital signs without significant proptosis should alert the clinician to the schirrhous form of carcinoma, metastatic to the orbit. Furthermore, in a review of 220 cases of carcinoma, Ferry and Font (1974) found 28 with metastases to the orbit. In these patients the primary site was:

Breast	8
Lung	4
G-U tract	4
Pancreas	1
Ileum	1
Undetermined	10

Thus, the largest single group comprised those cases in which the site of the primary lesion was unknown. The presence of a non-specific ill-defined orbital mass on CT scanning should raise discussion about the use of the CT whole body scan in the detection of a primary site (Fig. 3.34).

The site of orbital metastases is non-specific; they can be intra- or extraconal, or they can cause sufficient distortion of the normal retrobulbar structures for this distinction to be impossible. In distinction to the inflammatory lesions described previously, however, they are not in general multifocal, and the integrity of the anatomical structures is usually preserved. Neither the attenuation coefficients nor the behaviour with intravenous contrast medium are in any way specific, but CT often provides useful information for planning biopsy (Fig. 3.12, p.37).

Associated local bone destruction may be present, but does not necessarily indicate malignancy, since it can occur with granulomas. The presence of typical intracerebral deposits, or the history of prior malignant disease, are almost the only valuable differential diagnostic features.

Fig. 3.33 Orbital reticulum cell sarcoma. This woman had bilateral proptosis and ophthalmoplegia for 15 years, which was attributed to thyroid disease, though tests were abnormal on only one occasion. When seen at age 64, she showed tense orbits with conjunctival dilatation, proptosis, thickening of the lids and limited eye movements. There were also enlarged cervical nodes (a), and biopsy showed reticulum cell sarcoma. CT before (b) and after (c) intravenous contrast medium: the entire retro- and peribulbar spaces are occupied by soft tissue masses, showing considerable contrast enhancement and effacing the normal anatomy. The lamina papyracea bulges medially on both sides. The patient died one year later despite radiotherapy.

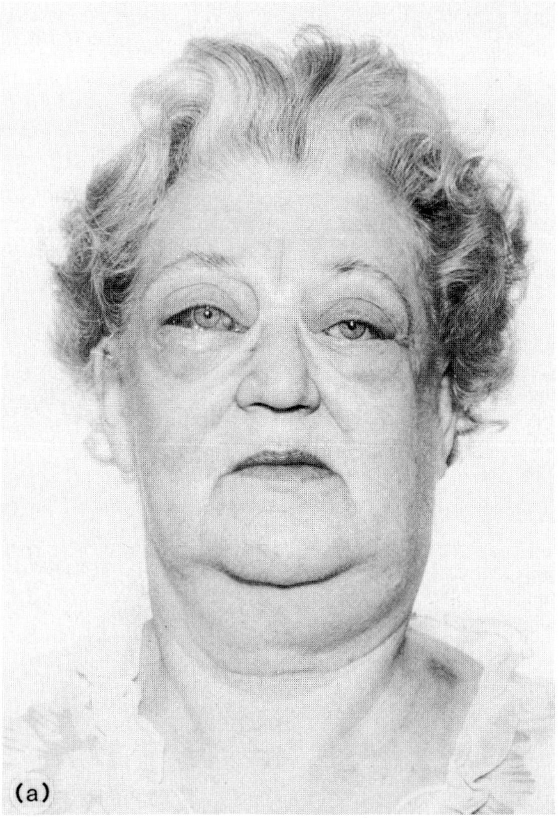

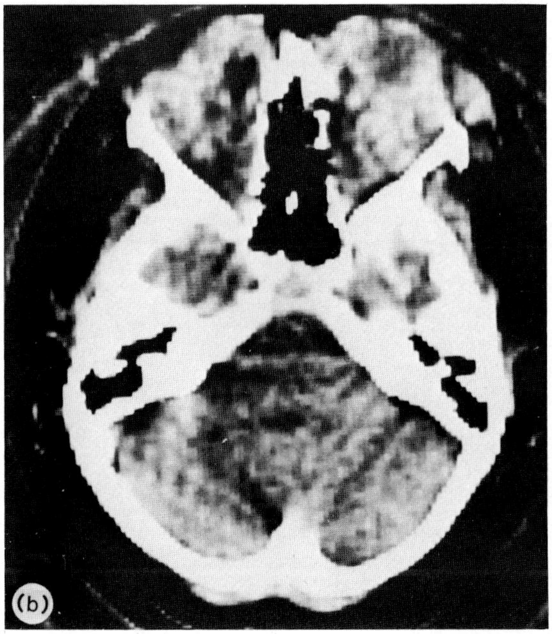

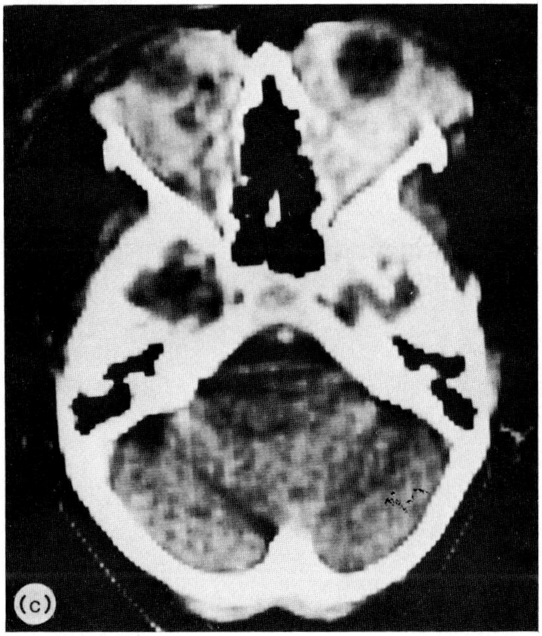

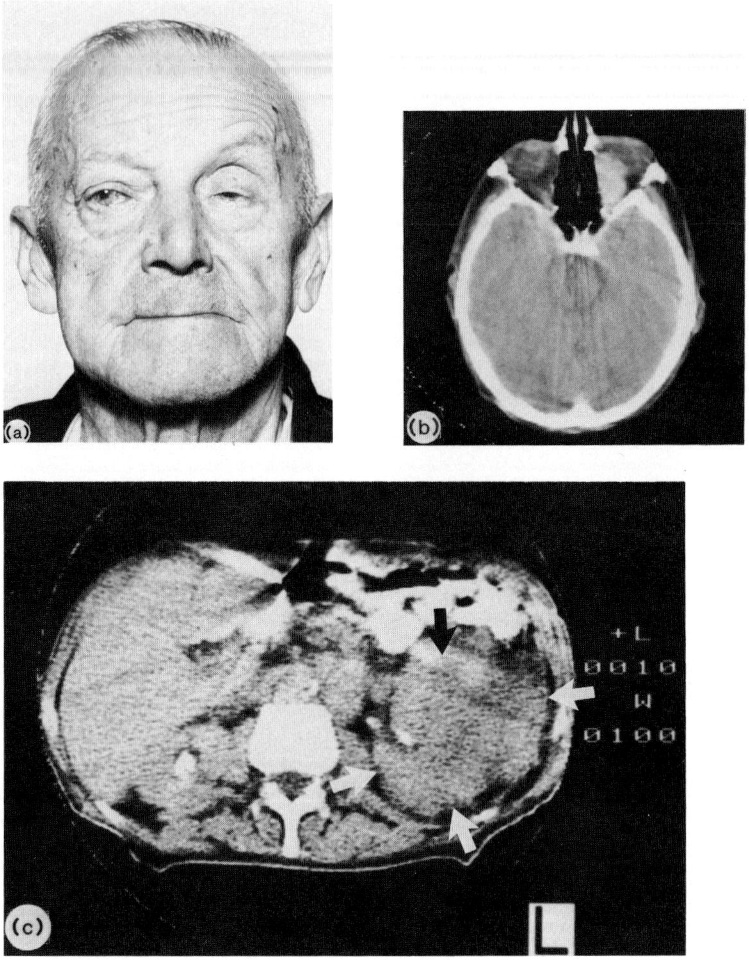

Fig. 3.34 Orbital metastasis. A 72-year old man presented with ptosis and diplopia. Ocular movements were limited on the right more than the left (a). CT showed a mass in the medial part of the right orbit (b) and other cuts showed infiltration of the left orbital apex. Biopsy showed a hypernephroma, and a whole body scan (c) demonstrated an enlarged left kidney (arrows), which was not clinically palpable.

Neuroblastoma. This tumour of the adrenal medulla and paraspinal neural tissues occurs in children and frequently metastasizes to the orbit or intracranially. Metastases are blood-borne and characteristically produce bony erosion. It is important to realize that although they generally occur late in the course of the disease, orbital manifestations may antedate recognition of the primary lesion, which in such cases is more commonly abdominal than intrathoracic.

3.3 VASCULAR LESIONS

The assessment of vascular lesions of the orbit (in the sense of congenital or acquired anatomical anomalies of the vessels, rather than atheromatous arterial disease) can call for a combination of clinical examination, plain radiography, angiography and CT. In many cases, however, particularly those in which no specific therapy is envisaged whatever the results of such investigations, such detailed work-up is not indicated. In the present section, therefore, the characteristic appearances will be described, and an attempt made to define the utility of the various investigations.

Congenital lesions are discussed in Chapter 7.

The only acquired lesion which need concern us is the *caroticocavernous fistula*, of which two main types can be distinguished, although there is some overlap between the two. *Traumatic* caroticocavernous fistulae are the result of head or facial trauma, usually severe, and result from a tear of the internal carotid artery (or one of its meningeal branches) within the cavernous sinus. There is a direct arteriovenous shunt, usually of high-flow type, but fed by a single artery. *Spontaneous* caroticocavernous fistulae do not follow any obvious antecedent, and may be the end result of a dural arteriovenous malformation, fed by the external carotid artery branches (or occasionally by a meningeal branch of the internal carotid), rupturing into the lumen of the cavernous sinus. Although the shunt may not be so voluminous, there may be several feeding vessels. Spontaneous closure is more common in this type.

The clinical features of caroticocavernous fistulae provide the best example of the ocular and orbital sequelae of hypoxia. The conjunctival and episcleral vessels are characteristic, with dilatation and arteriolization of the veins due to the high pressure arterial blood they contain. Chemosis, lid oedema, corneal changes, elevation of the intraocular pressure, and ischaemic uveitis and retinal vascular changes with venous decompensation may be seen (Sanders and Hoyt, 1969). Ophthalmoplegia, initially thought to be due to ocular motor nerve abnormality, may also be due to hypoxia of the extraocular muscles which are seen at CT to be enlarged. Pulsating exophthalmos is not usually a prominent feature. These clinical appearances may also be caused by other conditions in which orbital or ocular perfusion is precarious.

Diagnosis is usually not difficult, but in mild cases, presenting with a slightly red eye and failure of abduction, a bruit should always be listened for, in case a small dural shunt is present. CT plays a more important role in the cases in which the diagnosis is more obscure.

The natural history of this condition is poorly understood; a number of cases may close spontaneously, or closure may follow vomiting, carotid compression, or angiography. Angiography of the internal carotid artery and the branches of the external carotid is of diagnostic and nowadays of therapeutic value. Therapy which fails to close the fistula but reduces the arterial supply renders the globe and orbit even more hypoxic.

The CT appearances can be divided into primary, secondary and associated features. The primary abnormalities are the manifestations of the fistula *per se*: dilatation of the intraorbital veins, most strikingly of the superior ophthalmic vein, which may be up to 1 cm in diameter, and may be seen coursing obliquely through the upper part of the orbit, the flow being forwards from the superior orbital fissure (Fig. 3.35). Other veins, notably the inferior ophthlamic (best identified on coronal sections) and the angular (beside the nose), may also be dilated on one or both sides. The dilated veins show prominent increase in attenuation coefficients after intravenous contrast medium. There may also be marked enhancement representing the cavernous sinus and/or the vessel(s) feeding the fistula.

Secondary features are those caused by the presence of the dilated veins and the disturbance of the normal orbital haemodynamics. They include proptosis, often marked, and swelling, probably the result of venous engorgement and oedema, of such structures as the extraocular muscles; in severe cases the fat may also be seen to be oedematous. These latter abnormalities are more marked in the acute stages (Fig. 3.36).

Associated abnormalities are seen in patients with traumatic fistulae: evidence of old fracture and/or operation, post-traumatic cerebral defects, etc.

The primary and secondary abnormalities may disappear completely or regress following spontaneous resolution or therapeutic obliteration of the fistula (Fig. 3.36). Post-embolization control scans may show one or more contrast medium- or bismuth-filled balloons lying in the region of the cavernous sinus (Fig. 3.35).

3.4 INVOLVEMENT OF THE ORBIT BY DISEASE OF ADJACENT STRUCTURES

The paranasal sinuses

The orbits are closely related to the paranasal sinuses inferiorly, medially and anterosuperiorly; it is not surprising therefore, that sinus disease is a potent source of orbital complications.

Developmental lesions

Hyperaeration of one or more loculi of the ethmoid or frontal sinuses can occur. The diagnosis is usually evident from plain films, but CT may be very useful in demonstrating the exact extent of orbital invasion. Severe ocular problems are rarely associated.

Inflammatory disease

Inflammatory disease of the paranasal sinuses is extremely common, and although only a small percentage of patients develop orbital complications, the outcome can be serious. Acute infections of the sinuses may give rise to orbital cellulitis or

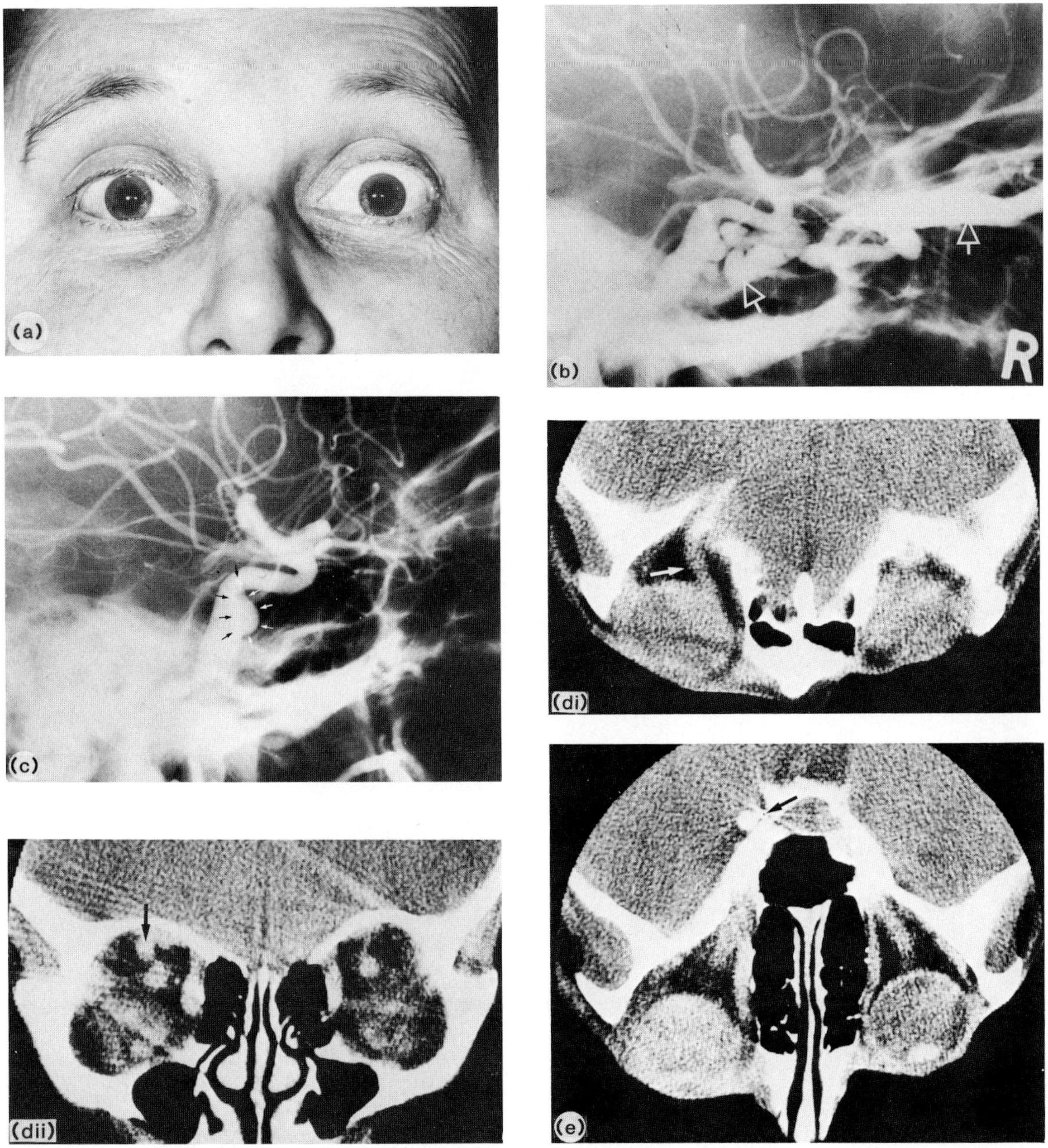

Fig. 3.35 *Caroticocavernous fistula.* No history of head injury preceded the onset of a bruit in this 47-year old woman. There was minimal right proptosis, with conjunctival hyperaemia (a), but the ocular fundus was normal. Carotid angiography (b) demonstrated immediate shunting to the cavernous sinus and superior ophthalmic vein (arrows). The fistula was closed with a detachable balloon catheter (c – arrows). Despite immediate improvement, subsequent CT (d) showed the persistence of a large superior ophthalmic vein (arrows). The silicone-filled balloon can be seen in (e) (short arrow).

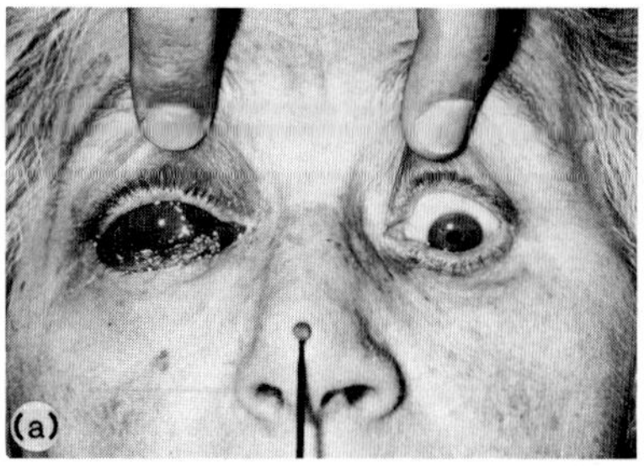

Fig. 3.36 Caroticocavernous fistula. This 72-year old woman with a known right middle cerebral artery aneurysm was seen during an attack of pain and swelling of the right eye. There was severe right haemorrhagic chemosis (a) with gross limitation of eye movements in all directions. Vision was normal and there was no bruit. CT(b) showed right proptosis, with herniation of the medial fat pad. The extraocular muscles were swollen; a dilated right superior ophthalmic vein was evident (arrowheads). (c) *Right* carotid angiogram: the middle cerebral artery aneurysm (open arrow) was seen but there was only very slight filling of the fistula (small arrows). (d) *Left* carotid angiogram: There was early filling of retrosellar meningeal branches (1, arrow), thence of the right cavernous sinus (2) and superior ophthalmic vein (3). After the angiogram, the clinical changes regressed and six weeks later the right eye was normal (e), as was the CT study (f).

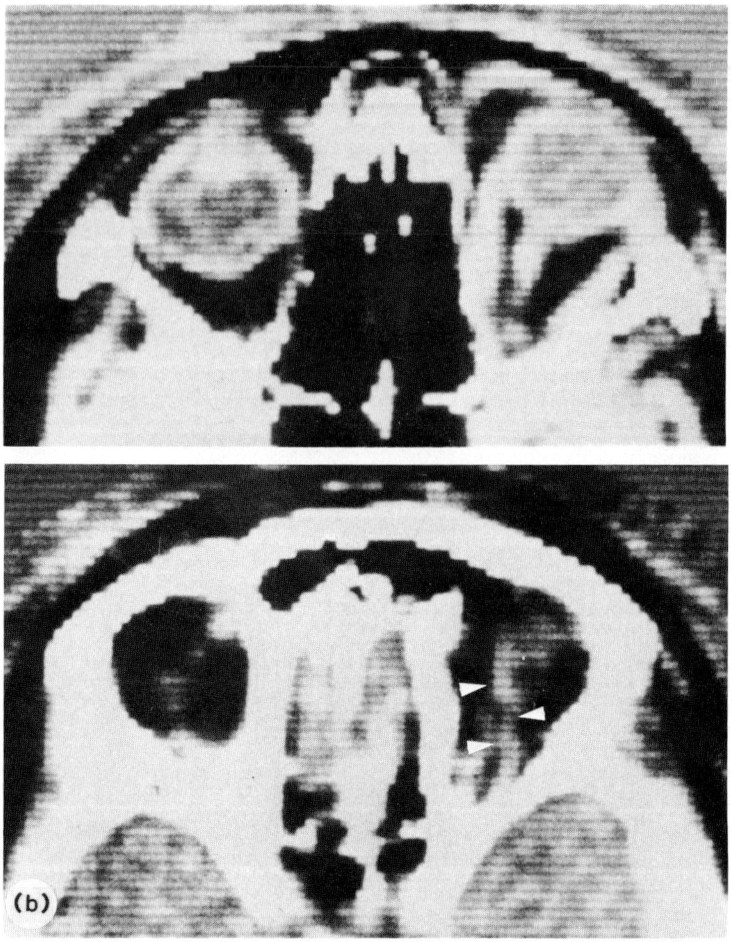

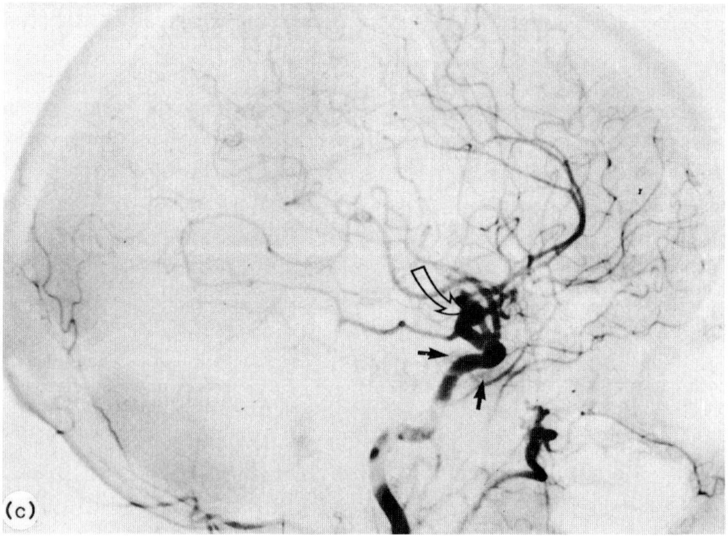

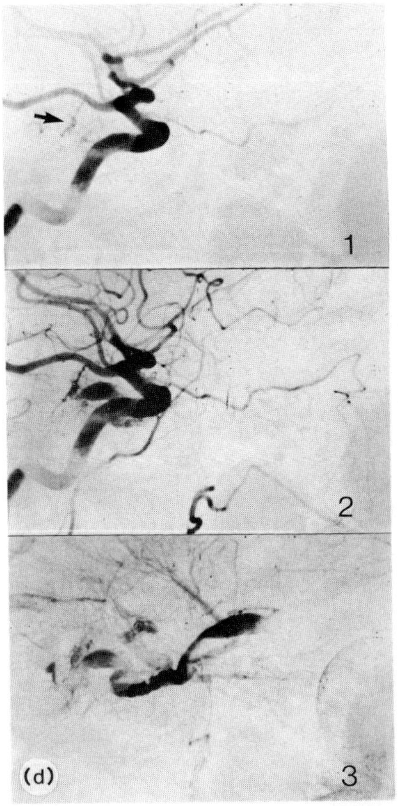

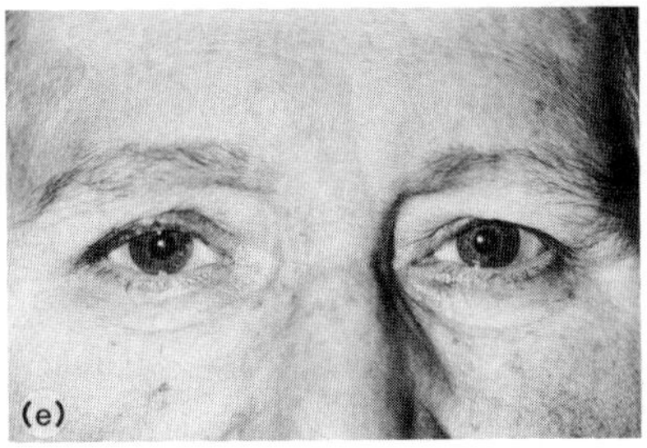

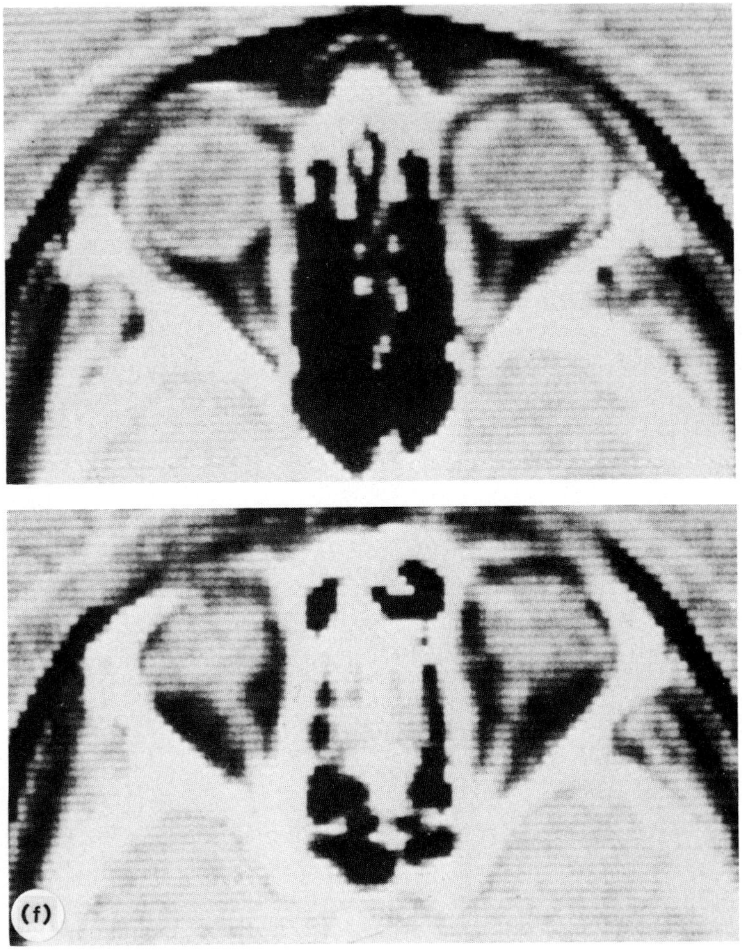

even frank suppuration; the CT changes are described above. The sinuses appear partially or completely opaque. This may be due to soft tissue swelling; if fluid is present, an air-fluid level can often be identified. When inflammatory changes are seen in both sinuses and orbits the primary lesion may be difficult to identify, but the source is almost invariably in the sinus.

Chronic inflammatory disease may be specific, e.g. Wegener's granuloma, but more commonly no aetiological factor is identified. Large soft-tissue masses are seen in the affected sinuses; their walls are often thinned and the sinus may be enlarged. The CT features may not allow the distinction between an ethmoid sinus expanded by pus, i.e. a mucocoele, and one full of soft tissue, as with a granuloma or exuberant polyposis. Low attenuation coefficients generally favour the former, and marked increase with intravenous contrast medium the latter, but these differences are not constant.

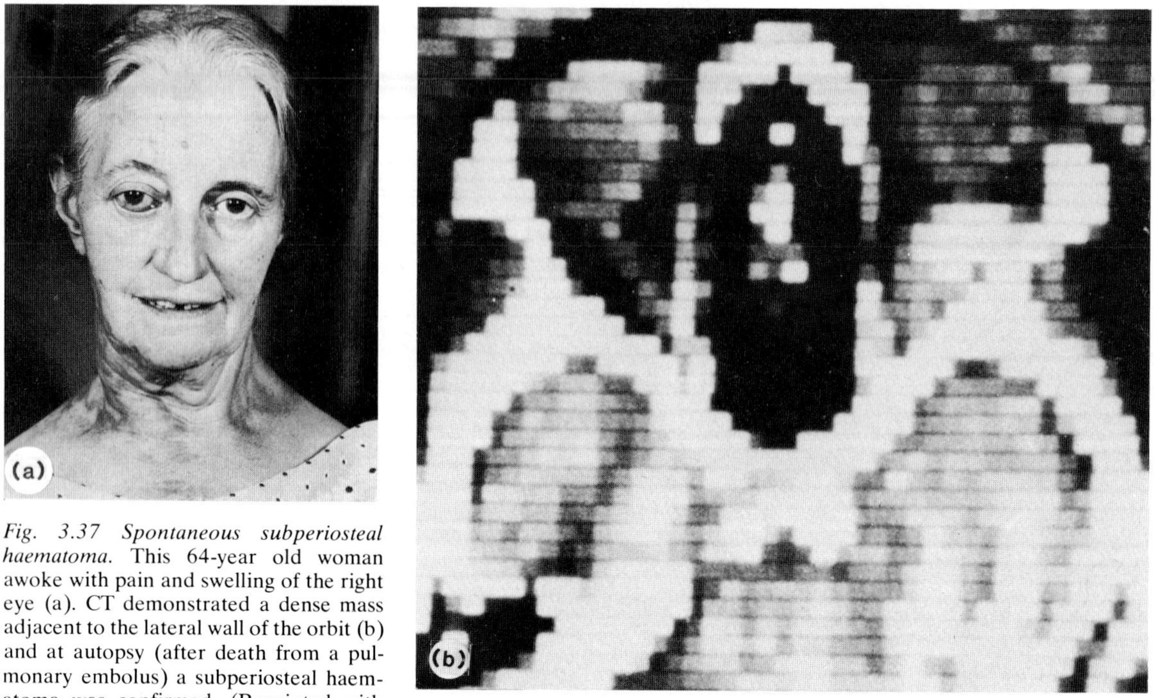

Fig. 3.37 Spontaneous subperiosteal haematoma. This 64-year old woman awoke with pain and swelling of the right eye (a). CT demonstrated a dense mass adjacent to the lateral wall of the orbit (b) and at autopsy (after death from a pulmonary embolus) a subperiosteal haematoma was confirmed. (Reprinted with permission. Previously appeared in 'Computer assisted tomography in orbital disease' *Br. J. Ophthal.*, 1974, **58** (6), 584 (Fig. 15a.)

Haematoma

Spontaneous intraorbital haematoma (Fig. 3.37) is a rare lesion, and may follow trauma or surgery to the lids or sinuses. Subperiosteal haematomata represent a new diagnostic entity with important therapeutic implications. We have only seen one case (Gawler *et al.*, 1974), but this condition has now been reported in other adults and indeed in babies with postnatal trauma.

Benign soft tissue tumours

Such tumours of the paranasal sinuses may be indistinguishable at CT from chronic inflammatory lesions. Ossifying fibroma present a different picture, with an extremely dense ossified mass within the sinus (usually the frontal sinus) (Fig. 3.38). In the advanced stages the sinus becomes expanded, and its walls may be breached.

Malignant tumours

The hallmark of malignant tumours of the sinuses, of which about 80% are primary carcinomas, is bone destruction, but once again there is significant overlap with the appearances seen in chronic inflammatory conditions and with benign neoplasm (Weber *et al.*, 1978). It should be noted that apparent bone defects in the lamina papyracea are commonly seen in the normal, and that bone destruction in this region should be diagnosed

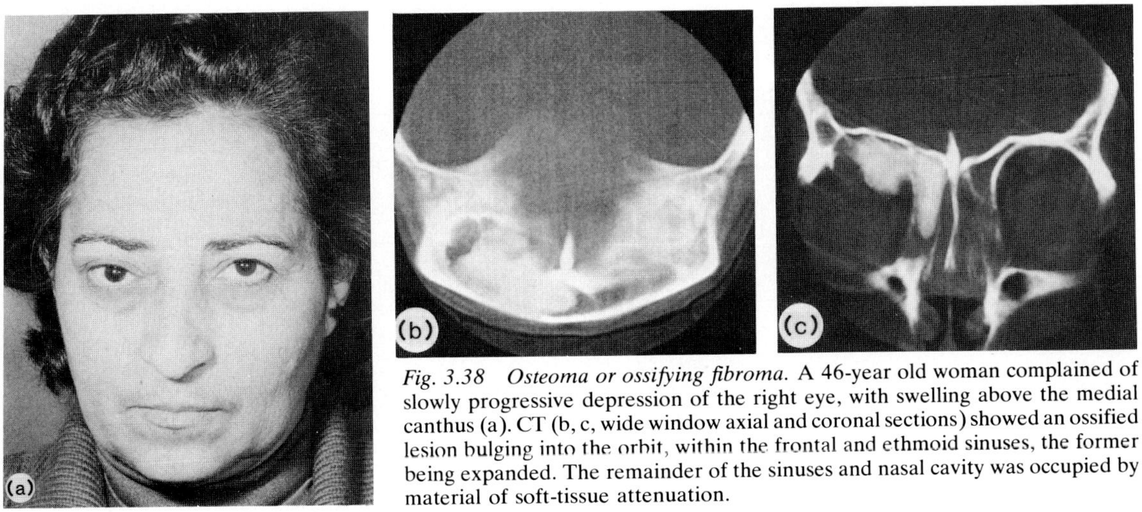

Fig. 3.38 *Osteoma or ossifying fibroma.* A 46-year old woman complained of slowly progressive depression of the right eye, with swelling above the medial canthus (a). CT (b, c, wide window axial and coronal sections) showed an ossified lesion bulging into the orbit, within the frontal and ethmoid sinuses, the former being expanded. The remainder of the sinuses and nasal cavity was occupied by material of soft-tissue attenuation.

with caution. In cases in which bone destruction rather than expansion of the sinus is the most salient feature, however, malignant neoplasm, usually carcinoma, is the most likely diagnosis. Such lesions usually arise in the ethmoid sinuses or adjacent nasal cavity. Direct invasion of the orbit is uncharacteristic; the tumour is often apparently resisted by the periorbita, so that a mass bulges into the orbit, displacing its contents, without directly involving them (Fig. 3.39).

Mancuso *et al*, (1978) compared the relative ability of CT and pluridirectional conventional tomography to determine the extent of orbital involvement by lesions arising in the paranasal sinuses. The latter technique gave a higher proportion of false positive results. CT gave accurate information as to whether the invading mass remained external to the periorbita in every one of 13 cases in which this was confirmed surgically. Such lesions are usually treated by radiotherapy, and CT in axial and coronal planes is the ideal method for planning radiation fields so as to spare the globe and optic nerve, and for the assessment of the effects of treatment. Obstruction of the ostia of the paranasal sinuses rapidly results in the sinus becoming opaque. Since CT does not distinguish between tumour tissue and trapped secretions, the demonstration of sinuses apparently full of soft-tissue attenuation material does not necessarily indicate spread of the disease to them. Unfortunately, even analysis of the CT attenuation coefficients before and after intravenous contrast medium does not resolve this difficulty. Contrast medium injection is, however, of value for the demonstration of intracranial extensions (Parsons and Hodson, 1979).

Similar remarks apply to malignant tumours spreading upwards from the nasopharynx (Fig. 3.40).

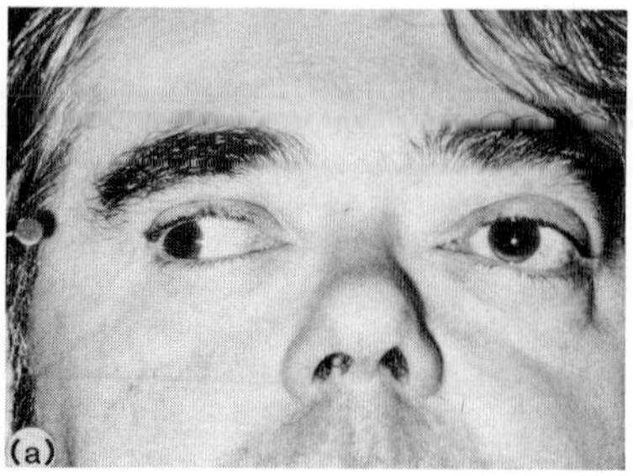

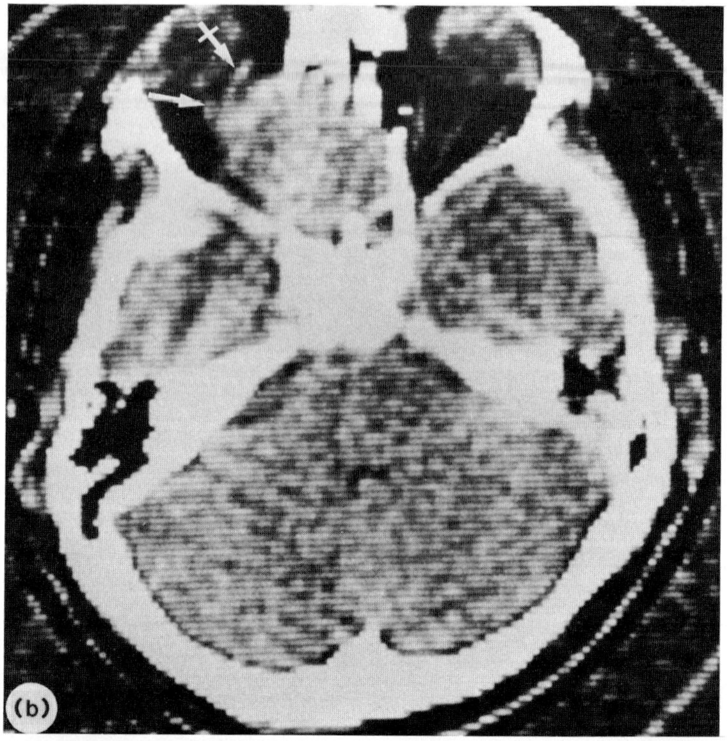

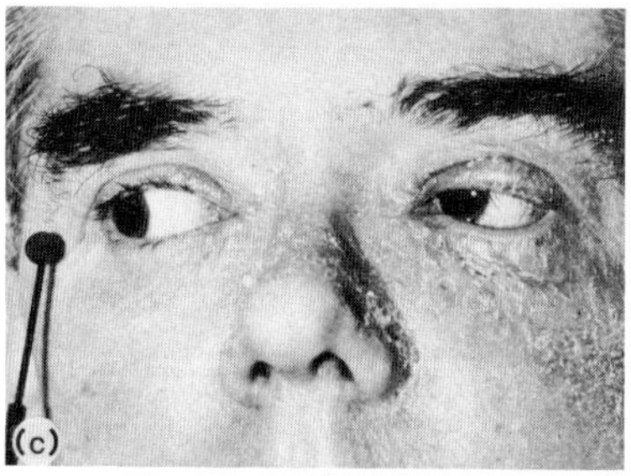

Fig. 3.39 Squamous carcinoma of ethmoid sinuses, with orbital extension. A 38-year old man was seen some months after surgery for a left ethmoidal carcinoma, with left visual loss, proptosis and ophthalmoplegia, principally failure of adduction (a). CT (b) showed a soft tissue mass extending from the ethmoid sinuses into the left orbit displacing the optic nerve (arrow) and medial rectus muscle (crossed arrow) laterally. One month later, following radiotherapy, the visual acuity was normal, there was no proptosis, and eye movements were virtually full (c). Repeat CT (d) showed considerable reduction of the mass. The left optic nerve and medial rectus muscle were now in normal position. Note that, without high spatial resolution, the integrity of the fine bony plates (e.g. the *right* lamina papyracea) cannot be assessed. (Reprinted with permission from Sanders and Gawler, 1975).

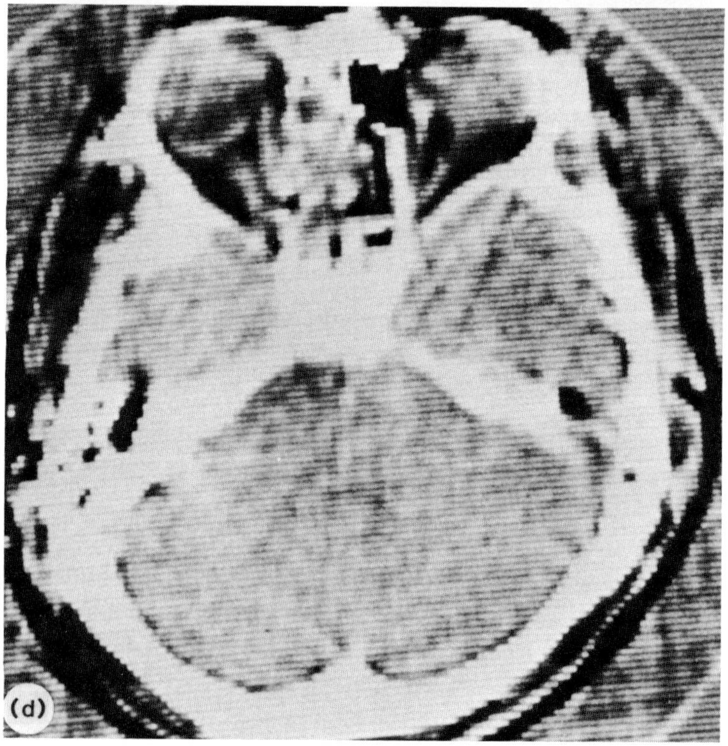

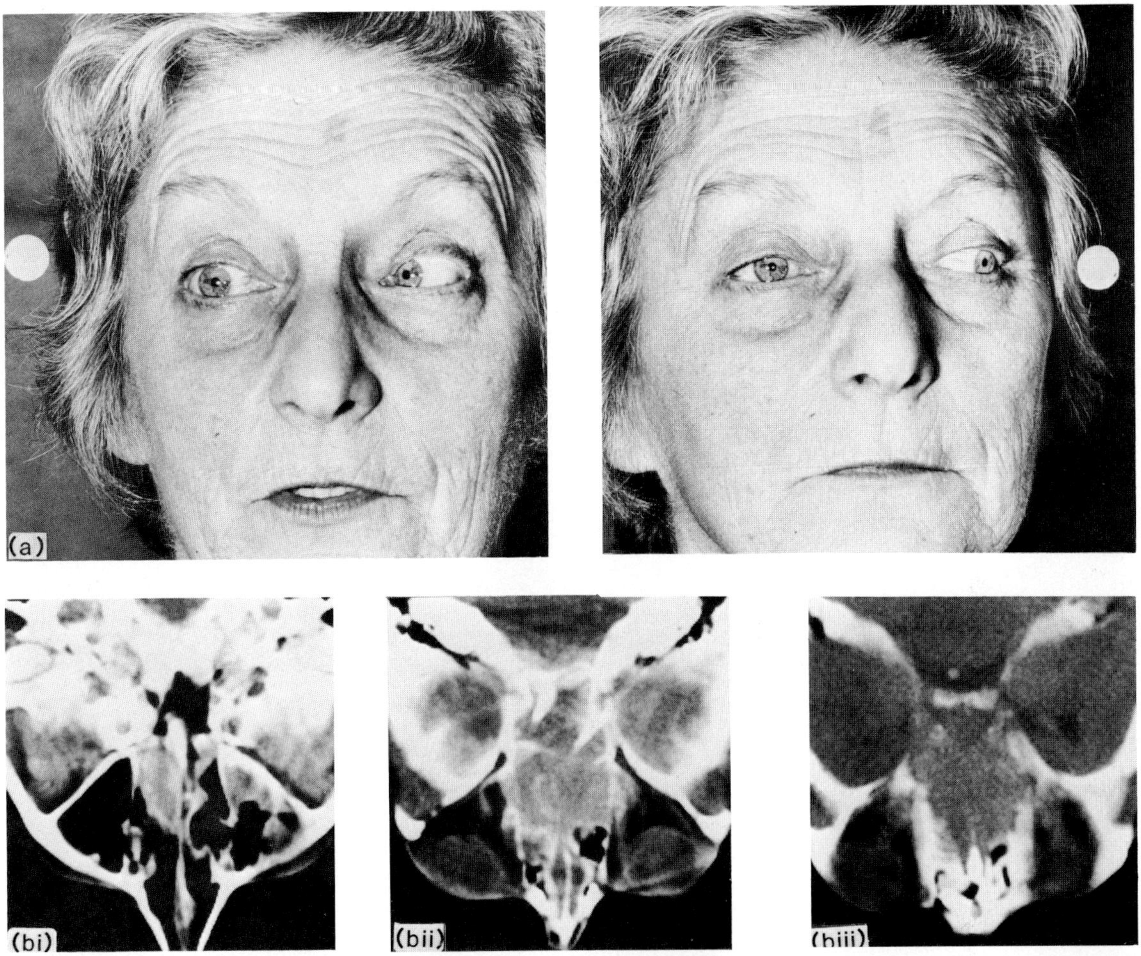

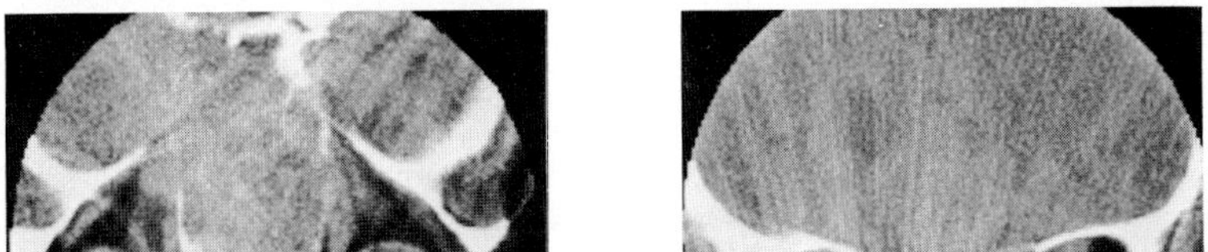

Fig. 3.40 Nasopharyngeal carcinoma. A 60-year old woman was seen with a history of headaches for six months, which were relieved by steroids. One week prior to the CT study she developed diplopia, with a right pupil-sparing IIIrd nerve palsy and a right VIth nerve palsy (a). CT (b) showed a mass in the nasopharynx, extending into the maxillary and ethmoid sinuses, infiltrating the right orbital apex and eroding the skull base. Histology showed a nasopharyngeal carcinoma, which progressed despite treatment (c).

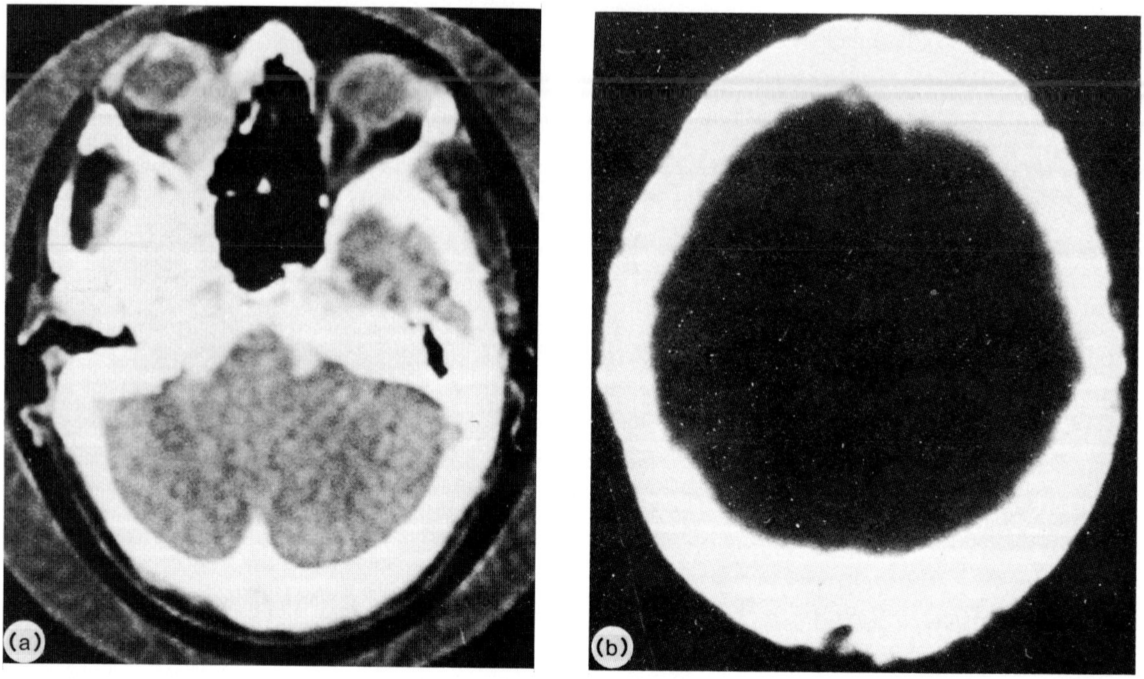

Fig. 3.41 Paget's disease of the skull in a case of orbital granuloma. A 71-year old woman, treated for some years for chronic sinusitis, developed a swollen, painful left eye. She was noted to have a reduced corneal reflex and impaired hearing on the same side. The head was large, hot and tender. An orbital phlebogram was thought to be normal. CT (a) showed a mass medially in the left orbit. The bones of the skull base appeared thickened and irregular, as did those of the vault, seen better with a wide window (b). The lesion was thought possibly to represent a fibrosarcoma arising in association with Paget's disease of the bone; surgery revealed a whitish tumour, which histologically was a granuloma.

The skull base

The bone of the skull base is subject to many of the diseases which affect bone elsewhere, and is indeed the site of election for certain diseases, e.g. fibrous dysplasia.

Developmental orbital defects

These are discussed in Chapter 7. Fibrous dysplasia is the commonest bone disease producing symptomatic orbital complications. CT shows expansion of the bone, with loss of the normal cortical and cancellous differentiation. Variable involvement of the base of skull and sphenoid may produce proptosis, by reducing the size of the orbital cavity, and visual loss may result from optic nerve compression.

Generalized thickening of the bone, with patchily increased density, may also be seen in osteopetrosis (Albers-Schonberg disease). In addition to exophthalmos and optic atrophy, reduction in size of the foramina by the thickened bone may give rise to ocular motor palsy.

Inflammatory conditions

Many other inflammatory or metabolic conditions, e.g. Paget's disease (Fig. 3.42) affect the skull base, but orbital problems are rare. Histiocytosis X may, however, produce bone, orbital and intracranial lesions. The CT appearances are described elsewhere.

Benign tumours

Benign tumours, in the form of osteomas, may bulge into the orbit, and very occasionally produce optic nerve lesions. They appear at CT as sclerotic condensations of the bone, frequently in the ethmoid region, but also in the frontal sinus (Fig. 3.38).

Primary malignant tumours and metastases

Primary malignant tumours of the skull base are infrequent (Fig. 3.42). Metastatic disease may, however, occur, with soft tissue extension into the orbit. The presence of erosive bone lesions, soft tissue masses and possibly of cerebral lesions is highly suggestive.

The brain

Invasion of the orbit by cerebral tumours is extremely uncommon, but very occasionally an invasive frontal glioma or optic

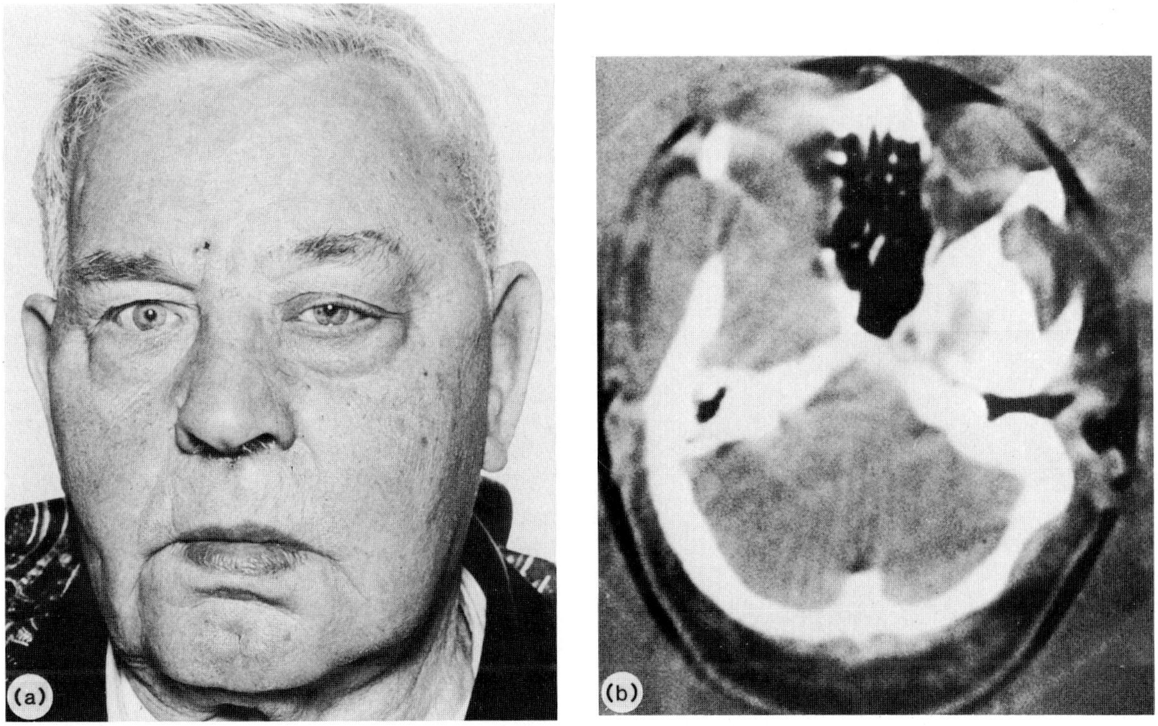

Fig. 3.42 Plasmacytoma. This 67-year old man had noted progressive, painless left proptosis. Visual acuity was decreased on the left, and there was proptosis, with inferomedial displacement of the eye and periorbital swelling extending to the left temple (a). CT showed a massive tumour involving the temporal and middle fossae in addition to the orbit (b). Biopsy revealed this to be a plasmacytoma; there was no evidence of systemic disease.

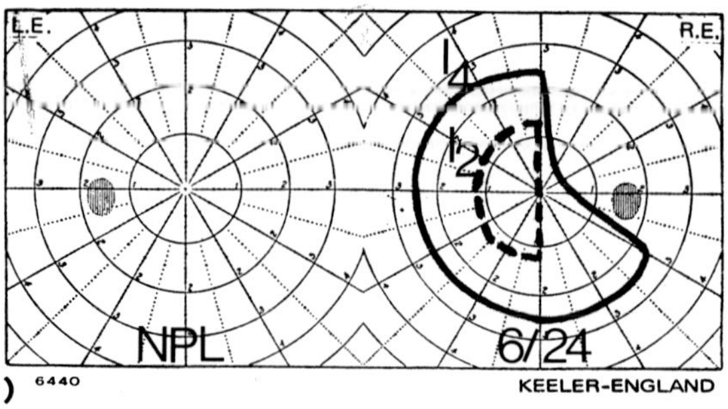

(a)

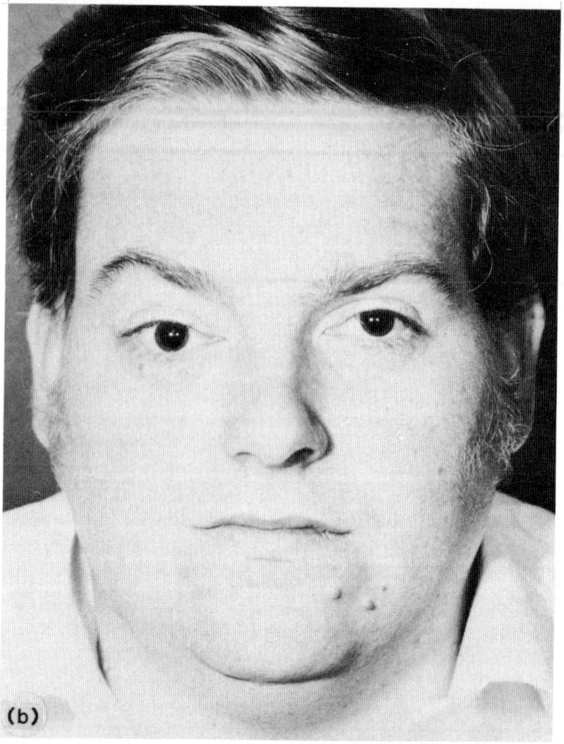

(b)

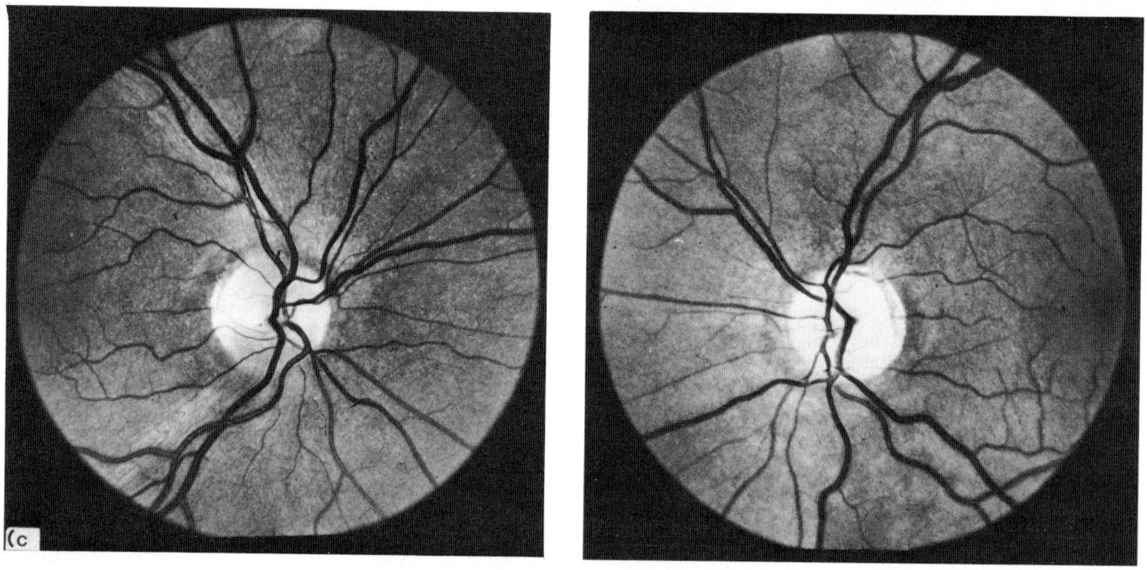

(c)

Fig. 3.43 Intracranial meningioma extending to orbit. A chromophobe adenoma compressing the chiasm and optic nerves was removed when this man was aged 13. He was subsequently treated by radiotherapy. Twenty years later he was unable to see with the left eye and there was slight deterioration in the right eye. He showed signs of hypopituitarism and examination of the right eye demonstrated vision of 6/24, with a temporal hemianopia denser above (a); there was no perception of light in the left eye. The right eye was depressed (b). Fundus examination showed gross loss of nerve fibres on the left, but on the right fibres entered the disc superiorly and inferiorly, to produce a 'bowtie' atrophy (c). CT showed a superolateral extraconal mass with hyperostosis of the lateral wall and roof of the orbit, depressing the globe (e). A large pituitary fossa was clearly visible (arrows f), containing material of CSF attenuation. A large enhancing mass was present in the right frontal region; there were areas of reduced density within the mass and surrounding it (g). A meningioma was removed, with improvement in the right visual field.

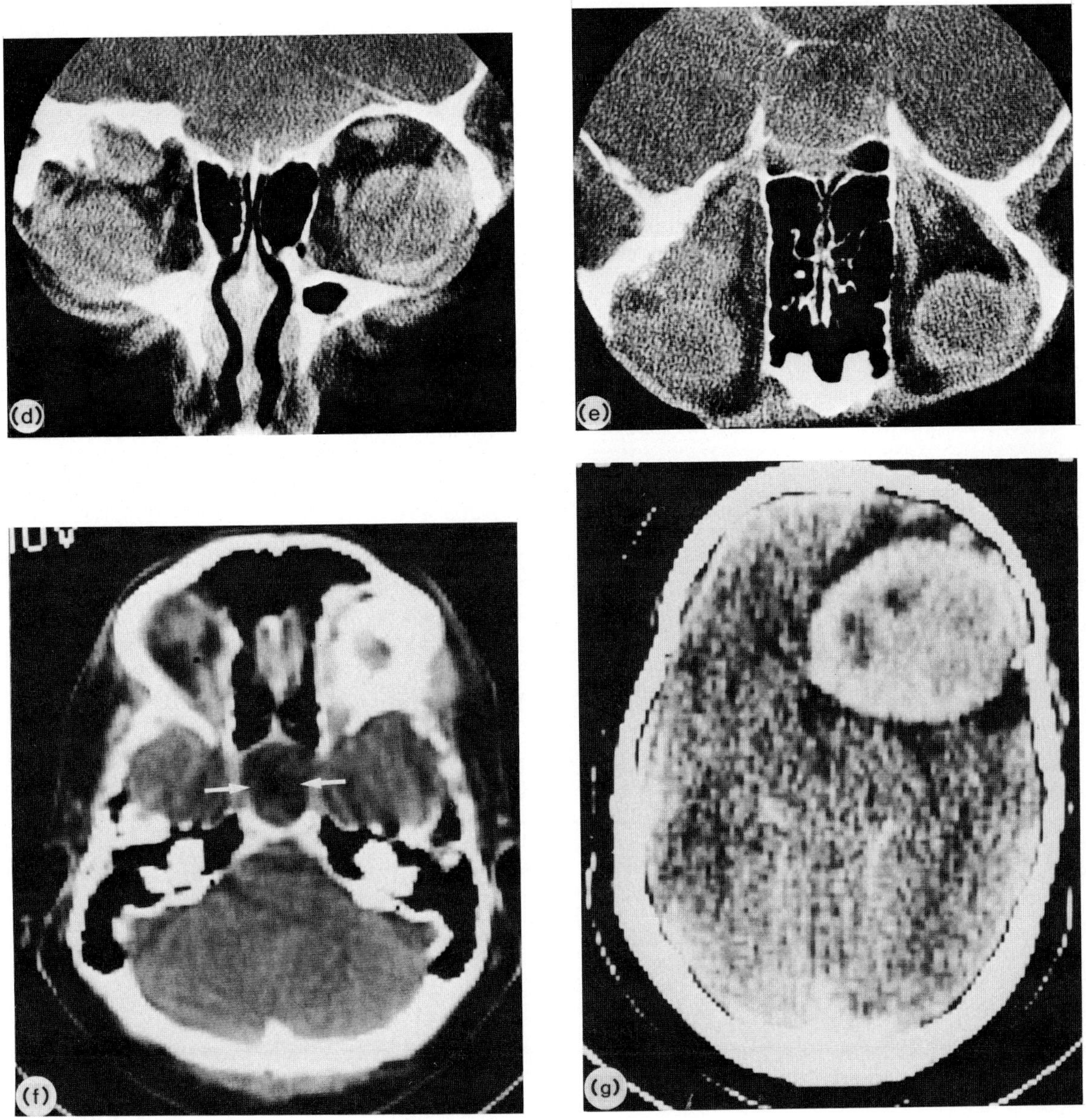

chiasm lesion may so erode the bone as to present in the orbit. When this is suspected clinically, CT examinations should if possible include coronal sections, since assessment of the condition and exact position of the orbital roof from axial sections or even from coronal and/or sagittal reconstructions is very difficult.

The intracranial abnormalities should make the diagnosis clear.

Meninges

Extension to the orbit of meningiomas arising in the adjacent structures is much less rare than the foregoing (Fig. 3.43). The results are often of visual failure and are therefore discussed further in Chapter 4.

The superifical tissues

Spread into the orbit of inflammatory skin conditions has already been mentioned.

Basal cell carcinoma of the skin around the orbit may spread deeply to involve the orbital tissues. This erosive, necrosing tumour is generally manifest by an irregular superficial defect; the bone may be involved. CT may be a useful way of determining the deep extent of the lesion.

REFERENCES

Alper, M.G. (1979), Computerized tomography (CT) in diagnosis of inflammatory orbital pseudotumour and Graves' disease. In: *Topics in Neuro-Ophthalmology* (ed. H.S. Thompson), Williams and Wilkins, Baltimore, pp.347–68.

Enriquez, P., Dahlin, D.C. Hayles, A.B. and Henderson, E.D. (1967), Histiocytosis X. A Clinical Study. *Mayo Clinic Proc.*, **42**,88.

Enzmann, D.R., Donaldson, S.S., Kriss, J.P. (1979), Appearance of Graves' disease on orbital computed tomography. *J. Comput. Assit. Tomogr.*, **3**, 815–19.

Enzmann, D., Donaldson, S.S., Marshall, W.H. and Kriss, J.P. (1976a), Computed tomography in orbital pseudotumour. *Radiology*, **120**, 597–601.

Enzmann, D.R., Kramer, R., Norman, D., Pollock, J. (1978), Malignant melanoma metastatic to the central nervous system. *Radiology*, **127**, 177–80.

Enzmann, D., Marshall, W.H., Rosenthal, A.R. and Kriss, J.P. (1976b), Computed tomography in Graves' ophthalmopathy. *Radiology*, **118**, 615–20.

Ferry, A.P. and Font, R.L. (1974), Carcinoma metastatic to the eye and orbit. *Archs Ophthal.*, **92**, 276–86.

Gawler, J., Sanders, M.D., Bull, J.W.D., Du Boulay, G. and Marshall, J. (1974), Computer assisted tomography in orbital disease. *Br. J. Ophthal.*, **58**, (6), 571–87.

Goldberg, F., Berne, A.S. and Oski, F.A. (1978), Differentiation of orbital cellulitis from preseptal cellulitis by computed tomography. *Pediatrics*, **62**, 1000–5.

Goldberg, L. and Danziger, A. (1977), Computed tomographic scanning in the management of retinoblastoma. *Am. J. Ophthal.*, **84**, 380–2.

Harris, G.J. and Jakobiec, F.A. (1979), Cavernous hemangioma of the orbit. *J. Neurosurg.*, **51**, 219–28.

Haynes, B.F., Fishman, M.L., Fauci, A.S. and Wolff, S.M. (1977), The ocular manifestations of Wegener's granulomatosis. *Am. J. Med.*, **63**, 131–41.

Hilal, S.K., Trokel, S.L. (1977), Computerized tomography of the orbit using thin sections. *Sem. Roentg.*, **12**, 137–44.

Howard, G. (1966), Amyloid tumours of the orbit. *Br. J. Ophthal.*, **50**, 421–29.

Jakobiec, F.A. and Jones, I.S. (1979), Introduction to ultrastructure, inflammation, and neoplasia. In: *Diseases of the Orbit*, (eds. I.S. Jones and F.A. Jakobiec), Harper and Row, Maryland, USA.

Jakobiec, F.A. and Tannenbaum, M. (1975), Embryological perspectives on the fine structure of orbital tumours. *Int. Ophthal. Clin.*, **15**, 85–110.

Keane, J.R. (1977), Alternating proptosis. *Archs Neurol.*, **34**, 642–3.

Mancuso, A.A., Hanafee, W.N., Winter, J. and Ward, P. (1978), Extension of paranasal sinus tumours and inflammatory disease as evaluated by CT and pluridirectional tomography. *Neuroradiology,* **16**, 449–53.

Moseley, I.F., Sanders, M.D. and Clavería, L.E. (1978), Diagnostic limitations of computerised tomographic examination of the orbit. *In: The Diagnostic Limitations of Computerised Axial Tomography* (ed. J. Bories), Springer, Berlin, pp.52–62.

Parsons, C. and Hodson, N. (1979), Computed tomography of paranasal sinus tumours. *Radiology*, **132**, 641–5.

Reese, A.B. (1956), *Tumors of the Eye and Adenexa*. Armed Forces Institute of Pathology, Washington.

Rosenberg, S.A., Diamond, H.D., Jaslowitz, B., and Craver, L.D. (1961), Lymphosarcoma. A review of 1,269 cases. *Medicine*, **40**, 31–84.

Sanders, M.D. and Gawler, J. (1975), Computerized tomographic Scanning (EMI scan) in neuro-ophthalmology. *Trans. Ophthal. Soc. UK*, **95**, 237–45.

Sanders, M.D. and Hoyt, W.F. (1969), Hypoxic ocular sequelae of carotid-cavernous fistulae. *Br. J. Ophthal.*, **53**, 82–97.

Skalka, H. (1978), Perineural optic nerve changes in endocrine orbitopathy. *Archs Ophthal.*, **96**, 468–73.

Spalton, D.J. and Sanders, M.D. (1981), Fundus changes in histologically confirmed sarcoidosis. *Br. J. Ophthal.*, **65**, 348–58.

Trokel, S.L. and Hilal, S.K. (1979), Recognition and differential diagnosis of enlarged extraocular muscles in computed tomography. *Am. J. Ophthal.*, **87**, 503–12.

Verness, M., Haynes, B.F., Favel, A.S. and Wolff, S.M. (1978), Computer assisted tomography of orbital lesions in Wegener's granulomatosis. *J. Comput. Assist. Tomogr.*, **2**, 45–48.

Weber, A.L., Tadmor, R., Davis, R., Roberson, G. (1978), Malignant tumours of the sinuses. *Neuroradiology*, **16**, 443–8.

Wing, S.D., Hunsaker, J.N., Anderson, R.E., Van Dyke, H.J.L. and Osborn, A.G. (1979), Direct sagittal computed tomography in Graves' opthalmopathy. *J. Comput. Assist. Tomogr.*, **3**, 820–24.

Wright, J.E., Stewart, W.B. and Kronel, G.B. (1979), Clinical presentation and management of lacrimal gland tumours. *Br. J. Ophthal.*, **63**, 600–6.

4 · Visual loss

4.1 SIGNIFICANCE OF VISUAL FIELD EXAMINATION TO ANATOMICAL ORGANIZATION

Testing of the visual fields is one of the most important diagnostic contributions an ophthalmologist can make. Simple techniques (e.g. confrontation and Bjerrum screen) and a careful observer are usually sufficient for accurate localization and diagnosis (Fig. 4.1). More sophisticated automated machines are often too complicated for patients with cerebral problems, though a Goldmann perimeter provides sufficient controls for accurate confirmation and continued observation.

Progressive unilateral visual failure with optic atrophy suggests optic nerve compression. Continued observation of the visual fields for progression is essential.

Neurological field defects respect the vertical meridian, so attention is concentrated on disparities, particularly to red targets in the two hemifields in relation to the vertical meridian. Chiasmal field defects are characteristically bitemporal, though it should be remembered that a pituitary tumour has to be large before it comes in contact with the chiasm, and even larger before compression and visual loss occurs.

Retrochiasmal lesions produce hemianopic field defects ranging from total hemianopia to subtle relative homonymous field defects and inattention defects. The visual acuity should be normal with an homonymous hemianopia. Clinical localization may be difficult; tract lesions tend to be incongruous; anterior temporal lesions tend to produce upper hemianopic defects due to the inferior retinal fibres being deviated in their course by the temporal horn (Meyers loop). Parietal lesions produce other signs of perceptual disorganization and optokinetic abnormalities, whereas cortical lesions tend to be more congruous.

4.2 ANTERIOR LESIONS

The main clinical ambition is to detect compressive lesions at an early stage and it should be appreciated that lesions which may compress the chiasm may also compress the optic nerve. The field defect of optic nerve compression is related to the site of

Fig. 4.1 (i) Anterior visual pathways. (a) Optic nerve lesions include central scotoma, altitudinal and arcuate defects, or combinations of these. (b) Junctional scotoma; clinically important for localization, this is due to a lesion involving the ipsilateral optic nerve and the inferior contralateral crossing fibres (dotted line). (c) Chiasmal lesions produce bitemporal hemianopic defects with additional features b) or d). (d) Tract lesions: incongruous hemianopic defects (N.B. the pattern in the lateral geniculate body).

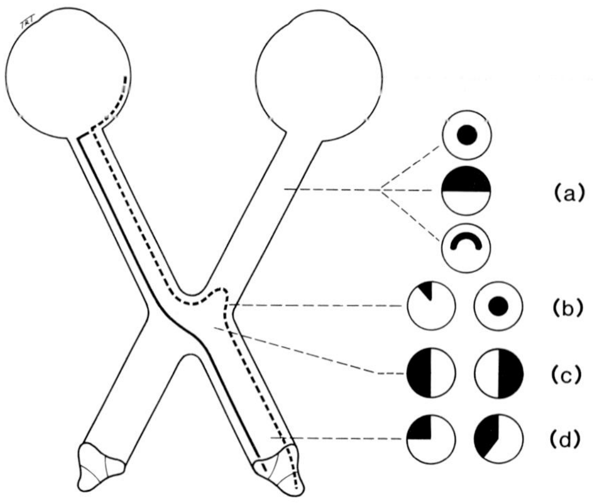

(i)

(ii) Posterior visual pathways

Upper fibres (left) Peripheral fibres (interrupted lines) pass from the medial portion of the geniculate to the upper anterior lip of the calcarine fissure. Lesions of the central and peripheral fibres produce a lower quadrantanopia (a). Homonymous hemianopia is due to involvement of upper and lower fibres (b). Small paracentral congruous homonymous defects may be seen with focal vascular lesions (c). Homonymous hemianopia is seen with lesions of the striate cortex and macular sparing is seen particularly with vascular disturbances (d).

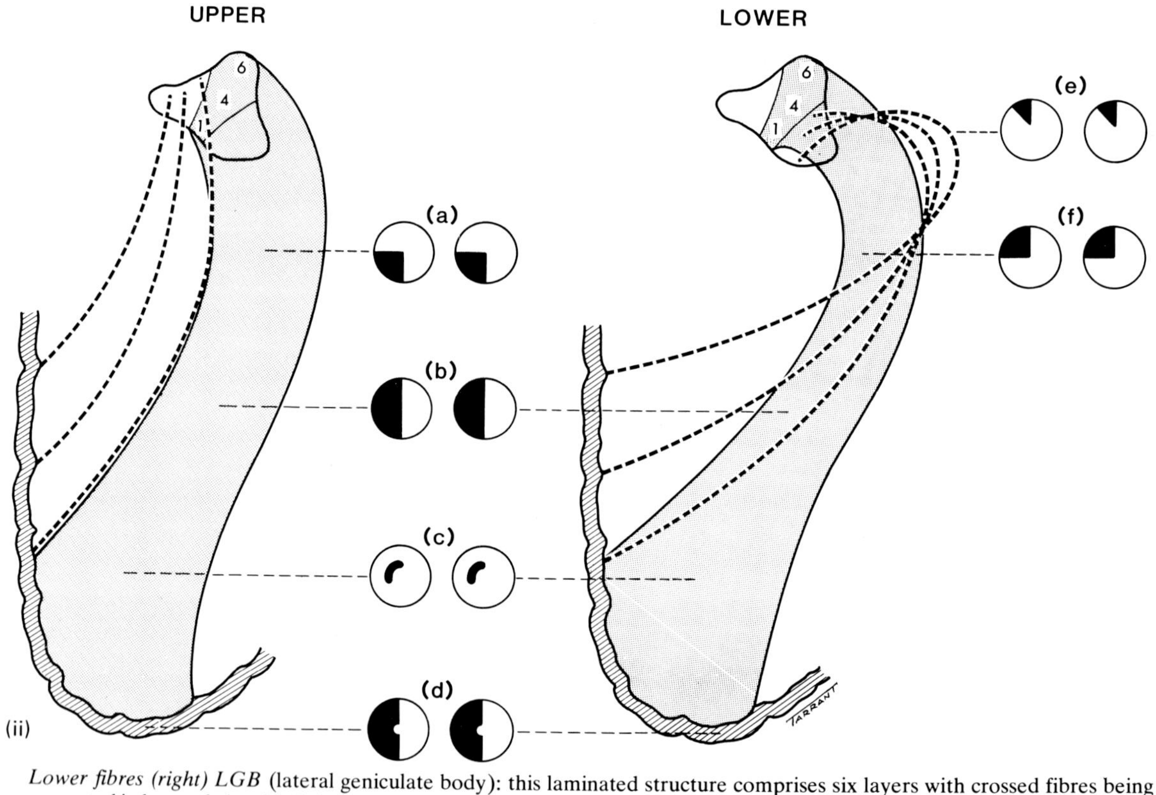

Lower fibres (right) LGB (lateral geniculate body): this laminated structure comprises six layers with crossed fibres being represented in layers 6, 4 and 1. Inferior fibres are lateral in the tract and inferolateral in the LGB passing anteriorly around the temporal horn of the lateral ventricle (stippled). Fibres subserving central vision (stippled) occupy the mid zone of the LGB and radition, with the central vertical meridian fibres passing from the apex of the LGB (layer 6) to the cortex at the 17–18 area border. Temporal lobe lesions produce a 'pie in the sky' defect (e) and lesions of central and peripheral fibres produce an upper quadrantanopia (f).

compression, the nature and direction of the compression, and the local peculiarities of blood supply to the site of compression. Thus central scotoma, arcuate scotoma and hemianopic defects may be the initial presentation, and progressive, inexorable visual loss the essential feature. Positive visual phenomena and Uhtoff's phenomenon may occasionally be described by patients with compressive lesions. Thus the ophthalmologist confronted with monocular visual loss due to optic nerve disease should at his initial examination of a patient include the following points:

1. Careful examination of the 'good' eye, for signs of a junctional scotoma.
2. Endocrine status – growth and development of a child, or abnormalities of skin appearance, frequency of shaving, temperature appreciation, sexual activity, polyuria or polydypsia.
3. Sense of smell.
4. Possible presence of café au lait spots, suggesting neurofibromatosis.
5. Ocular motor signs e.g. seesaw nystagmus, retraction nystagmus, cranial nerve palsies or pupillary signs (e.g. light/near dissociation).
6. Some aspects of the neurological examination, which may reveal signs of a posterior fossa lesion or of demyelination.

4.3 OPTIC NERVE LESIONS

Intrinsic lesions of the optic nerve are discussed elsewhere (Chapter 5) and as they are essentially not treatable by surgery, the main clinical emphasis must be placed on the detection of compressive lesions. The optic nerve may be compressed within the orbit, within the canal or within the cranial cavity.

Subtle clinical signs should be sought and these include:

1. A subjective dimness of objects.
2. Acuity may be 6/6 whereas the good eye is 6/5.
3. All the colour charts may be read, although the patient may say that they are dimmer with the affected eye.
4. Visual field testing may show a variety or combination of patterns of field loss, so that small targets on the Goldmann or small red targets on the Bjerrum screen are recommended.
5. Pupillary abnormalities provide objective evidence and a subtle afferent defect is a valuable finding, although pupillographic or neurophysiological tests may be necessary.
6. Examination of the optic disc demands red free light for assessment of nerve fibre pattern, and photography may be preferred to detect subtle differences in the two eyes.
7. Choroidal striae may be difficult to see with the ophthalmoscope, but readily seen with flourescein angiography.

Finally, the clinician's experience must dictate whether these signs are beyond the range of normal variation, and not associated with minor amblyopia. The detection of subtle optic nerve signs is a basis on which to document progression and this should be the prime objective prior to initiation of extensive investigations.

4.4 ORBITAL LESIONS

Orbital lesions producing visual loss (Chapter 3) are usually accompanied by proptosis, ocular motor signs, retinal signs or other features suggesting orbital disease. Proptosis may be minimal in long-standing lesions so that assessment of the resistance of the globe to retropulsion is an important additional clinical test, though interpretation may be difficult.

4.5 INTRACANALICULAR LESIONS

True intracanalicular lesions are rare and the authors have seen only one case of surgically confirmed intracanalicular cavernous haemangioma and one meningioma (Sanders and Falconer, 1964). Infiltrating meningiomas with diffuse dural spread are more common, and granulomatous infiltration also occurs in tuberculosis or sarcoidosis. Diagnosis may be determined by the clinical features and other investigations, as a wide variety of lesions may produce arachnoidal hyperplasia (see Chapter 5).

4.6 INTRACRANIAL OPTIC NERVE LESIONS

These may present initially with monocular loss, and again central, paracentral, arcuate, altitudinal or generalized reduction in all isoptres may be seen. Such lesions include pituitary tumours, craniopharyngiomas, meningiomas (Fig. 4.3, see also p. 116), metastatic tumours, aneurysms and lesions arising from the sinuses (Fig.4.2). These lesions will therefore be discussed in relation to their more common clinical presentation as a chiasmal syndrome.

4.7 BILATERAL OPTIC NERVE COMPRESSION

Any of the above lesions may produce bilateral optic nerve compression, though there is usually a chiasmal pattern to the field loss. Bilateral central scotomas, however, present a real diagnostic problem. In over 90% of cases they are due to nutritional or toxic amblyopias, hereditary optic neuropathy, demyelination or unexplained intrinsic optic nerve disease. We have seen three cases of bilateral optic nerve compression with bilateral central scotomas, without evidence of hemianopic disparities, in which CT provided important diagnostic information.

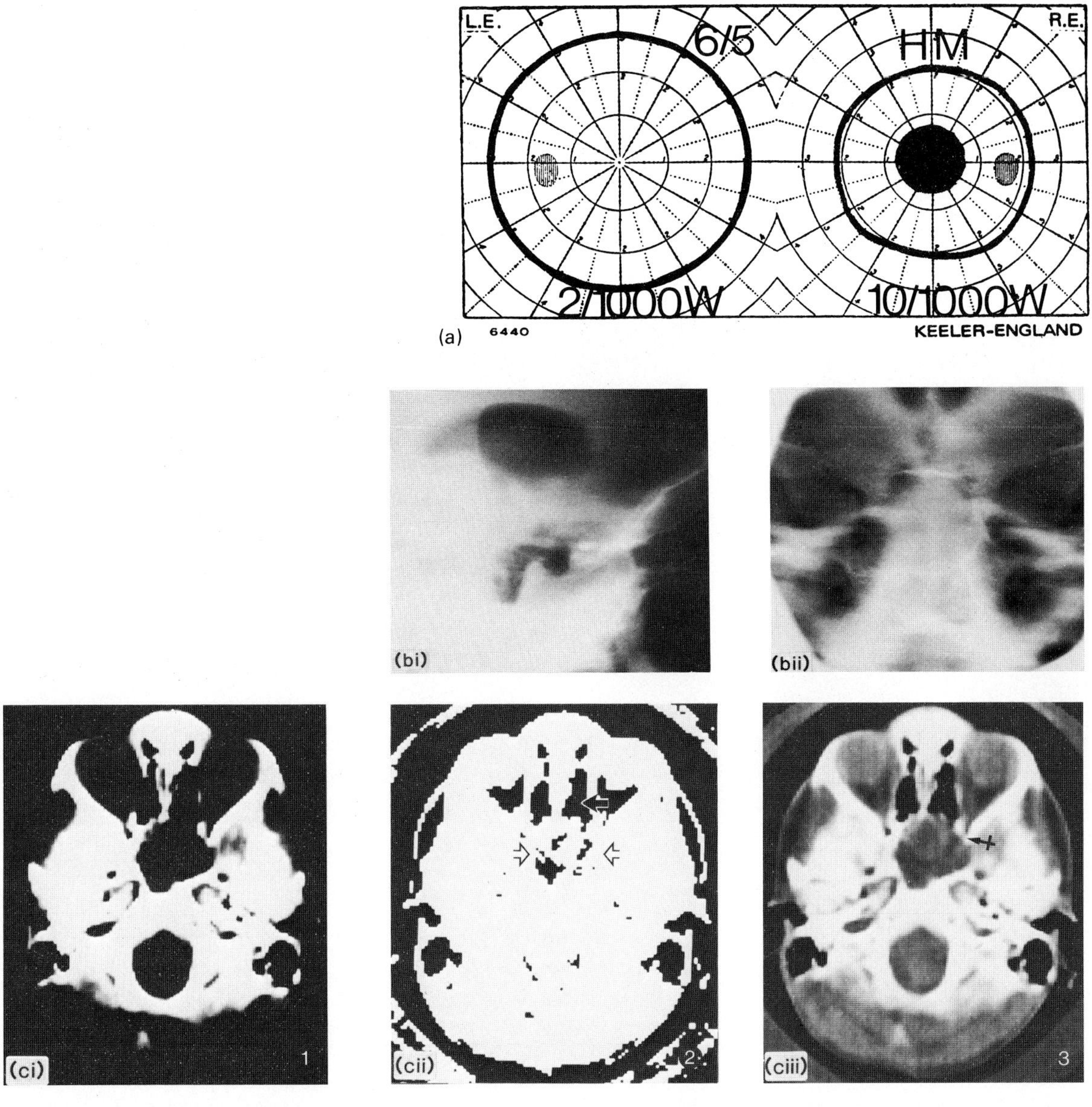

Fig. 4.2 Sphenoid sinus mucocoele. A boy of 16 had experienced recurrent episodes of visual loss in the right eye, associated with pain and was diagnosed as having optic neuritis. Ultimately vision was reduced to hand movements with a central scotoma(a). Pneumoencephalography (b, lateral and anteroposterior tomograms) excluded a suprasellar mass. CT of the skull base (c) appeared normal when viewed with the normal window for brain imaging (1), but with a window width of 1 EMI unit (2) it was clear that the contents of the sphenoid sinus (between open arrows) were denser than the air in the adjacent nasal cavity (arrow). A wide window image (3) showed the sphenoid sinus to be expanded, particularly towards the right optic canal (crossed arrow) and occupied by material of soft tissue attenuation, confirmed to be a mucocoele. Retrospective analysis of the air study also revealed the dense, expanded sinus. (Courtesy of Williams and Wilkins, Baltimore. Previously published in *Topics in Neuro-Ophthalmology* (ed. H.S. Thompson)).

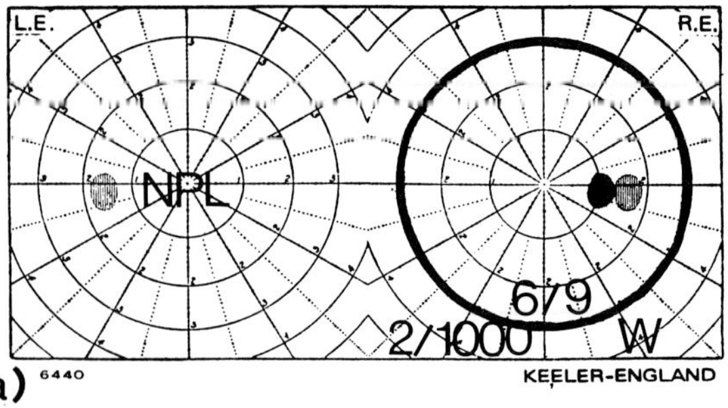

(a)

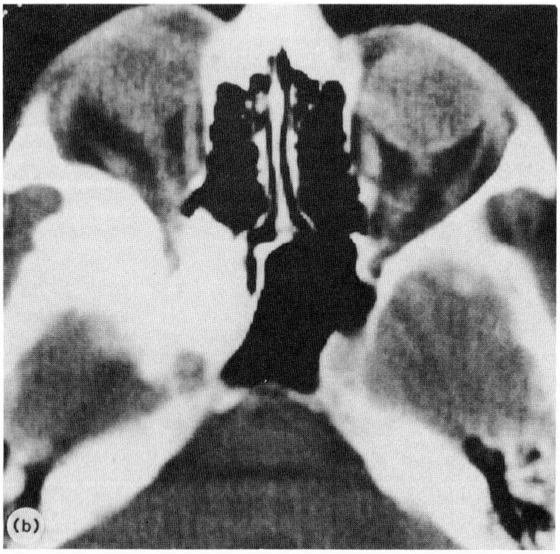

(b)

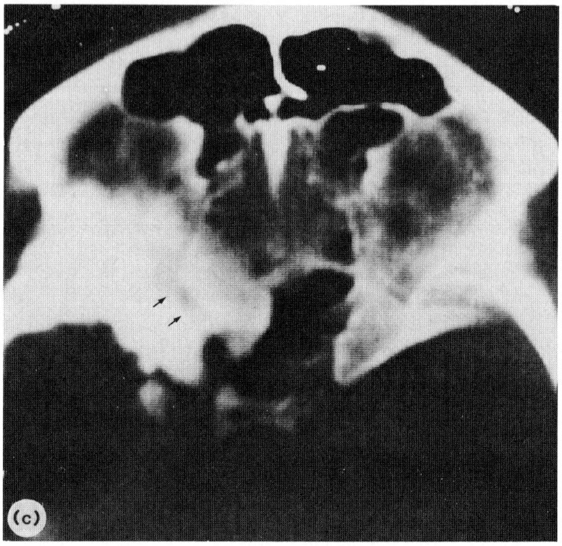

(c)

Fig. 4.3 Sphenoid wing meningioma. A man of 67 with a seven-year history of slowly progressive visual loss and left proptosis was blind in the left eye (a) and there was 5mm of proptosis. (b) CT shows gross hyperostosis of the left basi-sphenoid, extending from the sphenoid sinus to the malar region. The orbital contents are displaced anteromedially. (c) With a wide window (800 EMI units), the narrowed optic canal can be discerned traversing the thickened bone (arrows).

Case 1 (Fig. 4.4)
Progressive visual loss was the presenting symptom in a 9-year-old girl who had vision of counting fingers in each eye and bilateral central scotomata (Fig. 4.4a). The discs were of normal colour, with good nerve fibre visualization, and neurophysiological tests showed barely recordable visual evoked responses. Subtle ataxia was the only other neurological sign. CT (Fig. 4.4b) showed massive ventricular dilatation with a dilated third ventricle compressing the optic nerves and chiasm. A diagnosis of aqueduct stenosis was made. After ventriculoatrial shunting there was no improvement in vision and optic atrophy ensued.

Case 2 (Fig. 4.5)
A 36-year-old man presented with disabling frontal headaches initially diagnosed as migraine. Progressive visual loss prompted referral and reduced VERs and central scotomas were associated with vision of 6/60 in each eye (Fig. 4.5a). The optic discs were normal (Fig. 4.5b). CT demonstrated low attentuation areas with

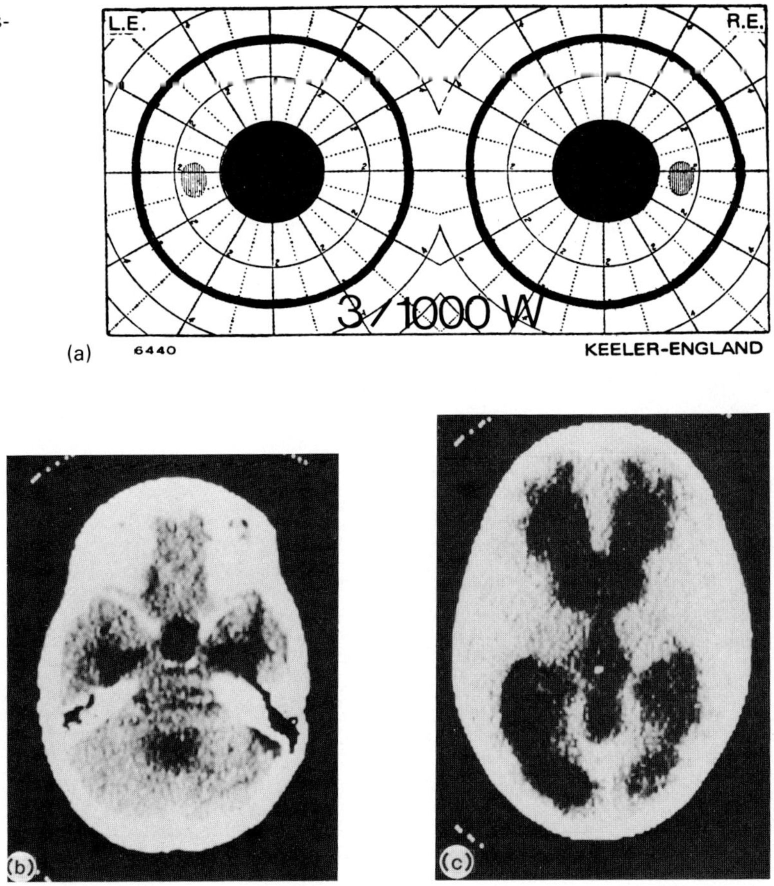

Fig. 4.4 Bilateral optic nerve compression in aqueduct stenosis. (Case 1.)

irregular contrast enhancement in the frontal lobes (Fig. 4.5c), and at surgery the intracranial optic nerves were seen to be compressed by the inferior gyrus rectus of both frontal lobes. Biopsy of this frontal lesion showed a genistocytic astrocytoma and despite radiotherapy vision failed to improve.

Case 3 (Fig. 4.6)
A young man presenting with bilateral visual loss and bilateral central scotomas (Fig. 4.6a) was shown at CT (Figs. 4.6 b-d) to have a pineal tumour, producing ventricular enlargement and dilatation of the third ventricle, compressing both optic nerves.

These cases, though unusual, indicate that compression may produce bilateral central scotomas, and though the precise mechanism is not understood we feel that the following circumstances may be necessary to produce this:

1. A post-fixed chiasm with long intracranial nerves.
2. Diffuse compression of the optic nerves by a soft mass.

Fig. 4.5 Frontal astrocytoma causing bilateral optic nerve compression. (Case 2).

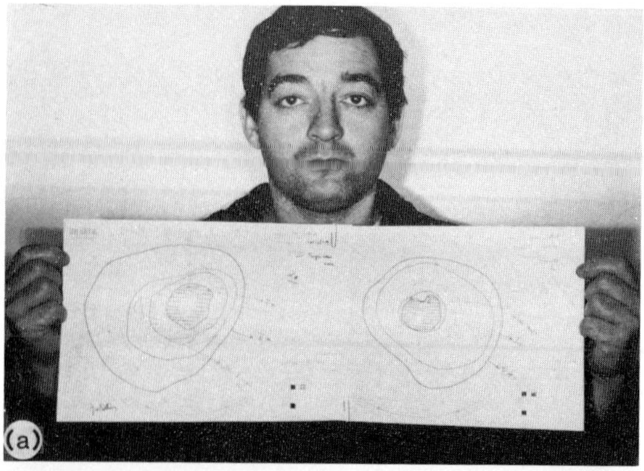

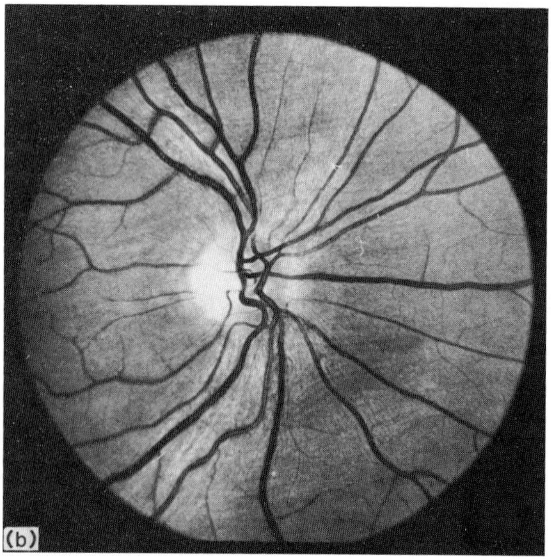

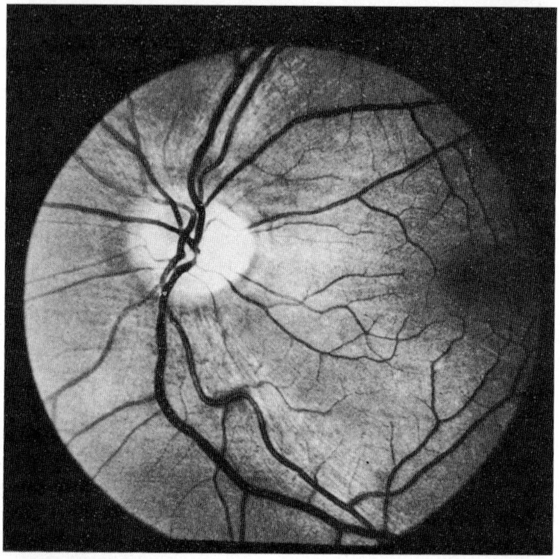

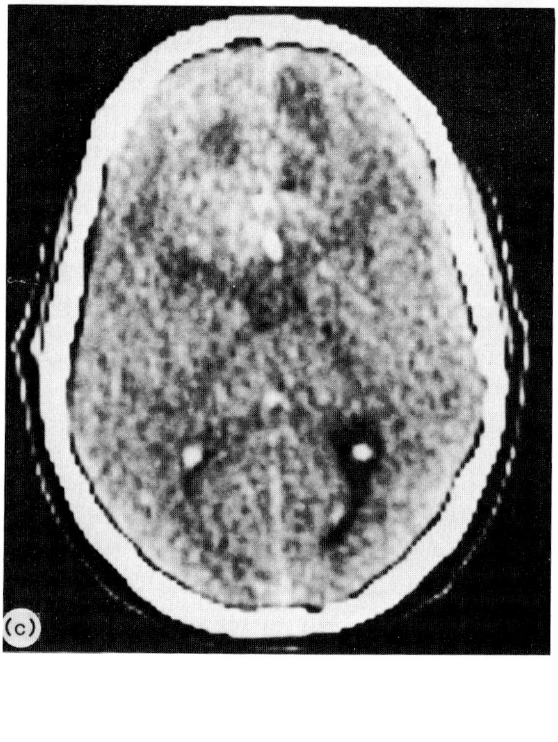

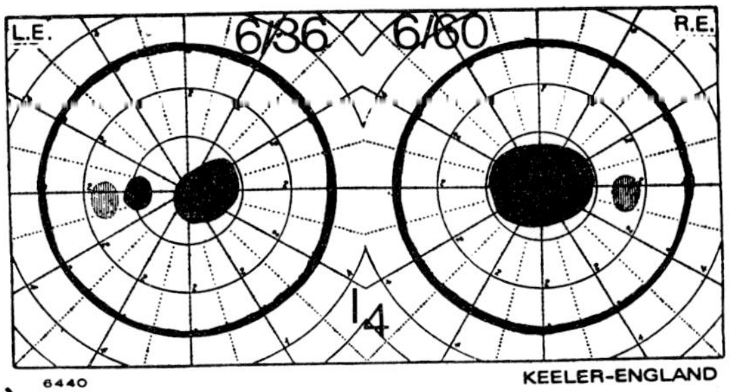

(a)

Fig. 4.6 Pinealoma causing bilateral optic nerve compression, via dilatation of the third ventricle. (Case 3).

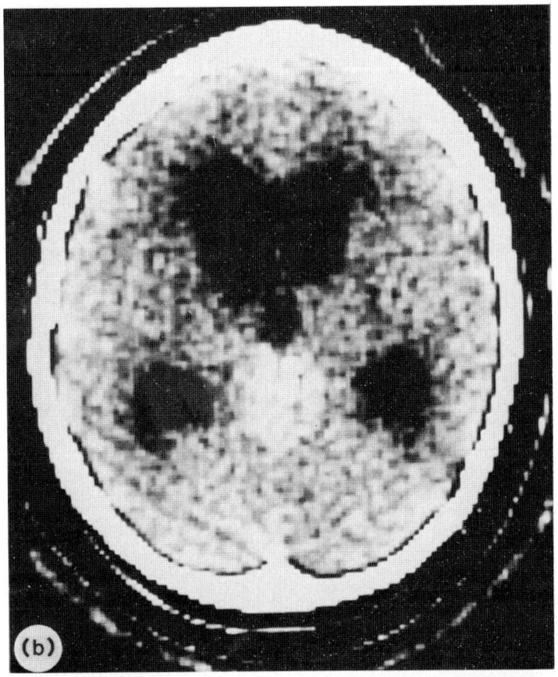

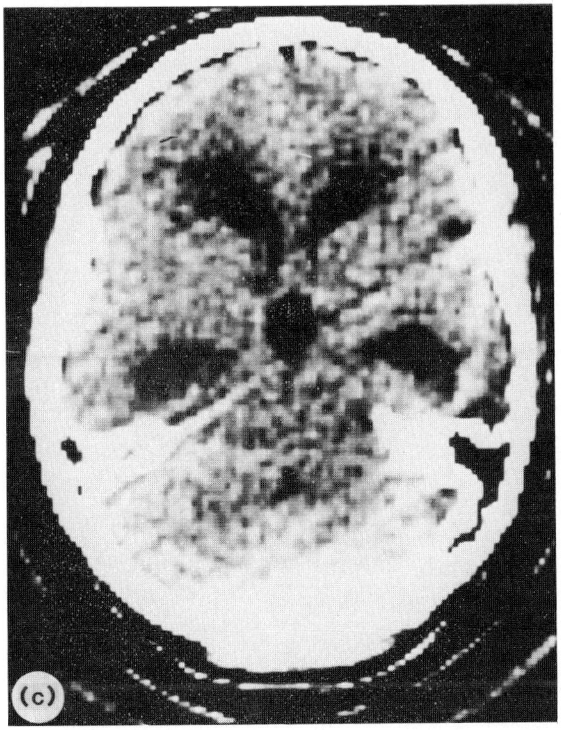

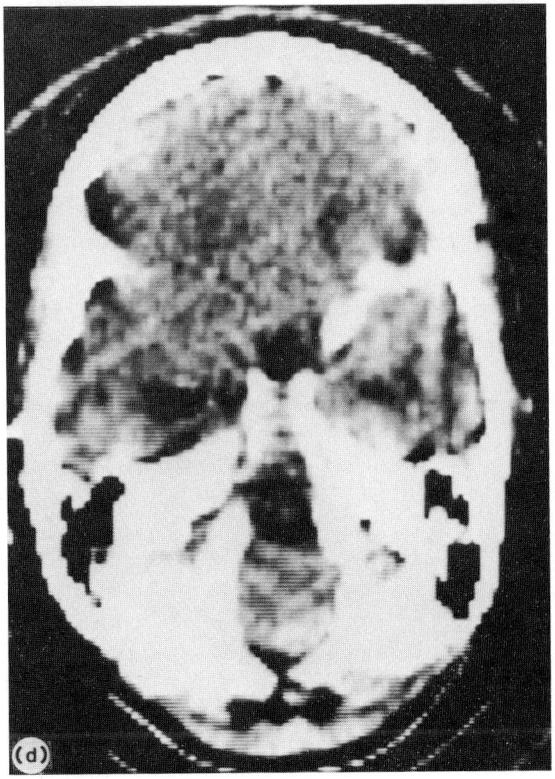

3. Compression occurring maximally in the central region of the intracranial optic nerves so that typical chiasmal signs are lacking, and the optic nerve is not asymmetrically compressed against the edges of the optic canal.

4.8 CHIASMAL LESIONS

Visual symptomatology

A dense bitemporal hemianopia is pathognomonic of chiasmal compression and may produce bizarre visual symptomatology. This is due either to blindness beyond the point of fixation, or to slipping of the two hemifields which produces horizontal diplopia (overlapping) vertical diplopia (hemifield slide) or disappearance of objects (hemifield separation). The transient nature of these symptoms means that patients rarely present with them directly, and are more likely to present noticing the temporal loss of vision in one eye on covering the other.

Specific examination

Accurate performance and interpretation of visual fields is nowhere as important as in the detection of chiasmal disease. The bitemporal nature of the field loss, even when involvement is asymmetrical, tends to show respect of the vertical meridian. This is a critical factor in the diagnosis of chiasmal compression, and red targets, large or small, should be used in conjunction with white targets in the careful investigation of the fields. If the field defect does not respect the midline, close scrutiny of the discs is necessary, as a temporal hemianopia not respecting the midline may be due to:

1. Tilted discs with nasal hypoplasia.
2. Severe myopic astigmatism.
3. Sector retinitis pigmentosa.
4. Large blind spots, usually in severe papilloedema.
5. Anatomical variation, with a large supraorbital rim or relative ptosis.

Examination of the optic disc is important, as an anomalous disc usually signifies a benign ocular developmental abnormality and obviates aggressive investigation. There is, however, some suggestion that congenital chiasmal lesions may in turn produce anomalous discs (see Chapter 7).

Confirmation of the presence of a chiasmal lesion is dependent on adequate radiology. The current clinical preference would be for a lateral skull X-ray supplemented by further projections if necessary and followed by CT.

Lesions producing chiasmal syndromes

Lesions affecting the optic chiasm usually produce visual loss as a result of compression. Primary vascular, neoplastic, and inflammatory disease of the chiasm are rare exceptions to this rule.

Chiasmal lesions can therefore be classified as follows:

1. Intrinsic.
2. Compressive, due to tumours or other structures with mass effect within or close to the sella turcica.
3. Traumatic.
4. Developmental (Chapter 7).

Intrinsic lesions of the optic chiasm

The commonest intrinsic lesion of the optic chiasm is the glioma. Chiasmal gliomas are more common than the isolated optic nerve glioma, and these hamartomatous tumours, often benign, characteristically arise in childhood, with an increased incidence in patients with neurofibromatosis (Oxenhandler and Sayers, 1978).

Chiasmal gliomas

Clinical presentation of chiasmal glioma can be extremely varied, and the diagnosis should be suspected in any young patient with visual loss, and in some cases associated ocular oscillations (Chapter 6). Extension of the glioma into one or both optic nerves produces visual field defects which are not characteristic of chiasmal lesions, while posterior extension of the lesion into the hypothalamus produces varying endocrine abnormalities. These include reduced growth and sexual maturity, precocious puberty, diabetes insipidus, obesity and, in the extreme form, severe wasting, reduced development and often vertical or rotatory nystagmus, the signs of Russell's diencephalic syndrome. Anorexia nervosa has been described in adult patients with hypothalamic involvement. An ocular motor abnormality may be seen which commences with monocular vertical or rotary small amplitude movements progressing to involve the second eye, *pari passu* with visual deterioration, and terminating in a picture resembling seesaw nystagmus (Fig. 6.17 p.208).

The tumour is seen at CT as a mass, often well defined, lying in the chiasmatic cistern and interpeduncular fossa (Fig. 4.7). Since the normal chiasm can be seen in many individuals, minor degrees of enlargement are difficult to detect and are more reliably demonstrated by air encephalography. Thin-section axial and coronal CT studies, possibly with intrathecal metrizamide, may eventually prove to be as accurate and less disturbing.

The tumour is generally isodense with the surrounding brain, or of slightly higher attentuation. Low attenuation lesions, which are probably cystic, are less common (Fig. 6.17 p.208). Optic chiasm gliomas show extreme variation in their behaviour with intravenous contrast medium, ranging from no change to dense

Fig. 4.7 Optic chiasm glioma (presumed) in neurofibromatosis. This 13-year old girl had poor vision since infancy. There were stigmata of von Recklinghausen's disease, including café au lait spots (a) and neurofibromata on the iris (b). The visual fields (c) were concentrically constricted and fundoscopy showed bilateral optic atrophy with loss of neurones and attenuation of retinal vessels (d). CT (e) demonstrated a rounded mass of slightly raised attenuation occupying the pentagonal basal cisterns; there was no enhancement with intravenous contrast medium.

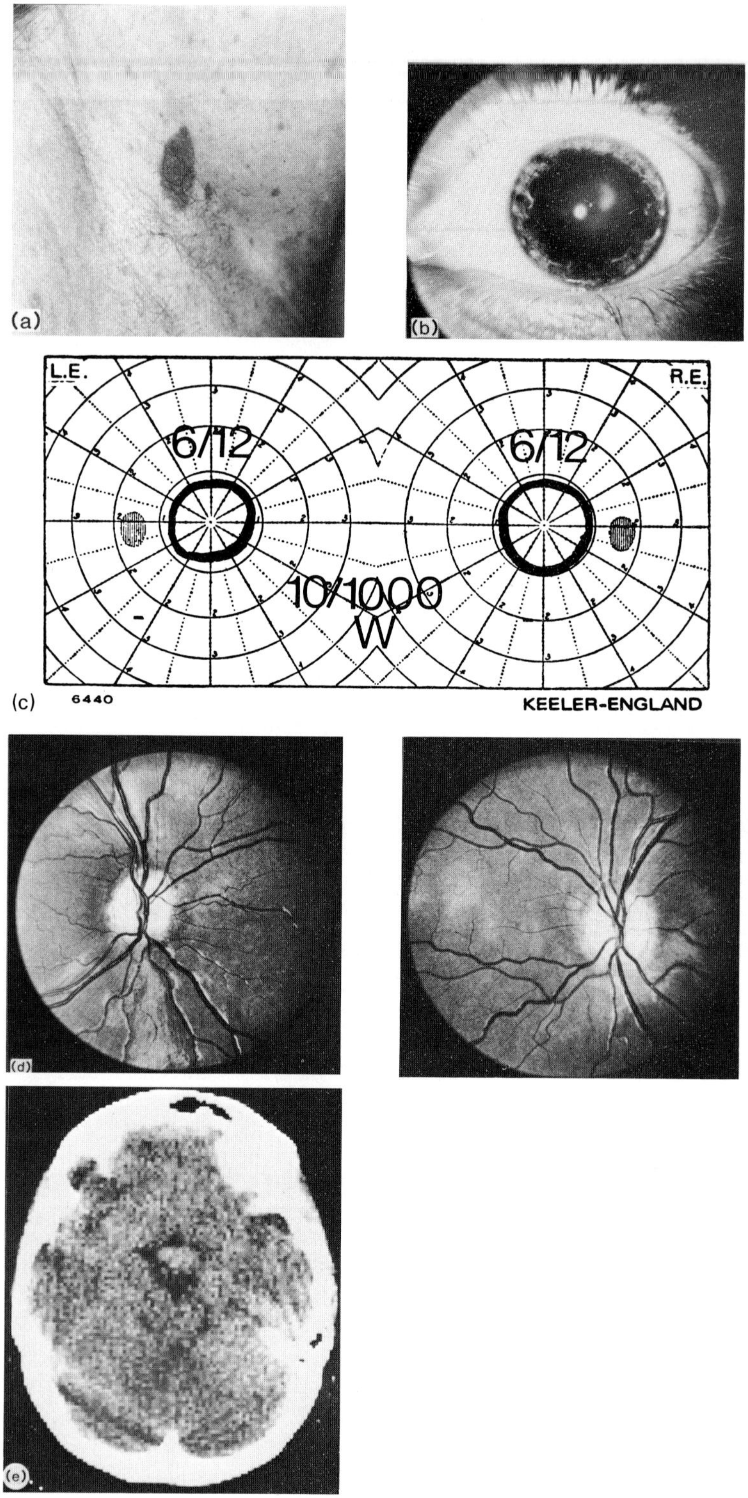

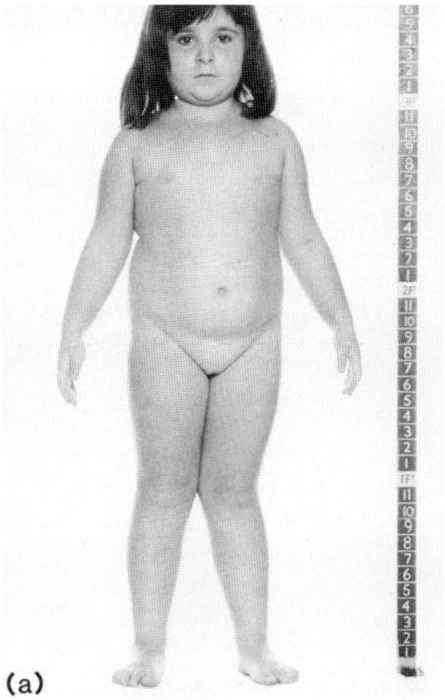

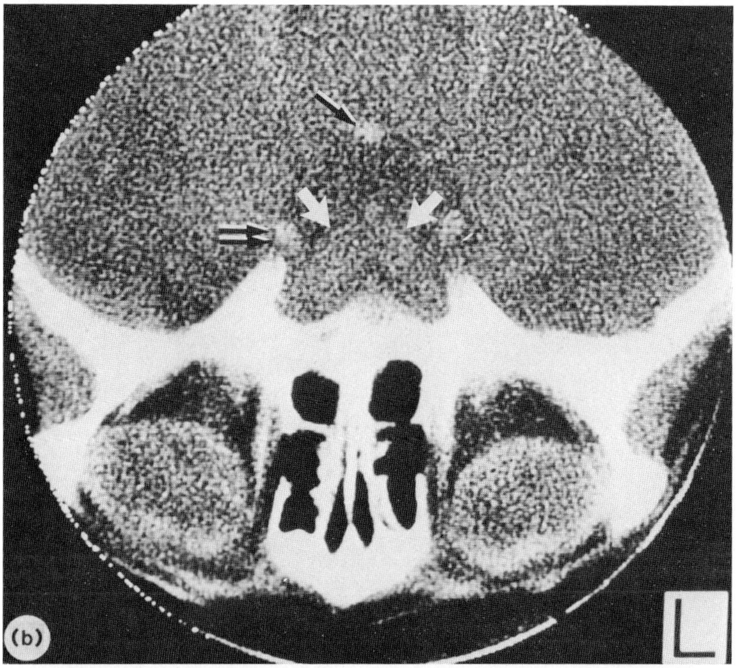

Fig. 4.8 Optic chiasm glioma with extension to optic nerves. This girl presented in 1970 with visual loss and precocious puberty (a). She had café au lait spots and a diagnosis of neurofibromatosis was made. Her vision was poor bilaterally, with bitemporal hemianopia. CT (b, c) showed enlargement of the intracranial optic nerves and chiasm (white arrows), and of the right intraorbital optic nerve (d – coronal section). The optic canals were enlarged (open arrows) and the region of the tuberculum sellae, between them, was eroded. Single arrow: basilar artery; double arrows: right internal carotid artery; crossed arrow: calcified tumour in right temporal lobe.

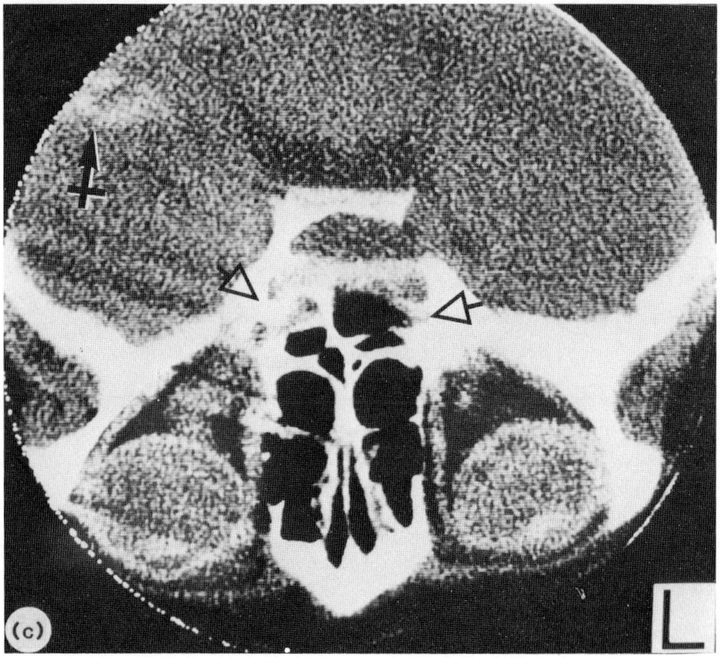

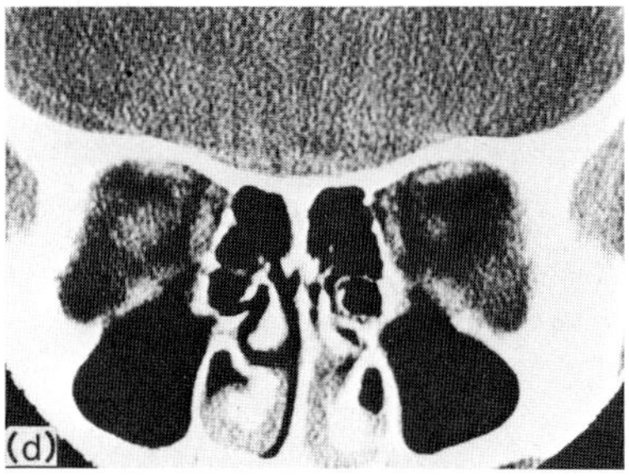

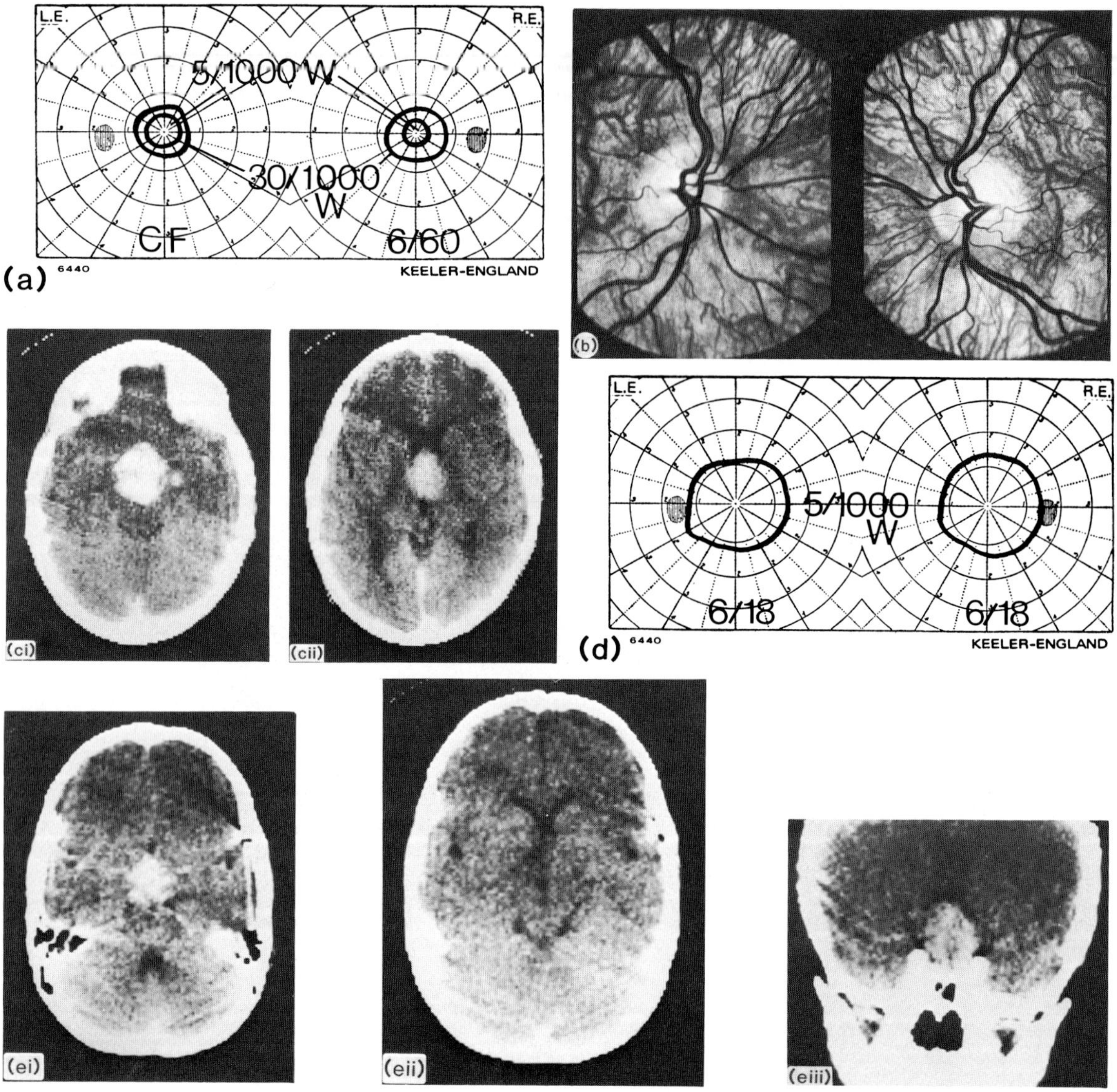

Fig. 4.9 Optic chiasm glioma. An 8-year old boy complained of failing vision, and was found to have severely reduced acuity and constricted fields (a). Fundoscopy showed no evidence of atrophy, the retinal vessels entered anomalously and there was paucity of pigment so the choroidal vessels could be visualized (b). There was no clinical evidence of neurofibromatosis. An enhancing suprasellar mass, bulging up into the third ventricle, was shown at CT (c); and biopsy confirmed a grade II astrocytoma. The patient was treated by radiotherapy and systemic steroids; ten months later there was significant improvement in vision (d) and reduction in size of the mass (e), although the coronal section revealed that considerable tumour tissue remained.

homogeneous enhancement; as yet these variations have not been correlated with the natural history or histological features of the individual tumour.

Spread of the glioma can take place forwards, into the optic nerves, or backwards into the optic tracts and the floor of the third ventricle. Forward extension is manifest by erosion of the planum sphenoidale, widening of one or both optic canals, of the optic nerve(s), and proptosis (Fig. 4.8). The orbits and optic canal regions should be examined carefully at any CT study in cases of known or presumed optic chiasm glioma. Posterior extension into the tracts can be more difficult to appreciate in tumours which show little or no enhancement with contrast medium; however, the prognosis seems to be worse and operative risks greater when such extension is present, so that CT, which is non-invasive, provides important therapeutic information.

Hydrocephalus is a not uncommon accompaniment of optic chiasm and third ventricle gliomas. If it is marked, the presence of the tumour may not be appreciated on the initial study; if clinical signs suggest a chiasmatic lesion, the scan should be repeated (with coronal sections) after ventricular shunting.

Development of CT has for the first time allowed the clinician to follow the progress of these lesions without repeated invasive studies. Whether deterioration is the result of malignant spread of a known lesion or of decompensation of adjacent tissue may hopefully be answered by this benign investigation. Furthermore, the effects of treatment (steroids or radiotherapy) may be assessed (Fig. 4.9). Repetition of identical absolutely comparable scans produces some difficulty, but this can usually be overcome. The extent to which repeated scans can be undertaken is perhaps limited by the effects of radiation.

Granulomatous disease

This may be non-specific, occurring as part of a basal arachnoiditis, or as a mass lesion involving the orbit, cavernous sinus, and parasellar region. Occasionally, specific granulomatous disease such as sarcoidosis or tuberculosis can involve the chiasm. This may be manifest at CT as partial or complete obliteration of the basal cisterns by material of soft-tissue intravenous contrast medium. As noted in the section on anatomy, the form and size of the chiasmatic and adjacent cisterns are sufficiently variable for the cerebrospinal fluid spaces to be poorly visualized on routine CT examination; multiple, thin, overlapping sections may be required. In cases in which the cisterns cannot be clearly shown, intravenous contrast medium injection may reveal that this is due to their being occupied by granulomatous material (Fig. 4.10).

Granulomata confined to the chiasm have not to date been identified as such by CT. However, CT demonstration of localized granuloma in this region shown by biopsy to be due to sarcoidosis (Decker *et al.* 1979) and histiocytosis (Tibbs *et al.*, 1978) has been recorded. One patient had a unilateral altitudinal defect and the second was blind in one eye, with temporal field loss in the other; both had endocrine disturbances. In both cases a mass of tissue isodense with the surrounding brain and showing marked homogeneous enhancement with intravenous contrast medium was seen (Fig. 4.11).

Other causes of intrinsic chiasmal disease include demyelination, rare primary tumours such as ganglioneuroma, and secondary infiltration by seeding from ectopic pinealoma, neuroblastoma, plasmacytoma etc.

It is of note that infarction of the chiasm is rare, difficult to document and defies radiological confirmation.

Compressive lesions

Extrinsic compressive lesions of the optic chiasm include:

(a) Tumours arising within the pituitary fossa.
(b) Suprasellar masses.
(c) Parasellar masses.

(a) Pituitary adenoma

Pituitary adenoma is the only common lesion to arise within the pituitary fossa. Refinement of endocrinological investigation in recent years had enhanced the diagnostic potential of these techniques, and a number of pituitary adenomas which were previously thought to be non-secretory have been shown to produce detectable quantities of pituitary hormones. Active tumours may produce growth hormone, leading to gigantism or acromegaly, prolactin (amenorrhoea and/or galactorrhoea), adrenocorticotrophic hormone (Cushing's syndrome), thyrotrophin (hyperthyroidism), or combinations of these. The ophthalmologist will tend in future to be confronted with those tumours which are endocrinologically silent and present with predominantly visual symptoms. However, with the potential early detection and drug treatment of hormonally-active tumours, the need for continued assessment of visual fields is unlikely to diminish and may even increase.

Prolactinomas are the most frequent form of secretory pituitary tumour, presenting in women with menstrual dysfunction, infertility and sometimes galactorrhoea, whilst in man the endocrine symptoms are loss of libido and impotence. Hyperprolactinaemia may be detected by radioimmunoassay and levels are usually higher than in other conditions involving the parasellar region (e.g. glioma, craniopharyngioma, meningioma etc). Treatment may be medical with bromocriptine, an ergot derivative with long-active dopamine agonist properties, and this may reduce the size of the tumour. Surgical treatment has now swung towards a transphenoidal approach, with microsurgical techni-

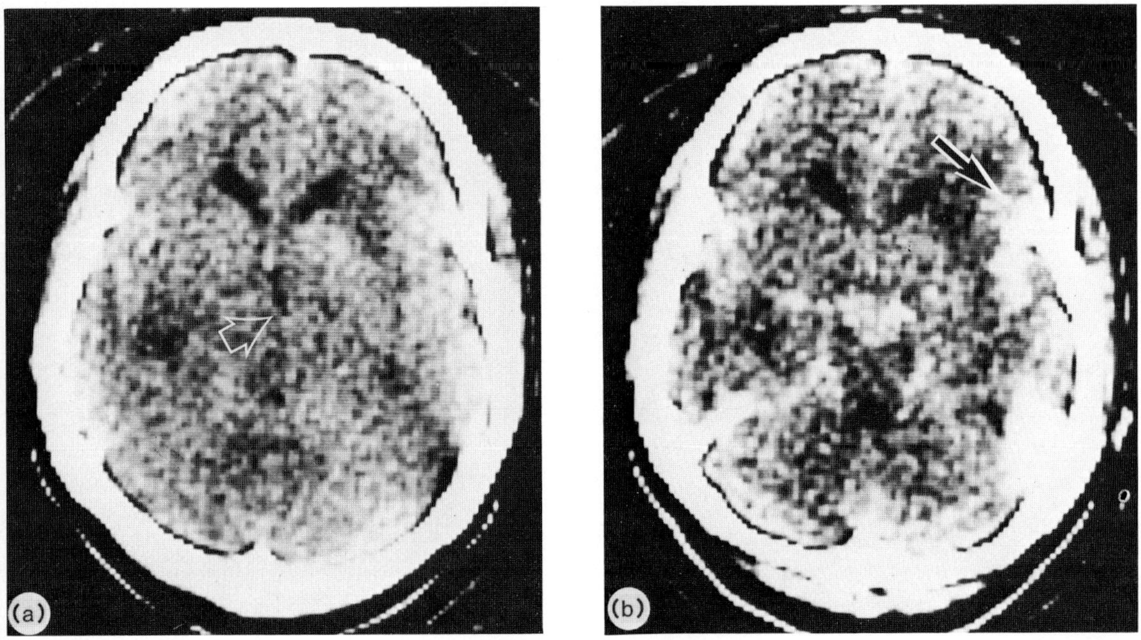

Fig. 4.10 Sarcoidosis causing basal meningitis. A 34-year old black Guyanese woman with chronic basal meningitis due to sarcoidosis. The basal cisterns are invisible ((a) open arrow indicates position of chiasmatic cistern). After intravenous contrast medium (b), they are seen to be occupied by enhancing inflammatory tissue. There is a granuloma in the right Sylvian fissure (arrow).

ques to remove a microadenoma, though larger tumours can also be removed by this route.

The following discussion of pituitary adenomas concerns those which cause visual or ocular motor disturbances.

CT appearances. The presence of visual loss almost invariably indicates that the tumour has extended beyond the sella turcica. Small suprasellar extensions – less than 1 cm in height – are very difficult to demonstrate reliably with axial CT sections. The earliest sign, referred to previously, is the inability to show the normal chiasmatic cistern and/or interpenduncular cistern. Coronal sections may be of some assistance, but with the limitation that when the section passes through the centre of an enlarged sella turcica, landmarks indicating the normal position of the diaphragma sellae may be lacking. Sagittal reconstructions may be more useful. Several groups of workers have indicated that lumbar or cisternal injection of Amipaque (metrizamide), a water-soluble contrast medium, may, by increasing the contrast between the cerebrospinal fluid and the adenoma, assist in delineation of the latter (Fig. 2.4 p.14). Amipaque, is, however not without toxic effects and its injection converts the CT examination into an invasive procedure: it can also be argued that conventional tomography following Amipaque injection may be

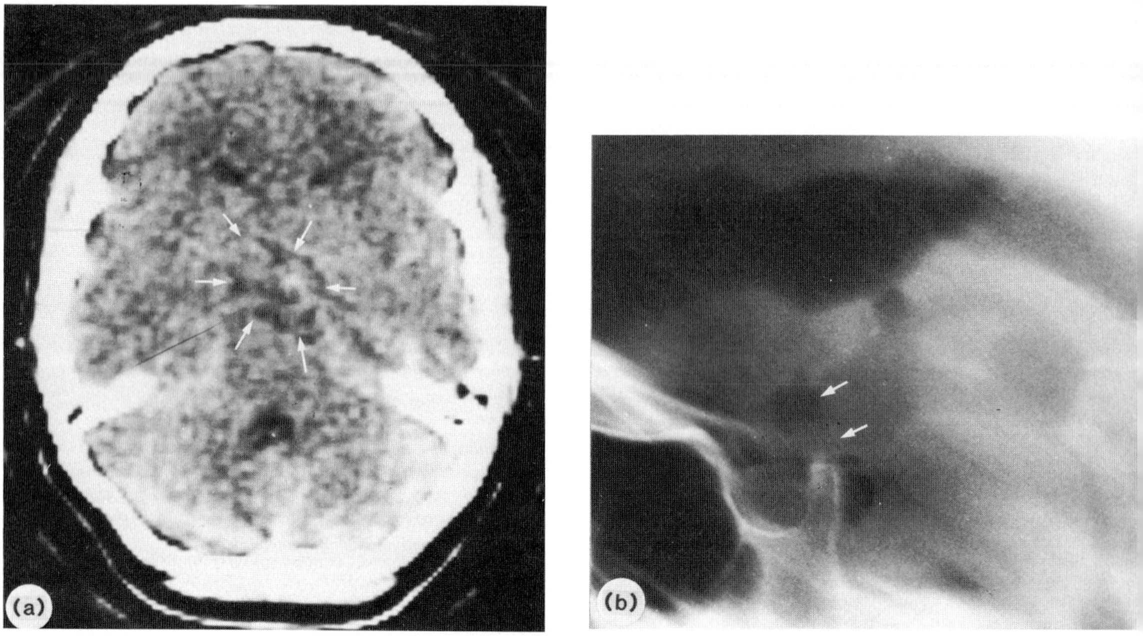

Fig. 4.11 Sarcoidosis involving optic chiasm. A 37-year old woman with known sarcoidosis suffered progressive visual loss Examination revealed signs of chiasmal compression. At CT (a) after intravenous contrast medium, a large irregular mass isodense with normal brain, was seen filling the suprasellar cisterns (arrows). The mass was not clearly outlined at pneumoencephalography (b), but the anterior recesses of the third ventricle (arrows) were truncated.

just as informative. Although the contrast medium can be used to outline the basal cisterns, it does not normally enter the ventricular system. Thus, if the surgeon requires to see the anterior end of the third ventricle preoperatively, in order to assess the position of the optic chiasm, it may still be necessary to carry out air encephalography.

Pituitary adenomas are usually rounded, although they are often lobulated, extending upwards to a variable degree; anterior, lateral or posterior extension can best be assessed by CT (Figs. 4.12, 4.14).

Attenuation coefficients of adenomas are usually rather homogeneous, being slightly higher than those of normal cerebral grey matter; hypodense or isodense tumours form about 20%. Calcification is seen in about 5%, and apparent cyst formation in a similarly small proportion. At least 90% of adenomas show homogeneously dense enhancement with intravenous contrast medium (Figs. 4.12, 4.13). A presumed pituitary tumour whose attenuation coefficients do not obviously increase after injection should be regarded with suspicion.

Although intravenous contrast medium may not be essential for detection of pituitary adenomas, it is very valuable in deter-

Fig. 4.12 Typical chromophobe adenoma. An upper temporal field defect (a) was discovered during a routine visit to an optician by a 49-year old man. The pituitary fossa was enlarged. CT (b, before, c–e, after intravenous contrast medium) confirmed the expansion of the sella, most marked on the left (arrows), and showed it to be filled by a mass of soft tissue attenuation, with homogeneous contrast enhancement (cf b, c). A relatively small, central, suprasellar extension (e) was closely applied to the adjacent major vessels (arrows).

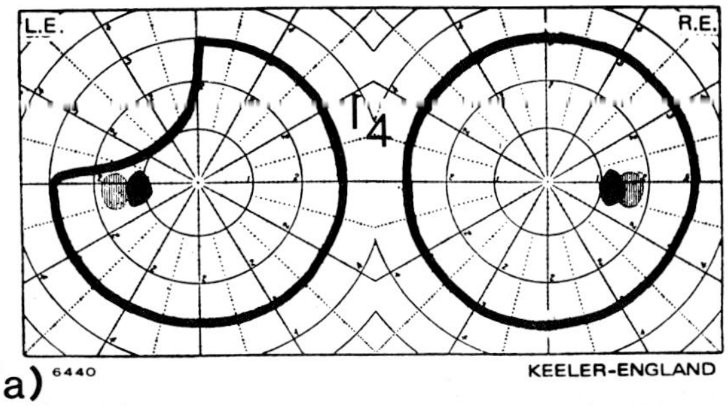

(a)

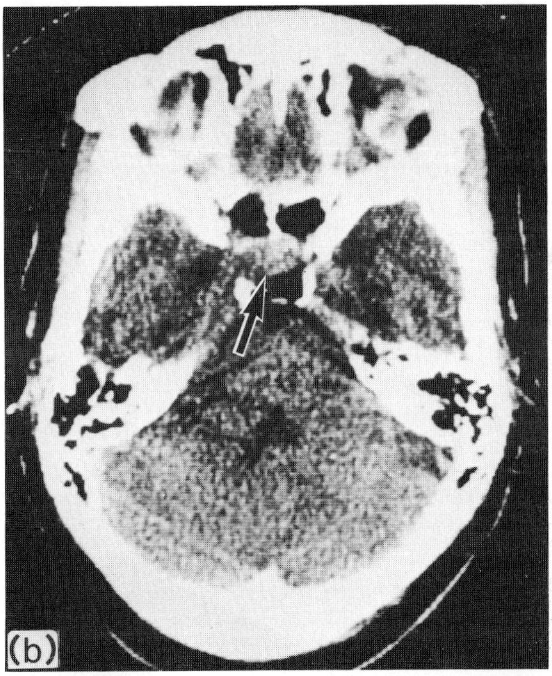

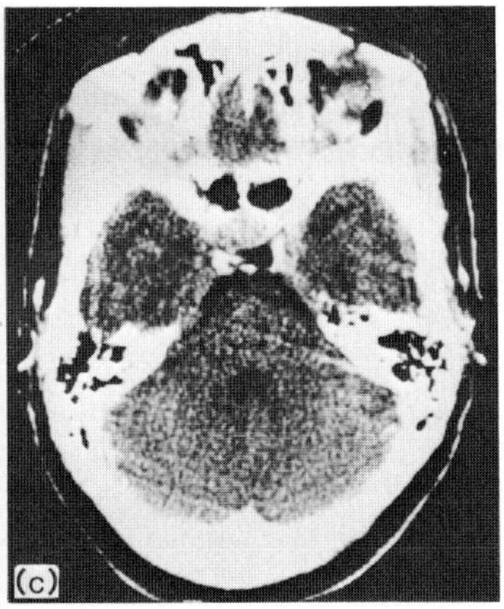

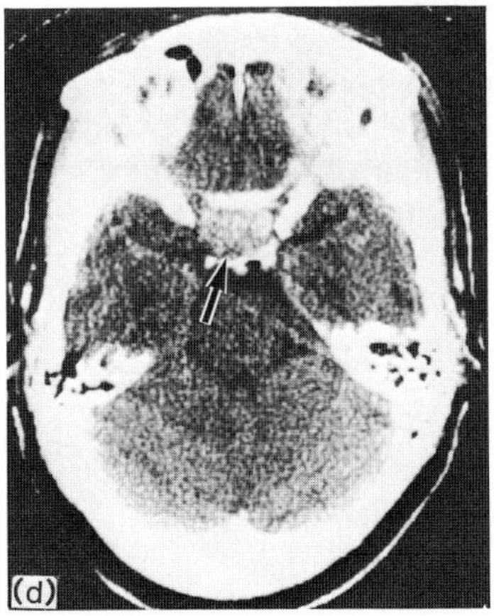

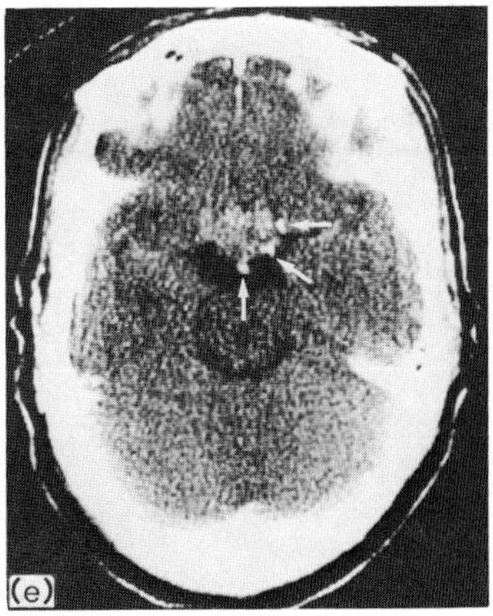

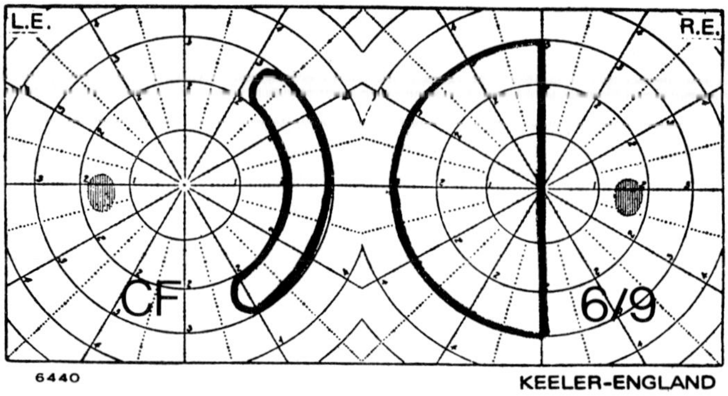

(a)

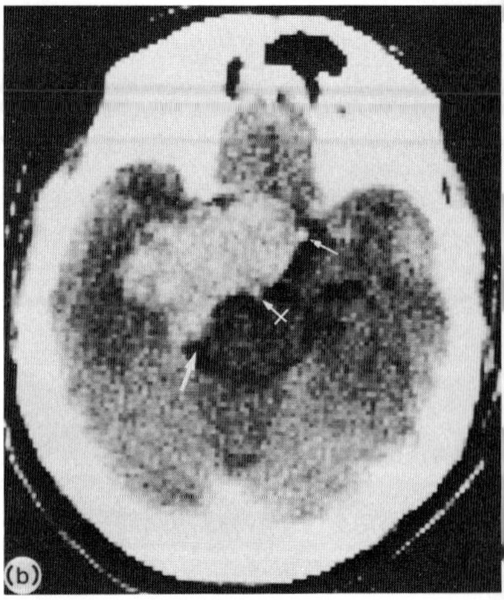

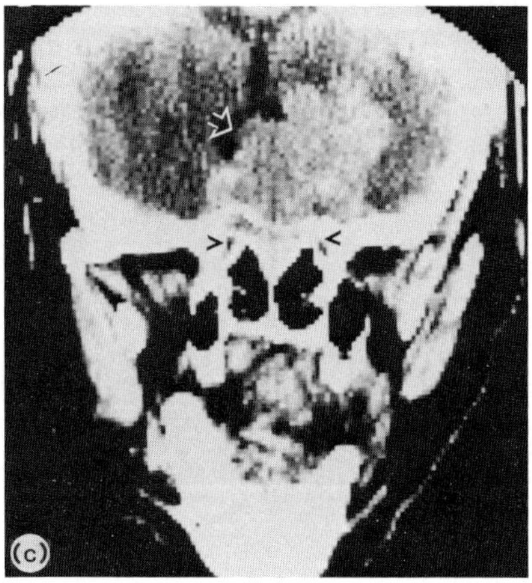

Fig. 4.13 Large chromophobe adenoma. A 54-year old man presented with a history of blurred vision in the left eye for two years and more recently loss of the temporal field in the right eye. On examination, vision was counting fingers in the left eye with a small residual area of nasal field. In the right eye there was a dense temporal hemianopia, but acuity remained 6/9 (a). CT (b,c) showed a large intra- and suprasellar mass extending upwards and to the left, into the middle cranial fossa. The axial slice (left) showed the left ambient cistern to be widened (arrow) as the brain stem was displaced to the right by the tumour. The right internal carotid (small arrow) and basilar (crossed arrow) arteries were closely applied to the tumour. Coronal section (right) showed the third ventricle (open arrow) to be draped over the mass, and there was extensive erosion of the basisphenoid (between black arrowheads), the tumour bulging into the upper pharynx.

mining the extent of the lesion; since the attenuation coefficients of the tumour are often not greatly different from those of the surrounding brain, the accentuation of the difference by contrast enhancement enables a much clearer assessment of the size of the tumour.

Correlation of CT and clinical findings. In a study of 40 patients with pituitary adenomas, of whom 35 had demonstrable field defects, the defects were noted to be bilateral in 27 (Moseley, *et al.*, 1979). There were 23 patients with temporal hemianopia, and this was symmetrical in nine. Five further patients showed quadrantic defects.

A correlation of the site of the lesion as indicated by the nature of the field loss with the extent of the tumour as demonstrated at CT was of some interest (Table 4.1). Of the 16 patients with a central suprasellar extension, 10 showed evidence of a chiasmal

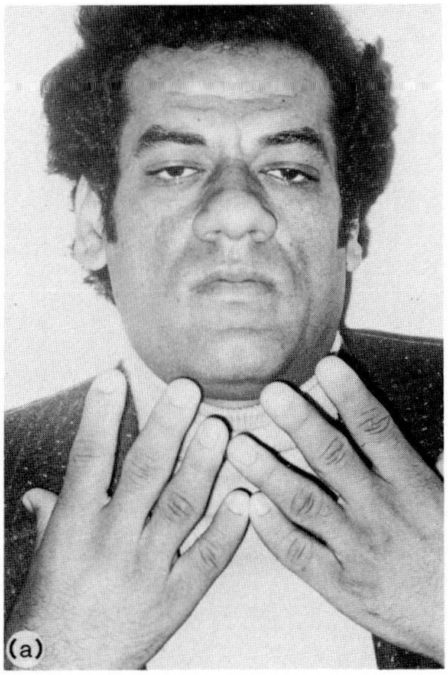

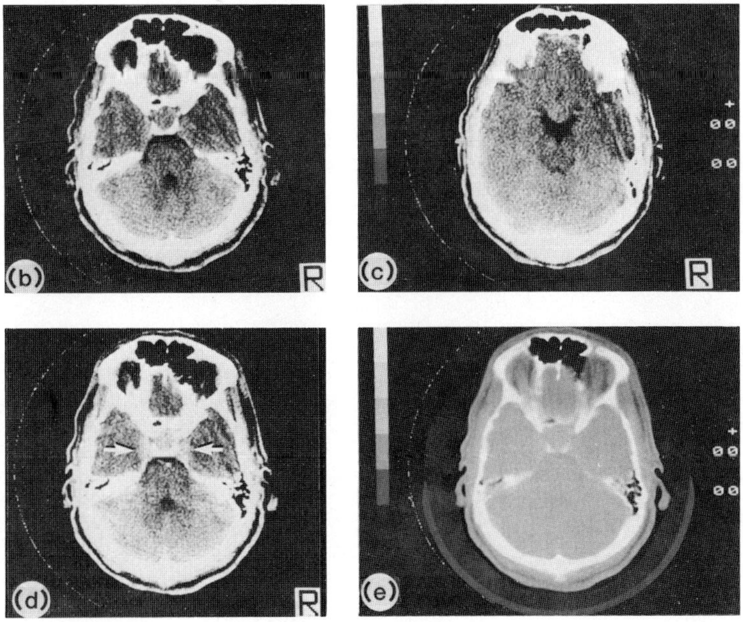

Fig. 4.14 Acromegaly. A 30-year old man was referred with increasing size of the hands, the feet and the soft tissues of the face (a). Endocrine investigation confirmed marked increase in growth hormone levels. Visual field examination was entirely normal, but CT showed an intrasellar tumour (b) with a substantial suprasellar extension (c). After intravenous contrast medium, there was marked enhancement, extending to the parasellar region on both sides (d, arrows). Wide-window imaging of the same section (e) shows the hypertrophic soft tissues, paranasal sinuses and external occipital protuberance.

lesion; two had evidence of optic nerve compression, and in three the field loss suggested an optic tract lesion, a feature seen in none of the nine patients with predominantly lateral extension. When the scan indicated an anterior extension of the tumour, five of the 12 patients showed optic nerve lesions, and only one gave evidence of optic tract disease, but both the patients in whom the scan showed a posteriorly extending mass had predominantly optic tract signs.

In the same study, there were eight patients with involvement of the trigeminal or ocular motor nerves. CT demonstrated a lateral extension of the lesion on the appropriate side (bilaterally in one case) in half this group.

Secondary effects of pituitary tumours demonstrated at CT include those resulting from the tumour mass and those caused by endocrine disturbances. Most important among the space-occupying effects are bone erosion and hydrocephalus.

Table 4.1 Comparison of clinical and CT localization of the compressive lesion in 39 pituitary adenomas.

Clinical localization	*CT* Central mass only	Lateral extension	Central + anterior	Central + posterior
Optic nerve (9)	2	2	5	0
Chiasm (19)	10	3	6	0
Optic tract (6)	3	0	1	2
None (5)	1	4	0	0

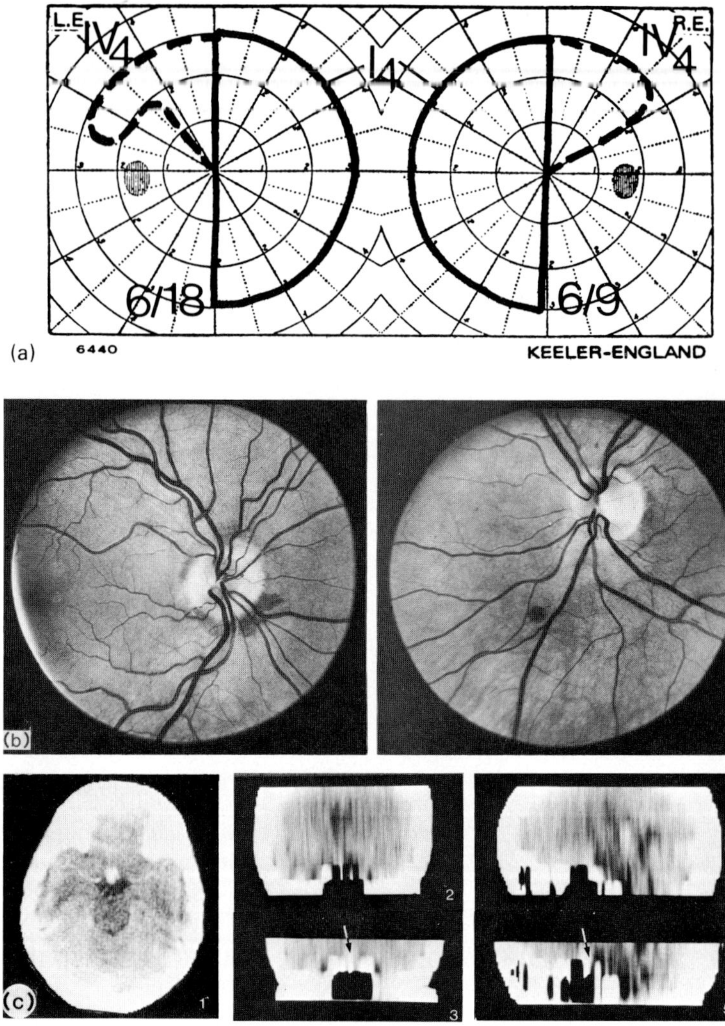

Fig. 4.15 Pituitary apoplexy (infarction). A 37-year old woman suddenly developed headache and blurred vision. She had noticed thirst and nocturia for three months and her periods had ceased seven months previously. She was found to have an atypical bitemporal hemianopia (a). The right optic disc was slightly anomalous with a peripapillary haemorrhage and there were nerve fibre and retinal haemorrhages in the left eye. There was no papilloedema (b). Skull radiographs were thought to be normal. CT (c)–1: axial post-contrast injection; 2, 3: coronal; 4, 5: midline sagittal reconstruction (before and after injection) showed a small, enhancing suprasellar mass (arrows), thought to be an aneurysm, but angiography was negative. At operation, a pituitary adenoma was found elevating and kinking the right optic nerve and chiasm. It was haemorrhagic and infarcted.

Bone erosion is an almost constant finding in pituitary adenomas producing visual problems. Enlargement of the pituitary fossa is a valuable confirmatory sign of the intrasellar origin of the tumour (Figs. 4.12, 4.14); extensive erosion of the skull base may also be seen (Fig. 4.13). Both patients with optic tract lesions referred to above showed erosion of the petrous apex. Extension into the sphenoid sinus is common, and a rare complication of pituitary adenoma is erosion into the air spaces, manifest at CT by the presence of air within the tumour or the cerebrospinal fluid.

Hydrocephalus is uncommon in pituitary adenomas, being seen in less than one quarter of cases. When it does occur, it is usually due to obstruction at the level of the foramen of Monro by a large mass. CT examination of large adenomas should thus always include sections to show the lateral ventricles. Distortion of the temporal horn of the lateral ventricle is not uncommon when the tumour extends into the middle cranial fossa. Cerebral oedema is not a feature of pituitary adenomas.

Endocrine disturbances, particularly acromegaly, may cause abnormalities which are evident at CT: thickening of the soft tissues, enlargement of the paranasal sinuses, bony protruberances etc., and thickening of the cranial vault (Fig. 4.14).

Pituitary apoplexy can be a manifestation of infarction or of haemorrhage into a pituitary adenoma (Fig. 4.15). Such changes may be beyond the powers of CT to demonstrate but haemorrhage into the adenoma itself, or into the subarachnoid space or cerebral substance can be demonstrated at CT. Weisberg (1977) described the CT findings in two cases presenting clinically as pituitary apoplexy. One showed high attenuation within the tumour, which was virtually unchanged by intravenous contrast medium; at operation, the haemorrhagic nature of the lesion was confirmed. In the other case, a high attenuation rim to the tumour became denser after contrast medium while the centre remained of lower attenuation than the surrounding brain. Surgery revealed a cystic lesion with minimal haemorrhagic and necrotic changes. Since haemorrhagic pituitary apoplexy can closely mimic subarachnoid haemorrhage, plain skull radiographs and CT studies can be of considerable value in the acute situation (Fig. 4.16). The late result of apoplexy may be an empty sella (see p.124).

(b) Craniopharyngioma

Clinical considerations. Arising from epithelioid remnants of Rathke's pouch, craniopharyngiomas represent the commonest suprasellar tumour. They can arise within the sella turcica itself, or lie virtually within the third ventricle, but typically they lie above the posterior half of the sella, between the diaphragma sellae and the optic chiasm. They usually present at a younger age than pituitary tumours, and may even be present at birth. Clinical presentation is variable, depending on the site of the lesion, and though visual loss is a prominent feature, most cases show endocrine signs suggesting hypothalamic involvement and almost 30% of patients have papilloedema due to posterior extension of a large mass, blocking the foramina of Monro.

Diagnosis is particularly important in children, who may endure gross reduction in visual acuity and field without complaint. Confrontation fields and routine X-rays will often make the diagnosis, but the history-taking must include direct questioning to elicit evidence of polydypsia, polyuria, disturbances of growth or sexual development, slipped femoral epiphyses etc.

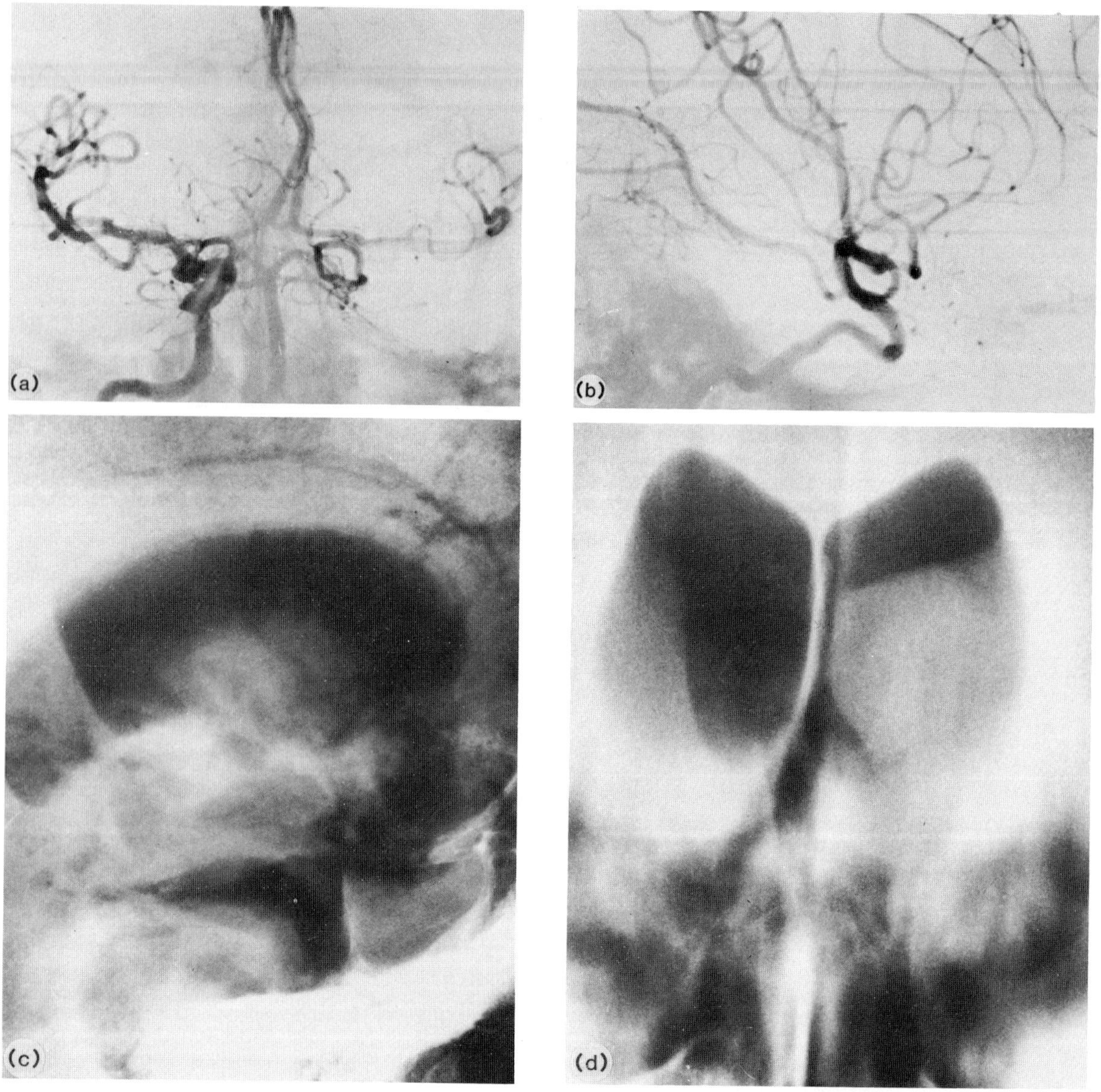

Fig. 4.16 Pituitary apoplexy (haemorrhage). A 67-year old man presented with sudden severe headache, accompanied by loss of consciousness and impaired vision. Lumbar puncture indicated subarachnoid haemorrhage. Plain skull radiographs showed ballooning of the pituitary fossa (c). Four-vessel cerebral angiography (a, b) did not reveal a source for haemorrhage, but midline displacement (a) indicated a right frontal mass, later confirmed by pneumoencephalography (c, d). The nature of the mass was made clear only by CT (e, left), which showed an intracerebral haematoma. At operation this was found to have arisen from a pituitary tumour. (e, right) Two weeks later, a post-haemorrhagic cavity is seen to lie alongside the right air-containing frontal horn.

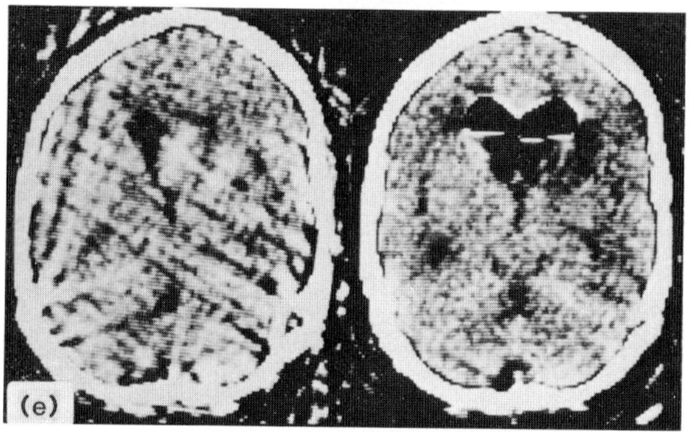

In adults the presentation is variable, with asymmetric field loss and endocrine signs. Bizarre presentations, however, include positive sensory phenomena such as flashing lights, episodic headaches resembling migraine and fluctuating visual loss. An intraventricular extension may rarely compress the optic nerve or chiasm from above.

Diagnosis can be more difficult than in pituitary tumours because the skull may appear normal on routine lateral radiographs. However, midline suprasellar calcification is characteristic and common, occurring in about 90% of children and up to 50% of adults. In typical cases the dorsum sellae is truncated, but this sign is difficult to assess. Signs of raised intracranial pressure may predominate, particularly in children.

CT appearances. CT demonstrates a suprasellar mass, usually midline, and frequently rather more posteriorly placed than the typical pituitary adenoma, filling the interpeduncular fossa. There may be some extension behind the clivus into the posterior fossa.

Calcification of the lesion is almost invariable in children, and is present in about 50% of adults. About one half of craniopharyngiomas appear cystic, i.e. they have a centre of reduced attenuation as compared with brain, surrounded by a capsule of brain attenuation or above, often calcified (Fig. 4.17). However, the range of appearances commonly encountered with craniopharyngiomas is much greater than with pituitary adenomas. About one third are of mixed attenuation; uniformly low attenuation is seen in about one quarter and a small proportion are completely calcific. There is only a general correlation between attenuation coefficients and the consistency of the lesion; tumours isodense with brain, for example, may be either largely fluid or completely solid.

Craniopharyngiomas are among the few tumours which often show little increase in attenuation with intravenous contrast medium. About one third show no enhancement, particularly in adults (Fig. 4.18), while in one half the enhancement is peripheral only, and may at least in part represent vessels stretched around the mass. Homogenous enhancement occurs in only 10–15% (Fig. 4.19), enhancement of the basal portion being more frequent. Thus, the classical craniopharyngioma is a rounded, posterior suprasellar mass of low attenuation centrally, with a calcified base or capsule; contrast medium injection produces basal or peripheral enhancement or is without effect. Fitz *et al.* (1978) suggested that the CT diagnosis of craniopharyngioma should be based on the triad of cyst/calcification/contrast enhancement, although only about 70% of the cases in their series showed these features.

Correlation of CT and clinical findings (Table 4.2). In a series

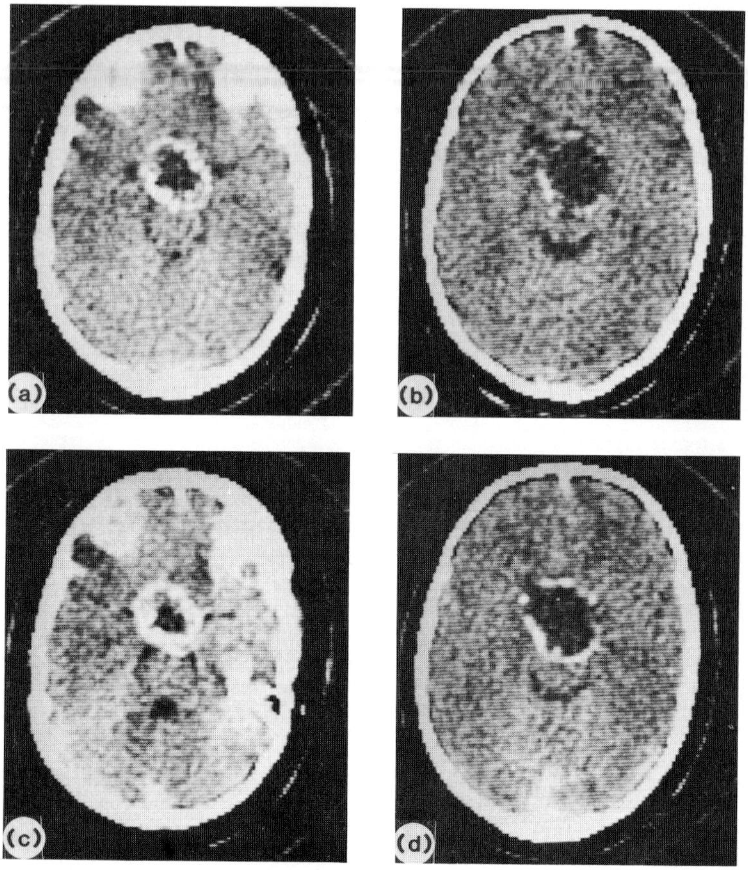

Fig. 4.17 Craniopharyngioma. An 8-year old boy, with visual loss and short stature. There was bilateral optic atrophy. CT (a,b) showed the typical appearances of this type of tumour: a rounded mass of low attenuation, with peripheral calcification, occupying the suprasellar cisterns. After intravenous contrast medium (c,d), any enhancement is confined to the capsule of the tumour (NB The sections are not strictly comparable).

Table 4.2 Comparison of clinical and CT localization of the compressive lesion in 21 craniopharyngiomas.

Clinical localization	CT		
	Central mass	Lateral extension	Central + posterior
Optic nerve (6)	5	1	0
Chiasm (12)	6	6	0
Optic tract (5)	2	1	2

similar to that of pituitary adenomas noted above, we found field defects in all of 21 patients with craniopharyngioma. These had hemianopic features in 13, which were bitemporal in seven. There were four patients with normal vision in one eye, of whom three showed relative defects in the other eye.

Of the twelve patients with a centrally situated mass at CT, six showed evidence of chiasmal compression, five of optic nerve lesions, and two also of optic tract disturbance (Fig. 4.20). Six of

Fig. 4.18 Craniopharyngioma. This 41-year old female complained of galactorrhoea and progressive visual loss. Examination showed a bitemporal hemianopia (a). The serum prolactin was 2560 μg/ml, but the skull radiographs (b) did not suggest a pituitary tumour. CT (c) showed a poorly-defined, lobulated mass lying on the right side, above the sella (arrowheads). This was confirmed by pneumoencephalography, and at operation, proved to be a craniopharyngioma.

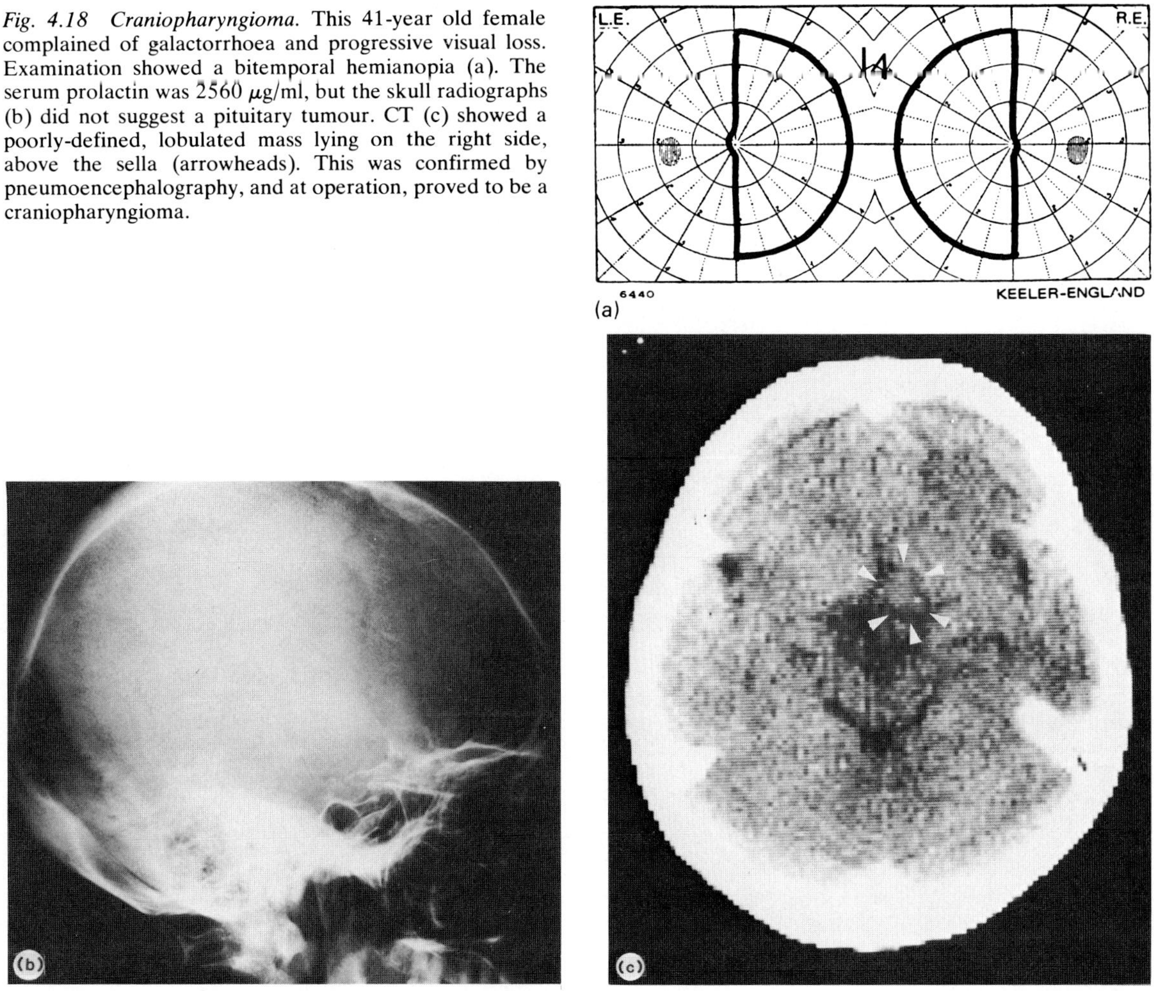

the seven patients with central and lateral masses showed chiasmal signs. Two members of this latter group in whom the lateral extension was particularly marked showed optic nerve lesions: in one, a unilateral hemianopic defect, and in the other a small defect in one eye with complete contralateral blindness. The only two patients with solely optic tract lesions both showed posterior extension of the tumour, and in keeping with the rather more posterior position of this type of tumour, there were none in whom an anterior extension could be correlated with optic nerve compression.

Bone erosion is not typically seen at CT in craniopharyngiomas, although a flattened sella turcica may at first appear enlarged.

Cerebral oedema is infrequent. Hydrocephalus is, however,

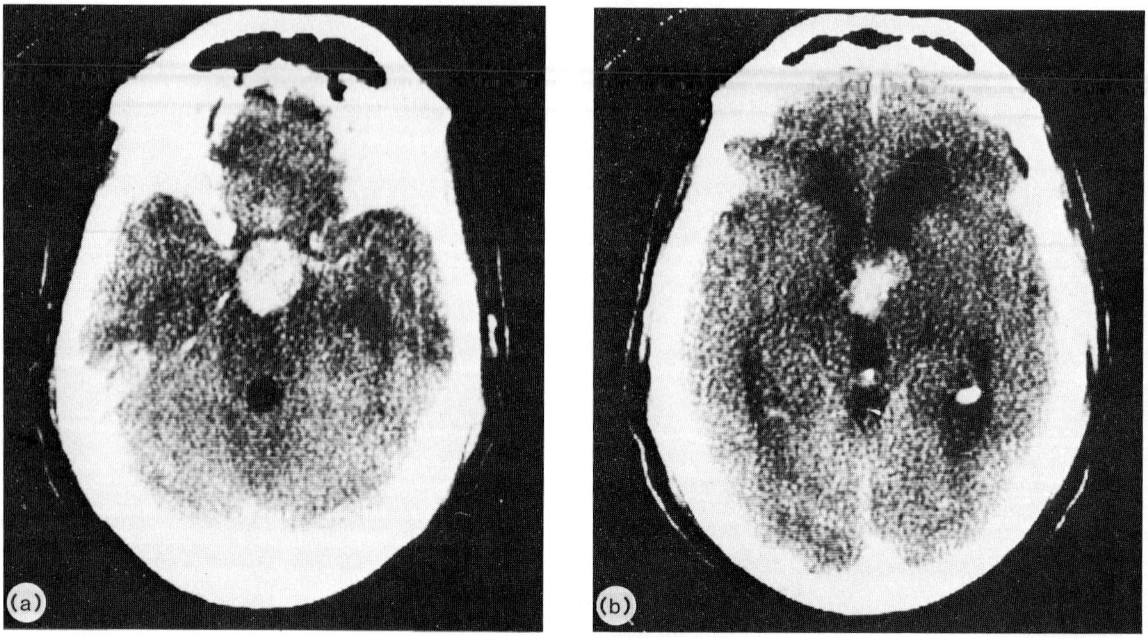

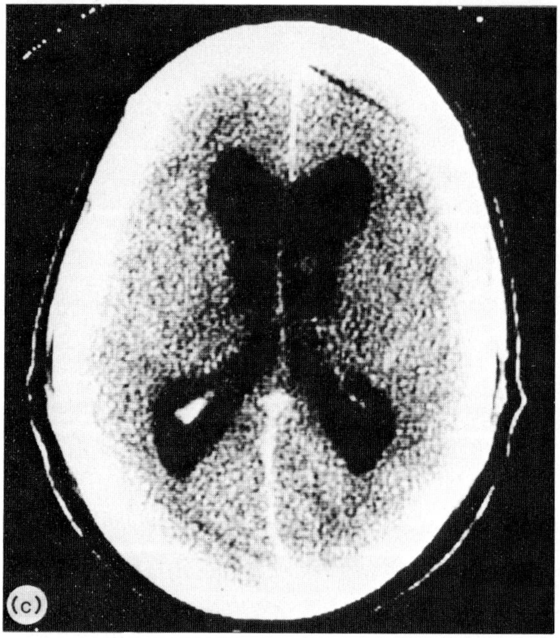

Fig. 4.19 Craniopharyngioma. A man of 42 years, presenting with headaches and visual impairment, was shown to have a classical bitemporal hemianopia. The sella was eroded, and CT (a–c, after intravenous contrast medium) showed a rounded suprasellar mass, which enhanced rather homogeneously. There was moderate hydrocephalus. Operation confirmed the presence of a large craniopharyngioma.

common, occurring in at least 50% of our patients, and in 60% of the series described by Naidich *et al.* (1976). Patients with severe loss of visual fields showed a high incidence of hydrocephalus (70%) in our series, while ventricular enlargement was seen in

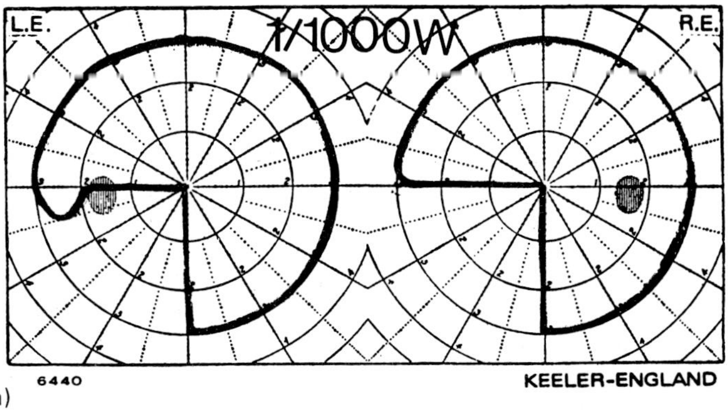

(a)

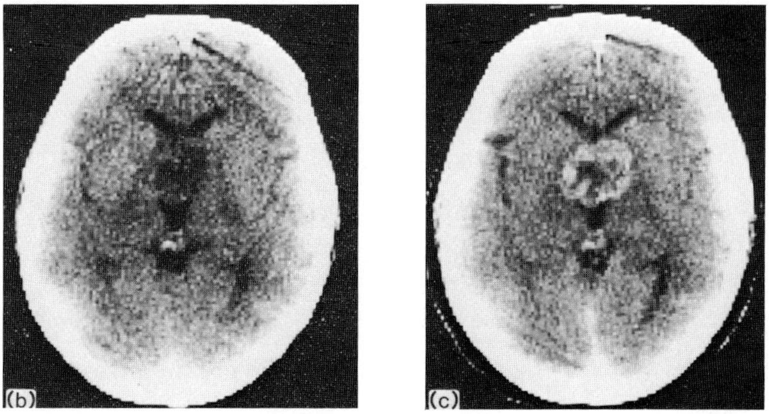
(b) (c)

Fig. 4.20 Craniopharyngioma. This 60-year old man presented with blurring of vision and personality change. He had a left inferior quadrantanopia (a). Prolactin level was 1300 units. CT showed a suprasellar mass of mixed, but generally low attenuation, obliterating the anterior end of the third ventricle, and causing mild hydrocephalus (b). After intravenous contrast medium there was peripheral enhancement, but a low attenuation centre remained, suggesting a craniopharynigioma (c). An initial attempt at subfrontal removal was unsatisfactory but a large craniopharyngioma extending into the third ventricle was subsequently removed completely via a transcallosal approach.

three of the four patients with ocular motor palsies.

Because of their more or less central location, craniopharyngiomas may obstruct one or both foramina of Monro (Fig. 4.19). CT is therefore of considerable importance in the follow-up of patients who are treated by ventricular shunting procedures, for the assessment of the efficacy of ventricular decompression.

Surgery is often necessarily incomplete, since the tumour may be markedly adherent to such structures as the optic chiasm or basilar artery. Recurrent tumour is generally similar in attenuation characteristics to the original growth; very rapid recurrence of the mass is frequently the result of cyst formation. CT is a much more sensitive non-invasive technique for assessing residual or recurrent tumour than plain film demonstration of calcification, the method previously employed in some centres.

Differential diagnosis

Hamartoma of the tuber cinereum and hypothalamus represents an important differential diagnostic consideration. This rare childhood tumour usually causes death by the second decade. It appears at CT as a more or less discrete mass, sometimes calcified, occupying the chiasmatic cistern or interpeduncular fossa (Lin *et al.*, 1978). Visual disturbance is, however, surprisingly infrequent.

Arachnoid cysts are generally congenital in origin. They occur in certain classical situations, notably in the suprasellar region, but also the quadrigeminal cistern, and the middle and posterior cranial fossa. Suprasellar lesions are often of considerable size, several centimetres in diameter, lying centrally above the sella. At pneumoencephalography the diagnosis may be rendered difficult by the fact that air does not enter the lesion; in theory, therefore, it could be a solid mass. CT diagnosis is also not straightforward, since the rounded collection of cerebrospinal fluid attenuation, often associated with marked lateral ventricular enlargement may simulate a hugely dilated third ventricle, leading to the erroneous diagnosis of aqueduct stenosis. Observations suggesting the correct aetiology are the disproportionate size of the 'third ventricle' – a diameter greater than 3 cm is in favour of a cyst – and its rounded shape, features which between them give rise to a typical 'Mickey Mouse' appearance. It may be evident that the posterior portion of the third ventricle is of normal size.

Acquired arachnoid cysts may arise in 'optochiasmatic arachnoiditis', a much disputed entity. There is general agreement that the condition may arise as the sequel to a number of chronic basal meningitides, e.g. tuberculosis, sarcoidosis. Its existence as a primary disease process is, however, controversial; in some centres it is diagnosed relatively frequently in patients who are explored after negative radiological investigations while in others the diagnosis is rarely if ever made.

We have seen a 28-year old epileptic woman, known for some years to have a left occipital porencephalic cyst. She complained of decreasing vision, and examination revealed a chiasmal pattern of visual loss, in addition to the anticipated homonymous hemianopia. CT studies showed the porencephaly, and an apparently prominent chiasmatic cistern (Fig. 4.21). Air encephalography showed an anteroposterior prolongation of the subarachnoid space into the sella turcica, with impaired filling of the cisterns anterior to this. A thickened arachnoid membrane was divided at operation, with relief of the chiasmal compression. It is tempting to suggest in this case that the original disease process causing the porencephaly had also resulted in chronic basal arachnoiditis.

Third ventricular tumours of any type may extend antero-inferiorly to compress or infiltrate the chiasm (Fig. 4.22). Such tumours are usually malignant, and the range of CT appearances is similar to that described above for optic chiasm glioma.

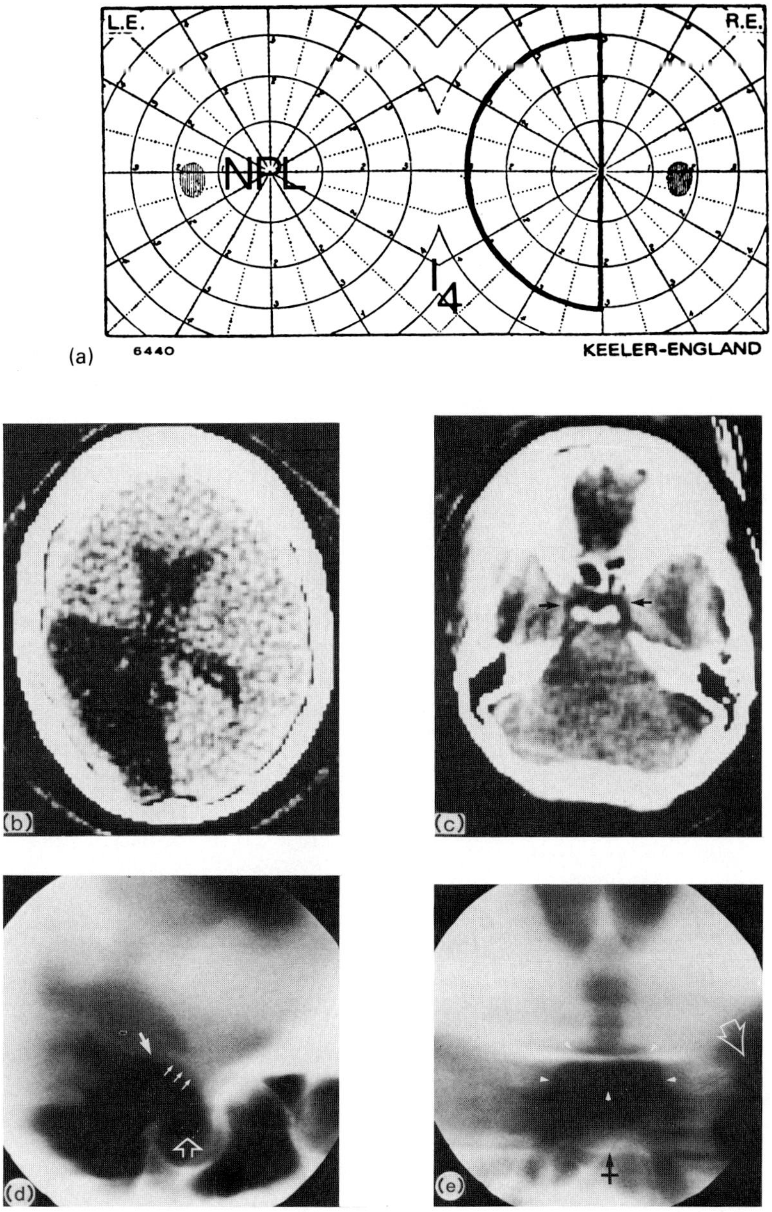

Fig. 4.21 Porencephaly and cystic arachnoiditis. No perception of light in the left eye and a temporal hemianopia in the right (a). CT: a large cavity communicating with the left lateral ventricle (b), and a rather prominent subarachnoid space extending across the midline between the tuberculum and dorsum sellae (c, arrows), The pathological nature of this fluid collection was confirmed by pneumonencephalography; (d) an apparently loculated fluid space filled the upper part of the sella (open arrow), truncated the chiasmatic recess (arrow) and bulged towards the optic chiasm (small arrows). A coronal tomogram (e) at the level of the floor of the sella (crossed arrow) showed the extent of the cyst (arrowheads). The open arrow indicates the porencephaly. (See text for details.)

Pressure on the chiasm by a *third ventricle* dilated as a result of distal obstruction, is a well-recognized cause of visual loss. Marked dilatation of the anterior end of the third ventricle is a feature of lesions causing obstruction either within the third ventricle itself, e.g. colloid cyst, or at its posterior end, e.g. aqueduct stenosis or pineal region tumours. The clinical features may thus include proptosis, ophthalmoplegia and visual loss indicative of optic nerve, chiasm or tract compression in addition

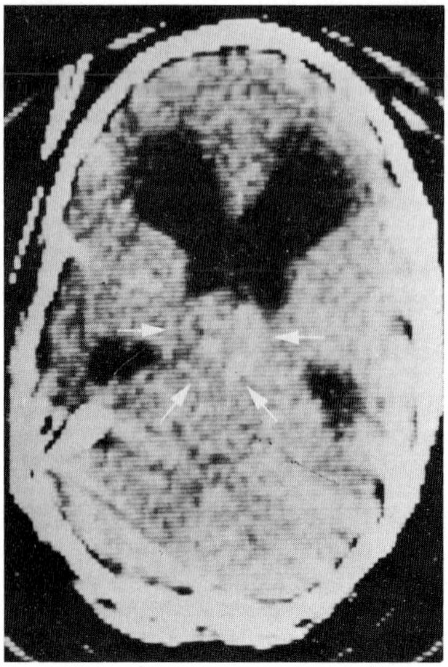

Fig. 4.22 Third ventricle astrocytoma. A 15-year old boy had complained of headaches, when over a two-week period, his vision decreased to no perception of light on the right and hand movements on the left. Skull radiographs showed evidence of long-standing raised intracranial pressure. CT demonstrated a dense, rounded mass in the region of the third ventricle (arrows) causing very marked hydrocephalus, with periventricular lucencies. There was no pathological contrast enhancement. At surgery the optic chiasm was compressed by a solid tumour originating within the third ventricle, which proved to be a Grade III astrocytoma.

to those of the primary lesions (Osher *et al.*, 1978). In such cases, skull radiography often shows truncation of the dorsum sellae and apparent enlargement of the sella turcica; chronic cases, typified by patients with aqueduct stenosis, show the classical J sella, with large anterior clinoid processes, a deep sulcus chiasmaticus, low tuberculum sellae, small sella and thin, anteflexed, truncated dorsum sellae. In our series of 33 patients with pineal region tumours, referred to in Chapter 6, there were two with bitemporal inferior quadrantanopia, indicating compression of the superior surface of the chiasm. In both, the CT scan showed considerable third ventricular enlargement. (Another patient showed a *homonymous* inferior quadrantic defect, thought to be related to ectopic pinealoma in the suprasellar region).

CT examination in axial, coronal or sagittal planes clearly reveals the abnormal anteroinferior extension of the dilated third ventricle, which occupies the anticipated position of the sella turcica.

Chiasmal compression is an uncommon complication of frontal lobe tumours, usually gliomas. CT establishes the diagnosis, although in some cases it may be difficult to determine whether a primary chiasmal lesion has extended upwards or vice versa. Coronal sections may be helpful in this context.

Meningiomas

Clinical features. No tumour in neuro-ophthalmology produces such gratification when diagnosed early, or such humiliation when the diagnosis is missed. Meningiomas conforming to the classical textbook sites provoke more rapid diagnosis than those lesions which infiltrate, arise from unconventional sites or are situated under bony crevices and remain sheltered from the X-ray beam (Sanders and Moseley, 1979). The clinician should therefore suspect a meningioma in any patient with progressive painless visual loss, progressive loss of retinal neurones, and a normal fundus. Reconsideration of the clinical facts, repetition of radiological tests and regular follow-up may be necessary to produce a definite diagnosis. Surgical treatment does not, however, invariably produce the dramatic recovery of vision seen with pituitary tumours or craniopharyngiomas, possibly because of the firmer consistency of meningiomas, and inability to remove the tumour entirely.

Tumours of this type arise in a number of characteristic sites around the sella turcica and may produce a variety of syndromes with visual loss and/or ophthalmoplegia. The authors have reviewed this subject in detail (Sanders and Moseley, 1979) and it will therefore be discussed more generally here.

Sites

1. Optic canal.
2. Anterior clinoid process.

Fig. 4.23 Suprasellar meningioma. This middle-aged woman presented with progressive painless right visual loss. There was a small area in the superior temporal quadrant in which she could appreciate hand movements (a). The left eye was entirely normal, with 6/6 vision and a full field. The pituitary fossa was normal on lateral skull X-ray. CT confirmed this (b), but showed a large, rounded suprasellar mass (c, after contrast enhancement). Enhancement was most intense in the region of the right orbital apex (arrows) (d: same image as (c), EMI number range 45–80 highlighted). Angiography (e) showed a typical tumour blush (arrows).

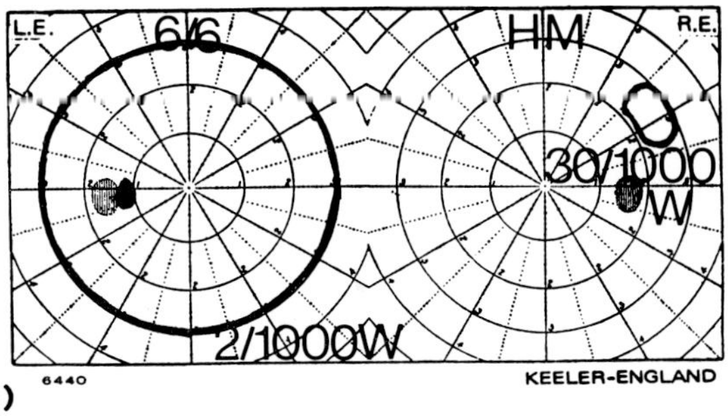

(a)

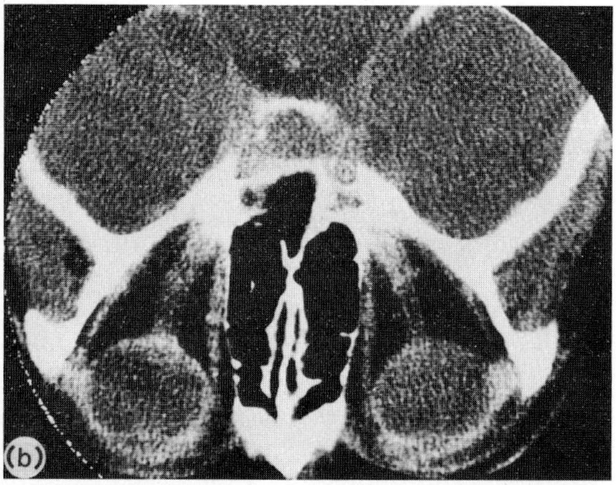

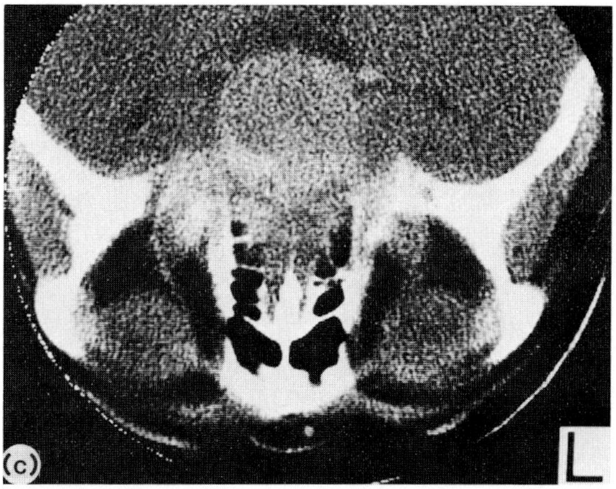

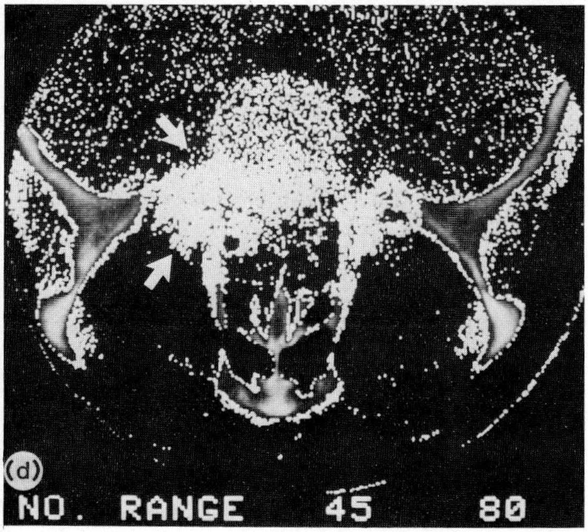

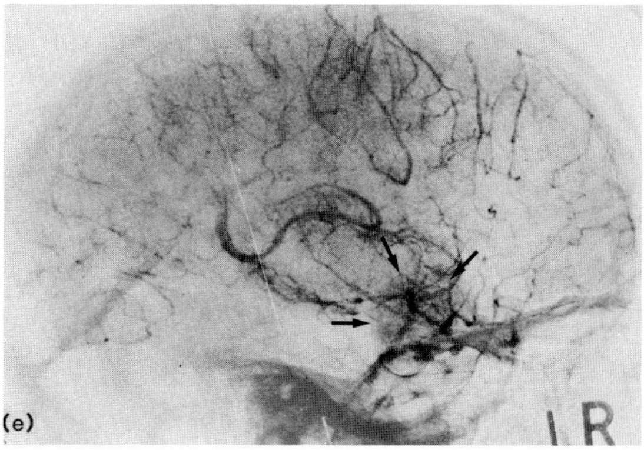

3. Tuberculum sellae/planum sphenoidale.
4. Greater wing of sphenoid, medial, lateral. (Fig. 4.3).
5. Diaphragma sellae.
6. Clivus.
7. Cavernous sinus.

Plain skull radiographs show hyperostosis or other changes (abnormal bone texture, blistering, erosion or calcification) in a high proportion of cases, although these abnormalities may be slight and only appreciated with conventional tomography or on retrospective analysis.

Basal meningiomas visible at CT are seen as rounded masses, generally with a smooth, slightly lobulated outline (Fig. 4.23). Surrounding low attenuation, representing oedema, is not a prominent feature of these basal tumours. When present, low attenuation affects mainly the white matter, in one or both frontal lobes, and this has been mistaken for the primary lesion. Backward displacement and splaying of the frontal horns may be the key observation; scans with and without intravenous contrast medium, and supplemented by coronal sections are essential for accurate diagnosis.

The attenuation coefficients of meningiomas vary from those of brain tissue to slightly above, thus covering almost the same range as those of pituitary tumours. This latter fact is often not appreciated, and may give rise to diagnostic confusion. Low attenuation and 'cystic' meningiomas may be encountered, but are rare. Calcification is neither common (occurring in up to 25%), nor is it usually extensive. Intravenous contrast medium produces a rather dense, homogenous increase in attenuation in the large majority of cases. This marked homogeneity is a suggestive factor in the differential diagnosis from pituitary adenomas, which tend to be slightly more variegated, and from large basal aneurysms, which may show filling defects, due to thrombus.

Hyperostosis and the other bone changes referred to previously may be visible at CT (Fig. 4.24).

Meningiomas in the parasellar region do not characteristically cause hydrocephalus.

Small lesions in several sites may be difficult or impossible to show at CT, or even with the complete range of current radiological techniques. Thus, small tumours in the optic canal/medial end of superior orbital fissure region may compress the optic nerve without producing any substantial mass. A tumour mass lying under the anterior clinoid process may easily escape detection, because the finite thickness of the CT sections does not allow it to be separated from the underlying bone. There is often considerable artefactual degradation of the CT images in this region. Changes within the orbit or in the orbital walls may be the clue to the presence of an adjacent meningioma (Fig. 4.25). *En plaque* lesions may be difficult to show in any situation, and this is particularly true of the planum sphenoidale/tuberculum

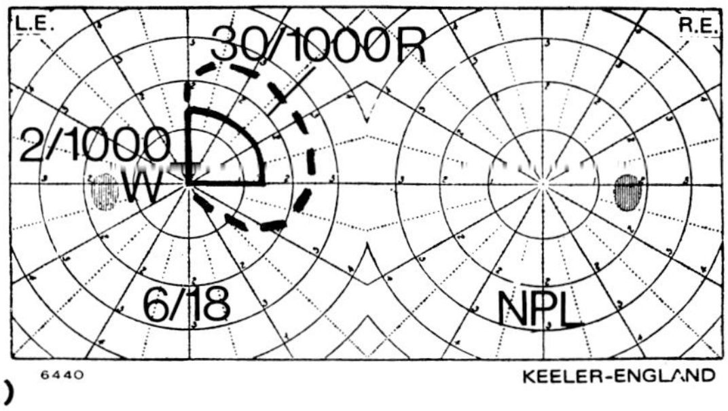

(a)

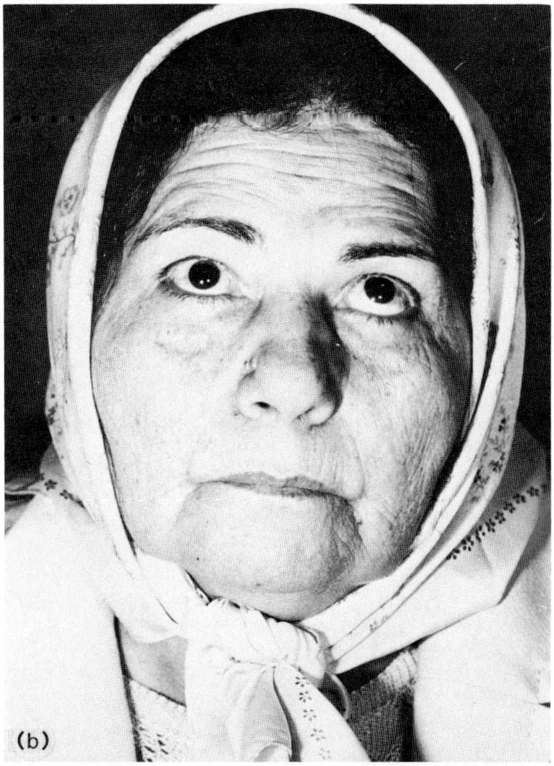
(b)

Fig. 4.24 Anterior visual pathway meningioma. A 58-year old woman had been blind in the right eye for 20 years; this was attributed to vascular disease, but over five months she was losing vision on the left. There was no perception of light on the right, and acuity on the left was 6/18, but limited to the upper nasal quadrant (a). Elevation and depression of the right eye were limited (b). The left disc was pale at the temporal margin, while the right showed opticociliary shunt vessels and extensive peripapillary pigment epithelial disorganization (c). Skull radiography demonstrated classical hyperostosis and 'blistering' of the planum sphenoidale. This was confirmed and shown to cross the midline by CT (arrows), which also showed a soft-tissue mass within the sinus, extending down into the upper part of the right nasal cavity (crossed arrow). Both optic nerves appeared dense and the right was unequivocally expanded. (d, e: axial and coronal sections at normal window settings; f, g: wide-window images to show bony abnormalities).

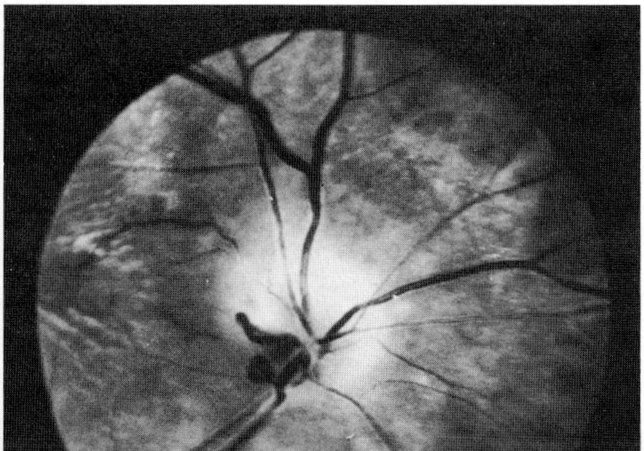
(c)

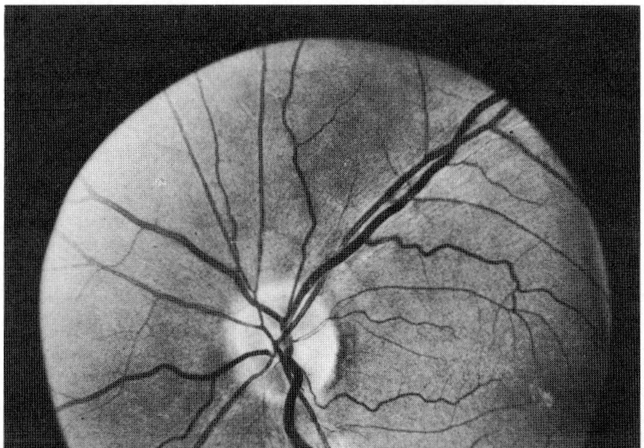

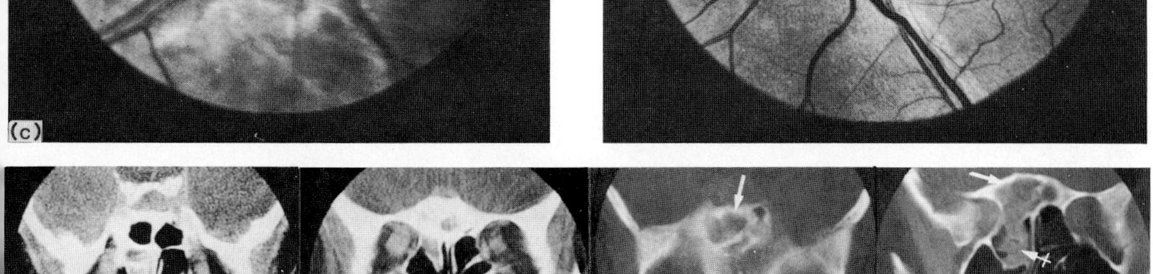
(d) (e) (f) (g)

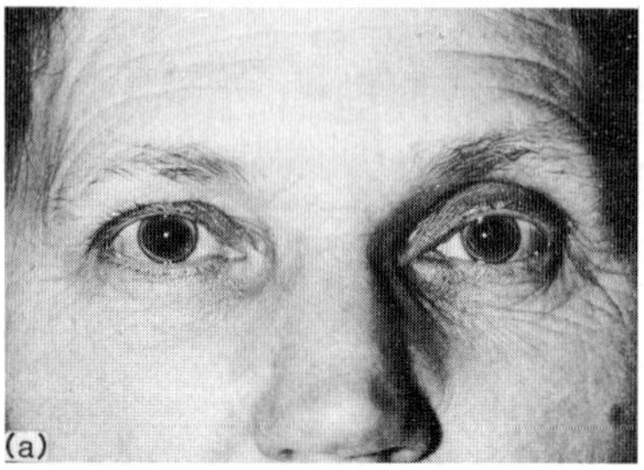

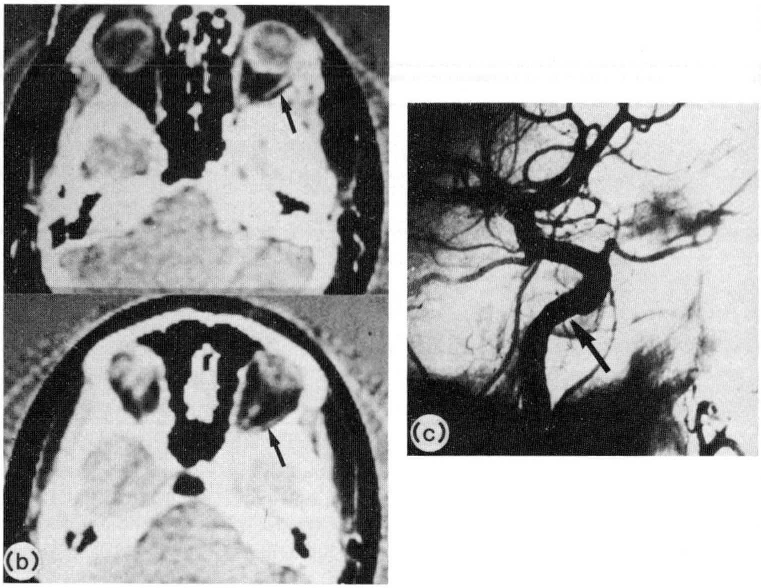

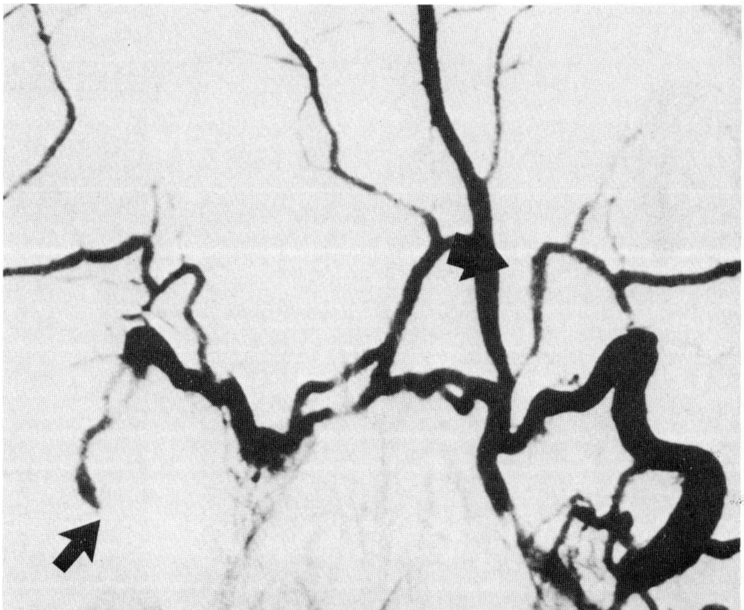

Fig. 4.25 Meningioma causing optic nerve compression. Numerous investigations had failed to show the cause of progressive right-sided visual loss in this 56-year old woman. She showed mild proptosis (a), slight limitation of abduction and right optic atrophy. CT (b) showed prominence of the right lateral rectus muscle (arrows); in all cuts, it was the most clearly seen of the external ocular muscles, as here. Minor constriction of the carotid siphon (c – arrow) was attributed (probably wrongly) to atheroma, but venography (d) clearly showed obstruction of the right superior ophthalmic vein (arrow) and possibly impaired filling of the ipsilateral cavernous sinus (open arrow). Surgical exploration revealed thickening of the right anterior clinoid process and adjacent sphenoid wing; there was meningioma in the cavernous sinus. The lateral rectus muscle was not involved by the tumour. (Courtesy of Williams and Wilkins, Baltimore. Previously published in *Topics in Neuro-Ophthalmology* (ed. H.S. Thompson), 1979).

sellae region. Axial CT sections may fail to show a flat tumour extending less than 1 cm above the planum, because it cannot be separated from the adjacent bone. Coronal sections may be useful in this respect, but are not infrequently degraded by artefact at the sphenoid sinus/bone interface. In such tumours examination of the skull radiographs is often valuable.

Cavernous sinus meningiomas are often of infiltrative type. CT may show unilateral erosion of the basisphenoid and adjacent enhancement after intravenous contrast medium, but while the former may be simulated or concealed by slight obliquity of the head, the latter is difficult to distinguish from the normal enhancement of the walls of the sinus and its contained blood.

Parasellar aneurysms

Parasellar aneurysms present few characteristic features to enable clinical diagnosis, but should always be considered as a cause of optic nerve or chiasm compression. The diagnosis is usually, but not invariably, resolved by angiography. Visual loss occurs particularly with aneurysms which arise from the terminal internal carotid artery, at the origin of the ophthalmic artery or more distally, although massive aneurysms at the anterior communicating artery may also be responsible.

Plain radiographs may show calcification, usually curvilinear, and erosion of the medial portion of the sphenoid bone, particularly the region of the anterior clinoid process and the lateral portion of the basisphenoid, including the pituitary fossa; it is essential to obtain frontal and/or basal projections, since these may show complete absence of the bone around the sella turcica on one side in cases in which the lateral film is apparently normal. Occasionally, the sella is enlarged in a manner strongly suggesting a pituitary adenoma. In many cases, none of these changes is present.

The CT findings are variable, depending on the exact site and size of the aneurysm and the degree of mural thrombosis and calcification. The attenuation coefficients of circulating, unclotted blood are slightly higher than those of cerebral grey matter, while thrombus is generally of higher attenuation. Thus, aneurysms large enough to be visible at CT tend to be of higher attenuation than the adjacent brain, although the difference may be minor. Large aneurysms frequently show calcification in the wall. The mass is usually well defined and rounded or lobular, but may be more elongated (Fig. 4.26).

The effects of contrast medium administration also depend on the degree of thrombosis. In smaller aneurysms, where mural clot is less developed, intense increase in attenuation of the entire lesion is seen; it may be evident that the lesion is in relation to a major vessel. In larger aneurysms the appearances may be similar, but intense partial enhancement of a high attenuation, possibly calcified lesion is the most characteristic picture. When

Fig. 4.26 Terminal carotid aneurysm. This 47-year old woman complained of visual disturbances and was found to have a bitemporal hemianopia (a). There was no endocrine abnormality and plain skull films were normal. A pneumoencephalogram performed at another hospital, however, showed a suprasellar lesion. CT confirmed the presence of a small rounded mass of increased attenuation showing marked contrast enhancement (b, axial, c, coronal sections); note unenhancing portion (arrow) in (b). Angiography (d,e) demonstrated this to be an aneurysm arising from the terminal carotid artery, which was successfully dealt with at surgery. Note the accurate portrayal of the form of the aneurysm (cf c and e).

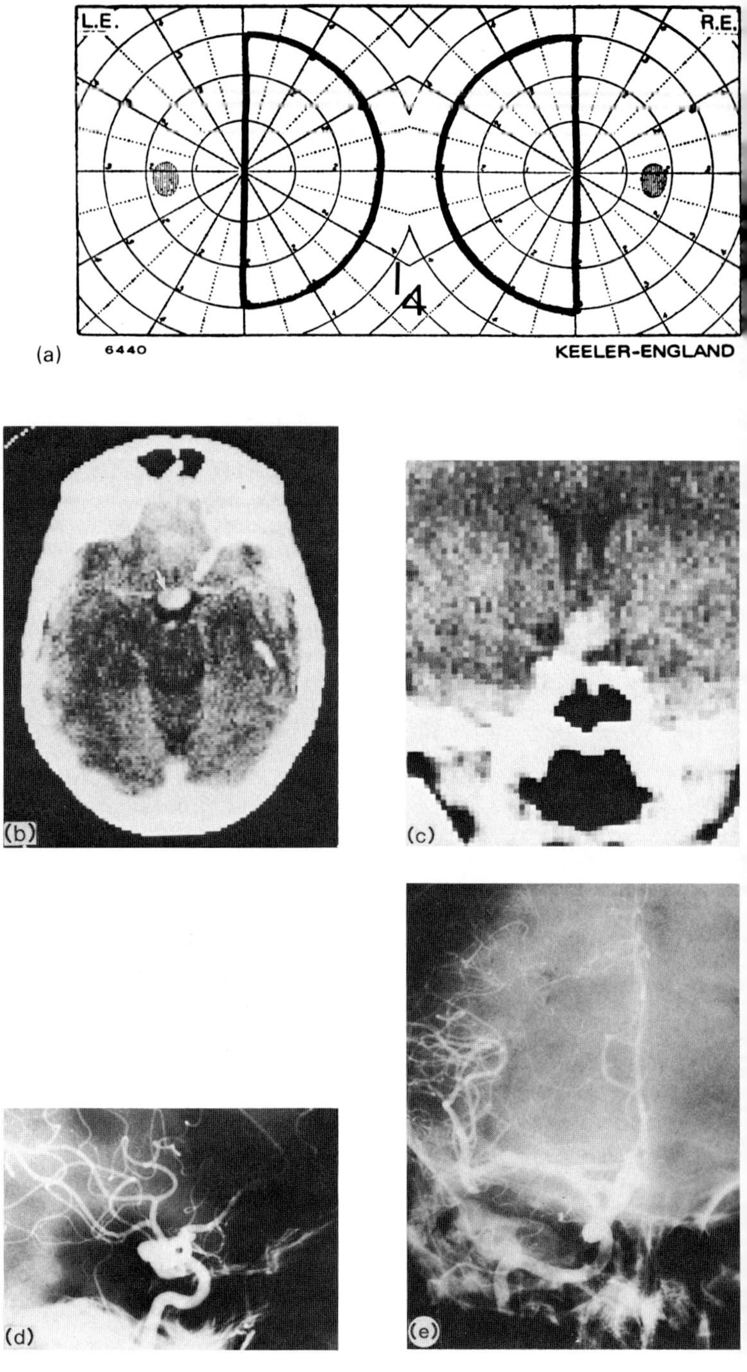

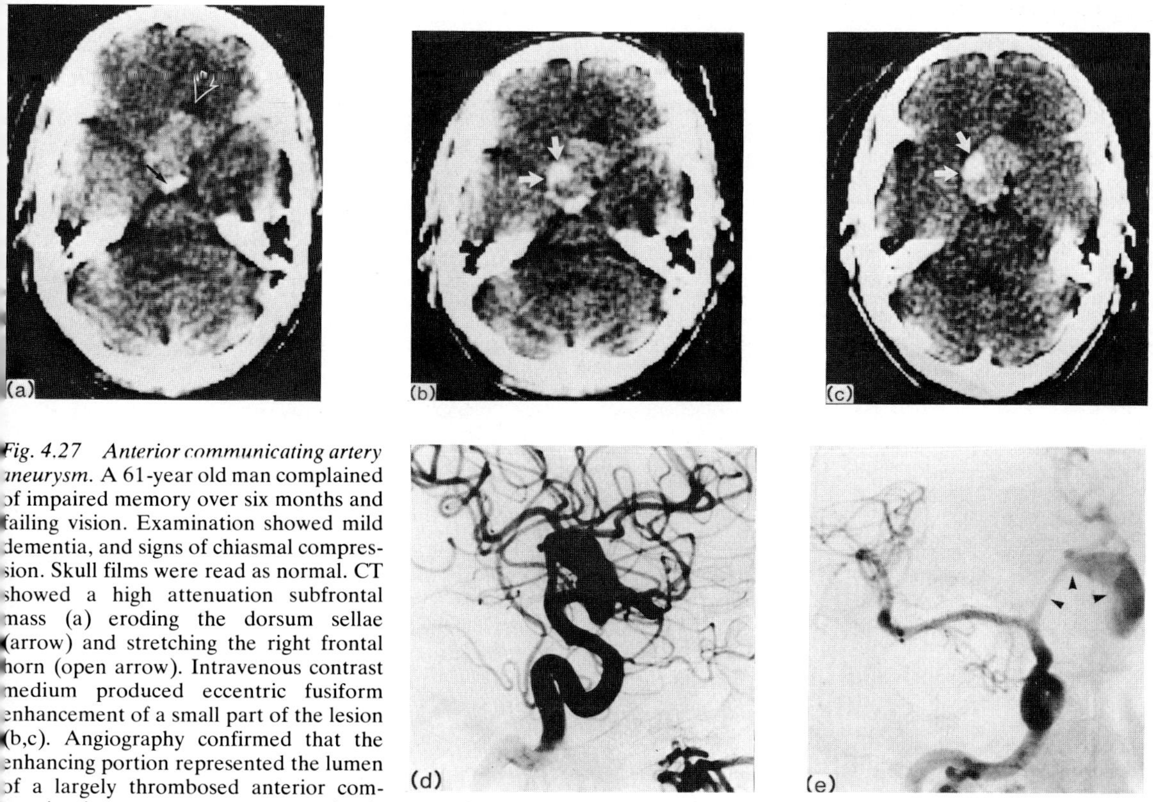

Fig. 4.27 Anterior communicating artery aneurysm. A 61-year old man complained of impaired memory over six months and failing vision. Examination showed mild dementia, and signs of chiasmal compression. Skull films were read as normal. CT showed a high attenuation subfrontal mass (a) eroding the dorsum sellae (arrow) and stretching the right frontal horn (open arrow). Intravenous contrast medium produced eccentric fusiform enhancement of a small part of the lesion (b,c). Angiography confirmed that the enhancing portion represented the lumen of a largely thrombosed anterior communicating artery aneurysm (d,e). Arrowheads show the elevation of the anterior cerebral artery, indicating the true size of the aneurysm.

the enhancing portion is seen on serial sections to be more or less tubular, there should be little doubt as to the diagnosis (Fig. 4.27).

Oedema is not typically seen around these large aneurysms, but bone erosion is occasionally visible. Hydrocephalus may be present; it usually involves the lateral ventricles only.

Chiasmal compression by ectatic internal carotid arteries is well recognized. The CT appearances are similar to those described above, with irregular, tubular, partially calcified masses on one or both sides of the sellar region, which show obvious increase in attenuation after intravenous contrast medium. Symmetrical lesions of both internal carotid arteries may be mistaken for prominent anterior clinoid processes. We have seen an apparently unique case in which chiasmal compression was due to a grossly ectatic basilar artery (Fig. 4.28).

Although they commonly present as mass lesions, these large aneurysms can, of course, give rise to subarachnoid haemorrhage. This is manifest at CT as conversion of the normally low-attenuation coefficients of the cerebrospinal fluid into those of blood, with streaky high attenuation more or less extensively distributed through the basal cisterns, and fissures. If the patient

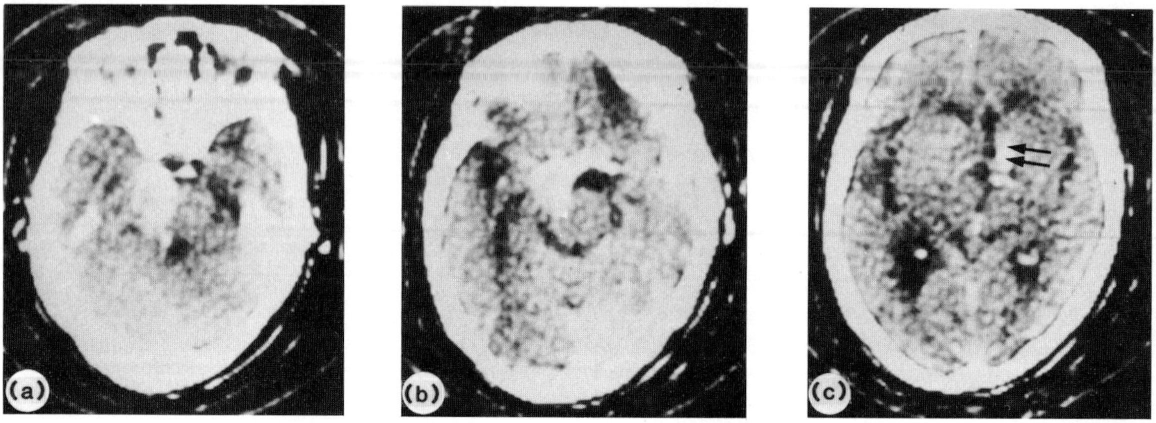

Fig. 4.28 Basilar artery ectasia. This 73-year old hypertensive woman presented with headache, dementia and visual loss. Examination showed anosmia, visual acuity was 6/24 in the right eye and 6/18 in the left eye with a bitemporal pattern of field defect (a). In addition there were bulbar and long tract signs. CT (a–c after intravenous contrast medium) showed a densely enhancing elongated mass extending from the left cerebellopontine angle (arrow) to the suprasellar region (b), where it can be seen to branch, to lie to the right of the third ventricle (two arrows). The diagnosis was confirmed by angiography.

is examined by CT within one week of the haemorrhage, such blood may be shown in about 90% of cases, but the detection rate falls markedly thereafter. Very occasionally, a large aneurysm may be seen as a filling defect in the coagulated blood.

It is self-evident that angiography is the definitive procedure for demonstration of the lesion, its relationship to the major vessels, etc. The only exception to this rule is for very debilitated patients in whom no active treatment would be planned regardless of the angiographic data. Rarely, however, aneurysms do not fill at angiography, and in these cases CT is particularly valuable in indicating the correct diagnosis. It is also useful for showing the full size of the lesion, i.e. not merely the lumen, and the presence of complications such as haemorrhage, hydrocephalus, etc.

Other rare primary tumours

Other *rare primary tumours* which may give rise to chiasmal compression include chordoma, chondroma/chondrosarcoma, certain hamartomas, and neuromas of the Vth nerve.

'Ectopic pinealoma' is a term frequently misapplied to primary suprasellar germinoma although spread of pineal region tumours to the anterior end of the third ventricle can occur. Primary suprasellar germinomas are equally common in boys and girls (unlike pineal lesions, which show a 6:1 male preponderance). Endocrine disturbance is the commonest presentation, but 80% of patients show reduced visual acuity or field loss, usually bitemporal, at some stage in the course of the disease. Takeuchi *et al.* (1978) described the CT findings in three cases: a suprasel-

Fig. 4.29 Metastasis involving chiasm. A 33-year old woman complained of polyuria and polydypsia prior to presenting with visual impairment, which rapidly progressed from an incomplete (a) to a complete bitemporal hemianopia. Plain radiographs were normal. At CT (b: before; c: after intravenous contrast medium) a small enhancing mass, isodense with brain, was seen in the chiasmatic cistern. This was confirmed by pneumoencephalography. Operation showed a solid mass intimately connected with the optic chiasm. It was thought to be a craniopharyngioma, but histologically was a metastatic papillary carcinoma, probably of pulmonary origin. The patient's vision improved only temporarily, and she died soon afterwards.

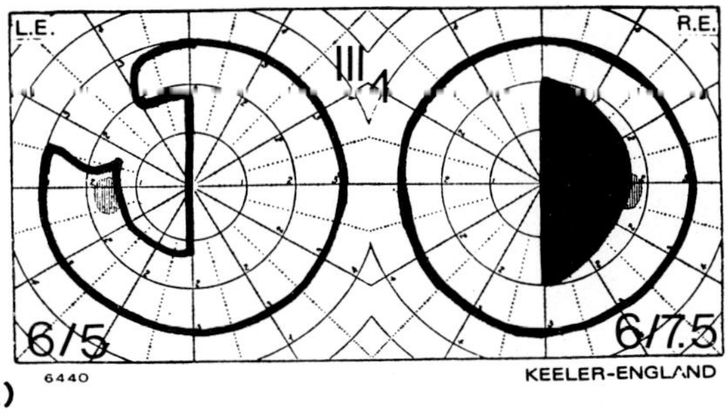

(a)

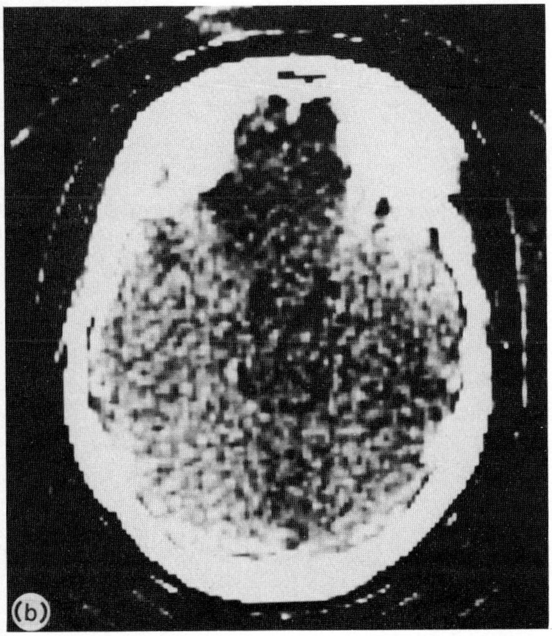
(b)

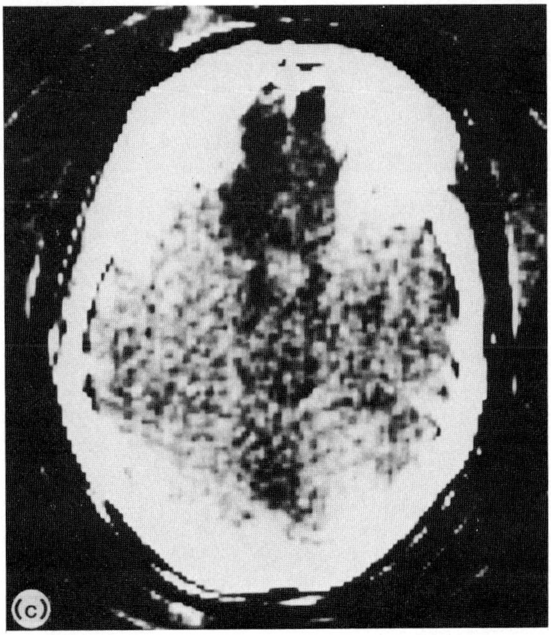
(c)

lar mass isodense with brain or of slightly increased attenuation, showing marked homogeneous contrast enhancement. They suggested that the diagnosis should be considered when any such mass with 'no clearly defined margins' is seen, but the example in their paper, and those published by other workers, show a well-defined rounded mass. The Japanese authors also noted complete disappearance of the tumour after a relatively small dose of radiation (1000–2000 R) and suggested that CT may be valuable in enabling the use of smaller doses than would previously have been applied.

Very extensive *carcinomas* arising in the sphenoid sinus/nasopharyngeal region may simulate pituitary adenomas, but usually show more marked bone destruction.

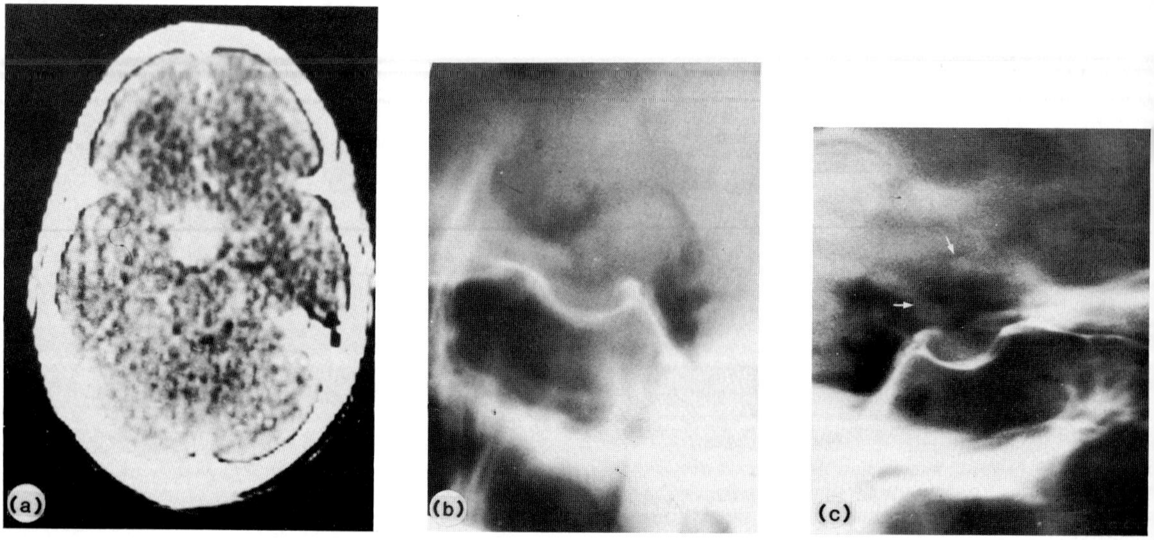

Fig. 4.30 Pitfalls in Diagnosis: meningioma of diaphragma sellae. A young woman who presented with a bitemporal hemianopia was shown by CT (a) to have an enhancing suprasellar tumour, which was thought to be a pituitary adenoma despite the fact that prolactin levels were normal and that the sellar changes were not typical of this type of tumour (b – pneumoencephalogram; arrows indicate tumour). A trans-sphenoidal hypophysectomy was carried out, showing what was thought to be 'chromophobe adenoma'. Further studies (c) revealed however, that the tumour was still present; a meningioma was subsequently resected at craniotomy.

Table 4.3 A Comparison of the original CT and pathological diagnoses (91 cases).

CT Diagnosis	*Pathological diagnosis*					
	Pituitary adenoma	Cranio-pharyngioma	Meningioma	Optic chiasm glioma	Other tumour granuloma	Aneur
Pituitary adenoma	33	2	1	–	1	1
Craniopharyngioma	1	15	–	–	2	–
Meningioma	–	–	8	–	1	–
Optic chiasm glioma	–	1	–	3	–	–
'Tumour'	6	2	3	1	3	–
Aneurysm	–	–	–	–	1	3
Normal	1	–	–	–	–	1

Secondary tumours

These tumours, from any source, may develop in the suprasellar or parasellar regions (Fig. 4.29). Metastases to the pituitary show a predilection for the more vascular neurophypophysis, and clinical suspicion should be aroused by signs suggestive of a chromophobe adenoma associated with marked polydipsia and polyuria.

Non-neoplastic disease of the basisphenoid is an important, though uncommon, cause of chiasmal syndromes. Most of the

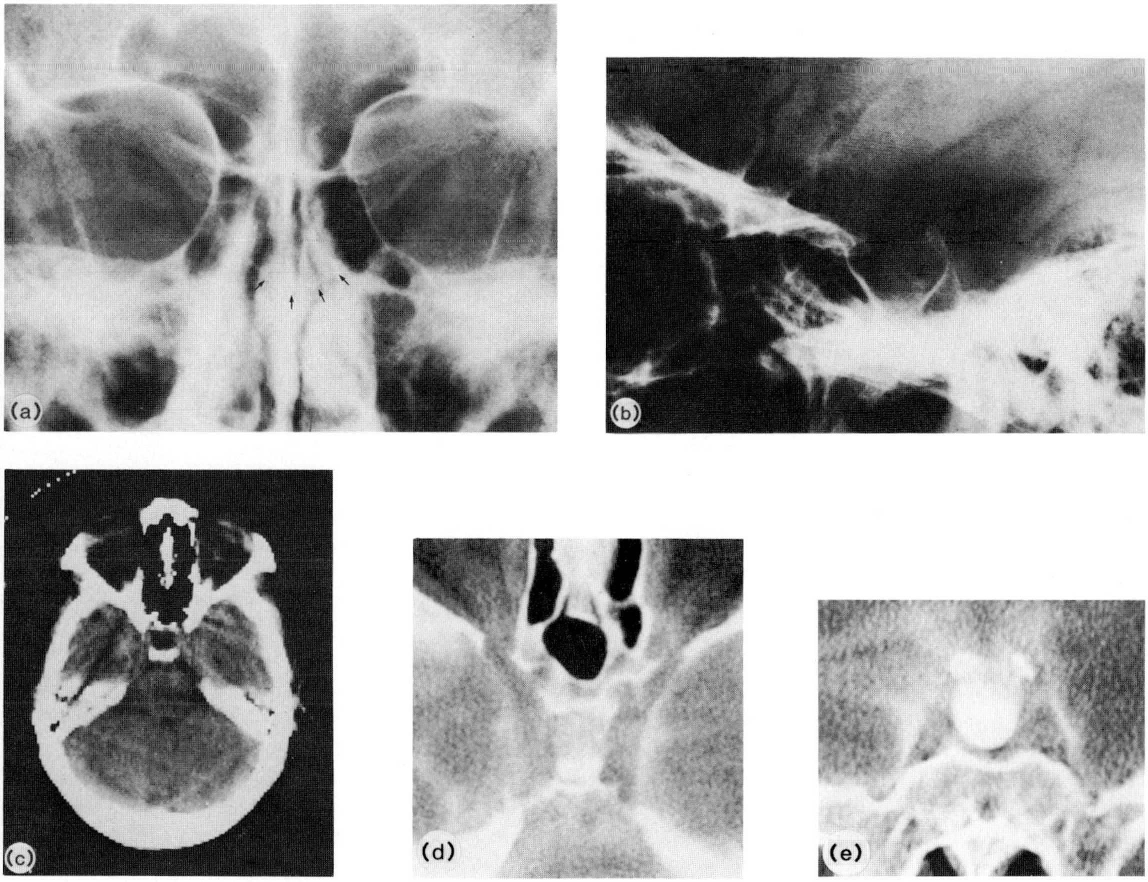

Fig. 4.31 Empty sella. This 51-year old woman had lost vision in both eyes for about two weeks following the birth of her fifth child 27 years previously. She recovered completely and had further uneventful pregnancies. Visual acuity and fields were normal on admission, and though there was mild disc pallor the VERs were normal. Plain radiographs (a,b) showed enlargement of the sella (arrows indicate the floor in the frontal projection). CT confirms this, and shows its contents to be of CSF attenuation (c). Involution of a pituitary adenoma would seem to be a plausible explanation of the 'empty' sella in this case. (d,e) Axial and coronal CT sections after intrathecal metrizamide in a case of Nelson's syndrome. The contrast medium tends to layer in the dependent portion of an empty sella; this is more marked in the axial section (with the patient supine).

primary bone diseases, e.g. osteopetrosis, fibrous dysplasia etc., cause expansion of bone and compression of the optic nerve rather than the chiasm, as does expansion of the sphenoid sinus by a mucocoele (Fig. 4.2).

The accuracy of CT in the diagnosis of the nature of parasellar lesions

Table 4.3 shows the CT and pathological (or in the case of aneurysms, radiological) definitive diagnosis in a group of 91 patients with lesions in the sellar region. If the groups in which the radiologist did not specify the nature of a tumour are included with those in which the CT diagnosis was correct, it will be seen that CT can offer a high level of diagnostic accuracy. This is increased still further when the findings at plain skull radiography are taken into account since the large majority of pituitary tumours and many other parasellar lesions will show characteristic features (Moseley *et al*., 1979). The combination of plain film,

CT and, where necessary, angiographic data should enable accurate diagnosis in most cases, and avoid errors such as that illustrated by Fig. 4.30. The CT characteristics of the principal lesions in this region are summarized in Table 4.4.

The 'empty sella syndrome'

Positive clinical features for diagnosis of this entity are lacking, and visual symptoms are uncommon; in the vast majority of cases the 'empty sella' is not associated with chiasmal compression. There is, however, considerable overlap in the clinicoradiological approach to patients with this condition and those with pituitary tumours. Discussion is therefore appropriate at this point.

The 'empty sella' is not a single entity, and may result from pituitary disease, from intracranial disease, or as a primary phenomenon, possibly related to a deficient diaphragma sellae. Pituitary tumours may undergo spontaneous involution, with necrosis, the superior part of the tumour then being replaced by an extension of the subarachnoid space. Similar changes may occur in patients who have had surgery or radiation treatment to the pituitary. This group of patients would seem to be the principal one in which downward herniation of the chiasm into the sella

Table 4.4 CT appearences of parasellar lesions.

Type	*Position*	*Shape*	*Attenuation*	*Calcification*	*'Cyst'*	*Enhancement with I.V. contrast*	*Changes in bone*	*Hyc cep*
Pituitary adenoma	Intra- and suprasellar may be parasellar	Rounded or nodular	Raised isodense	Rare	Uncommon	Uniform centred on sella	Erosion	Unc
Craniopharyngioma	Supra- and retrosellar may appear intrasellar	Rounded	Extremely variable	Common	Common	Marginal or uniform Many show no change	May erode sella	Cor
Meningioma	Variable	Rounded, nodular or plaque	Slightly raised	Not uncommon	Rare	Uniform	Erosion and/or hyperostosis	Rar
Aneurysm	Suprasellar or superolateral	Rounded or nodular	Raised	Not uncommon	No	Uniform or eccentric, tubular	May erode bone	Not unc
Optic chiasm or hypothalamic glioma	Suprasellar	Rounded – may extend into nerves or tract	Slightly raised	Rare	Rare	Uniform, but often slight	Optic canals enlarged; planum eroded	Not unc
Arachnoid cyst	Suprasellar	Rounded	CSF	Rare in this site	Constant	None	May erode bone	Cor

turcica, possibly as the result of adhesions, is associated with visual loss.

In benign intracranial hypertension, and very rarely in other conditions typified by prolonged increase of intracranial pressure, the subarachnoid space may herniate into the sella turcica, compressing the pituitary gland (Foley and Posner, 1975). Patients in whom this occurs may present with cerebrospinal fluid rhinorrhoea if the subarachnoid space eventually comes into continuity with the sphenoid sinus.

Many patients with an 'empty sella' have no evident cause for the herniation of the subarachnoid space into the sella. It has been suggested that in these individuals the diaphragma sellae is defective; although this theory itself has defects, no satisfactory alternative has as yet been proposed.

The commonest mode of discovery of this latter group is as the result of skull radiographs obtained from some unrelated purpose, e.g. investigation of headache or skull trauma. In many cases the form of the sella turcica, which is symmetrically deepened in the vertical plane without major increase in width or anteroposterior diameter, is sufficiently characteristic to indicate the correct diagnosis. In other patients it is more suggestive of ballooning, and would be compatible with a pituitary tumour, but again is typically symmetrical.

CT examination of the idiopathic group shows essentially normal intracranial structures. The sella turcica may appear slightly enlarged, and is occupied by material with attenuation coefficients of cerebrospinal fluid; this may be confirmed by coronal and sagittal sections or reconstructions (Fig. 4.31). However, with thick CT sections, e.g. the standard 13 mm slice, it is frequently impossible to be sure that only the sellar contents are being displayed, and that the attenuation coefficients are not being determined largely by suprasellar cerebrospinal fluid or by air in the sphenoid sinus. Thin (e.g. 5 mm) axial and coronal sections are required to make the diagnosis certain. It is almost impossible to demonstrate unequivocally that the sella is empty in patients in whom it is not enlarged. Parera (1978, personal communication) has suggested that if a series of adjacent sections through the sella is obtained, the image of the floor – 'the sellar ghost' – can be seen as a fine line on one section, and that the sellar contents are posterosuperior to this line. Newton (1977, personal communication) has observed cystic intrasellar pituitary adenomas simulating an empty sella. A firm diagnosis of empty sella can be made when the infundibulum is visible passing down into the fluid-filled pituitary fossa.

We believe that in patients without endocrine or visual disturbance in whom a typical 'empty sella' is discovered by chance, no further radiological investigation other than a CT study demonstrating the changes described here is required, and that it is important to reassure such patients of their normality. We have seen a professional soldier, aged 40, in whom a classical empty sella was shown on skull radiographs obtained during investigation of episodic hypertension. He was told that he had a silent pituitary adenoma, and it was only after this he became impotent and developed bizarre constriction of the visual fields. CT confirmed an empty sella.

These principles do not apply to patients having endocrine disturbances, since it is well recognized that a pituitary 'microadenoma' may occur in conjunction with an empty sella.

The CT demonstration of an apparently empty sella in patients being followed after pituitary surgery or radiotherapy may, also, not be adequate, since small tumour recurrences, or the development of adhesions (or internal carotid artery aneurysms following radiotherapy) may necessitate other modes of investigation. This is particularly likely, since the presence of postsurgical artefacts not infrequently renders the CT images difficult to interpret.

The CT findings in benign intracranial hypertension are discussed in Chapter 5.

4.9 TRACTS – RADIATIONS

Clinically, there may be few features which enable precise anatomical localization of lesions affecting the retrochiasmal optic pathways. However, if the field defect is grossly incongruous, showing homonymous, hemi- or quadrantanopic features, the tract should be suspected. Incongruous, wedge-shaped defects may suggest vascular lesions in the region of the lateral geniculate body. Sector atrophy of the optic disc provides further evidence of tract involvement, as do pupillary signs; Wernicke's and Behr's pupillary signs are clinically impractical though an afferent defect may be present in the eye with the temporal field defect (Bell and Thompson, 1979). Relative sparing of perception for moving targets (Riddoch's phenomenon) was originally described with occipital lobe lesions, but may also be demonstrated in chiasmal or tract lesions.

Pathological processes involving the tract, lateral geniculate body or the posterior limb of the internal capsule rarely affect the optic pathways in isolation. Similarly, the lesions which affect the pathways in their various sections are not usually specific: malformations, vascular accidents, trauma, infections and primary or secondary neoplasms can all exert their effects on one or more portions of the optic pathways. The following discussion will therefore deal briefly with each section, from optic tract to visual cortex, indicating where specific lesions may occur.

A Japanese study of the CT findings in 53 patients with homonymous hemianopia or cortical blindness revealed positive findings in 44 (85%) (Kan and Matsubayashi, 1978). The optic tract was the site of the lesion in one case of craniopharyngioma;

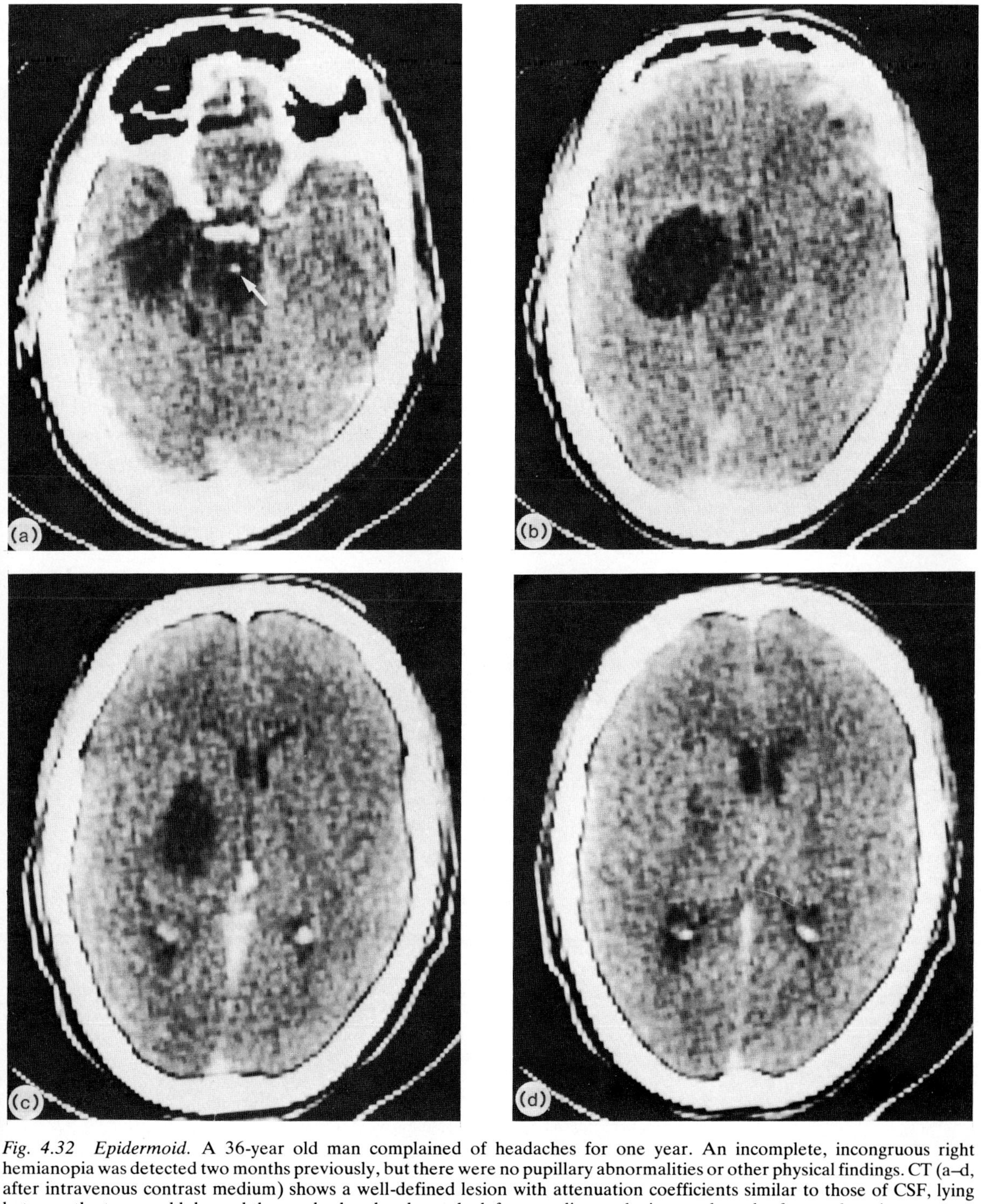

Fig. 4.32 Epidermoid. A 36-year old man complained of headaches for one year. An incomplete, incongruous right hemianopia was detected two months previously, but there were no pupillary abnormalities or other physical findings. CT (a–d, after intravenous contrast medium) shows a well-defined lesion with attenuation coefficients similar to those of CSF, lying between the temporal lobe and the cerebral peduncle on the left, extending to the interpeduncular fossa, where it appears to surround the basilar artery (arrow). There was no pathological contrast enhancement. At operation an epidermoid was found, compressing the left optic tract.

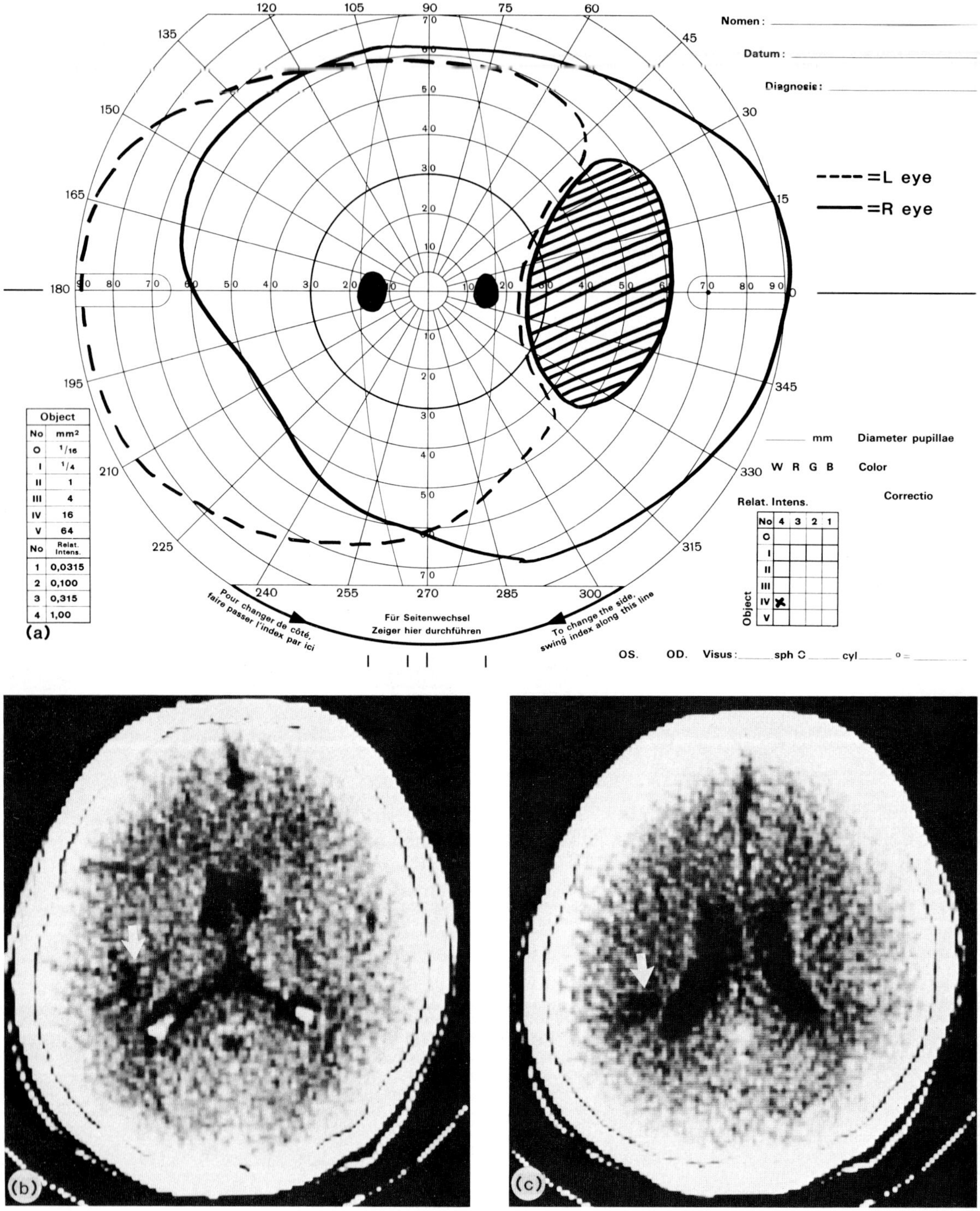
Nomen:
Datum:
Diagnosis:
----=L eye
——=R eye
Object
No mm²
O 1/16
I 1/4
II 1
III 4
IV 16
V 64
No Relat. Intens.
1 0,0315
2 0,100
3 0,315
4 1,00
mm Diameter pupillae
W R G B Color
Correctio
Relat. Intens.
No 4 3 2 1
O I II III IV V
Object
Pour changer de côté, faire passer l'index par ici
Für Seitenwechsel Zeiger hier durchführen
To change the side, swing index along this line
OS. OD. Visus: sph cyl
(a)
(b)
(c)

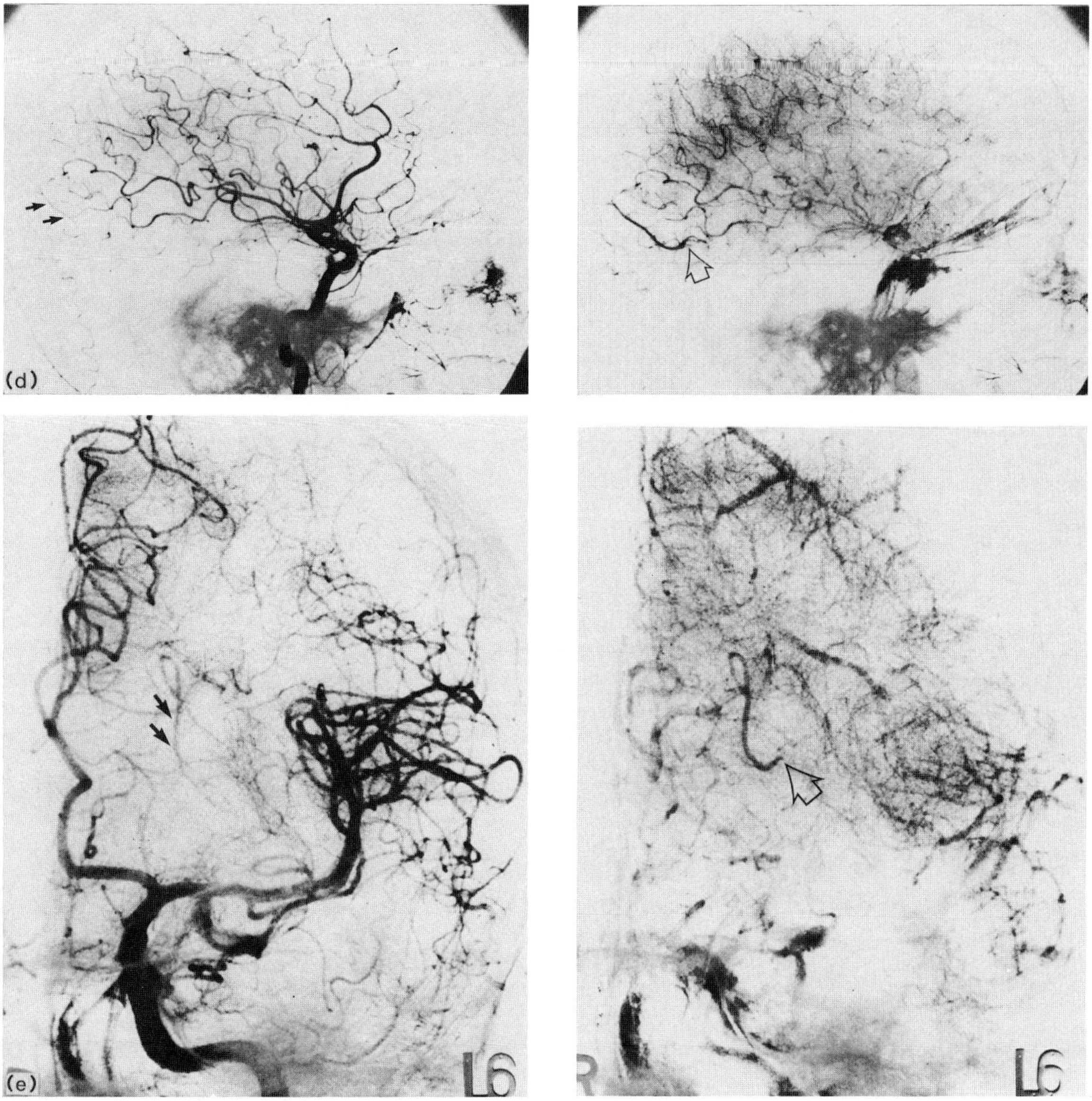

Fig. 4.33 Cerebral infarct. Seven years before the CT study, at age 25, this man had had an attack of diplopia, which lasted for two weeks. Six years later, he hit the right-hand curb while driving and was found to be dysphasic and to have difficulty using the right hand. CT at that time was normal. Three days before the present CT, he had a sudden 'sensation' in the head and found that he could not see on the right side; next day objects on the right were distorted. He showed an incongruous field defect (a), with a nasal defect extending to the periphery on the left and a large scotoma lateral to the blind spot but not reaching the periphery on the right. CT (b,c) revealed a low-attenuation lesion near the posterior limb of the left internal capsule suggesting proximal involvement of the optic radiations. Angiography (d–e) showed evidence of embolic disease: late filling of a posterior cerebral artery branch (arrows), which was blocked distally (open arrow). He was subsequently found to have raised blood triglycerides and lipoproteins.

there were no cases of lateral geniculate body lesions, but the optic radiations were affected in 22 cases, while the occipital lobes were involved (together with the posterior optic radiations) in 20. Perimetry in eight of the nine patients with normal CT scans showed homonymous hemianopias with and without macular sparing, and quadrantanopia; all patients with cortical blindness showed bilateral occipital lesions.

Optic tract lesions. The optic tracts may be compressed by aneurysms arising from the internal carotid or posterior communicating arteries; this is uncommon. The blood supply of the tract is derived from numerous adjacent vessels: the internal carotid, posterior communicating, middle cerebral and anterior choroidal arteries anteriorly and the posterior choroidal and thalamoperforating arteries posteriorly. Infarction of the tract is relatively uncommon, perhaps as a result of this multipedicular vascular supply, and usually occurs only with extensive interruption of the blood supply; this may be the mechanism in traumatic lesions.

Intrinsic tumours of the optic tracts are rare, but posterolateral extension of a chiasmal glioma may occur. Compression by extrinsic tumour is usually the result of pituitary adenoma or craniopharyngioma (Tables 4.1 and 4.2) which affect the anterior half of the tract (Figs. 4.30 and 4.32). The posterior half is much less commonly involved by thalamic, third ventricular or temporal lobe neoplasms, which are usually malignant gliomas or ependymomas.

Demyelination may affect the optic tract, but CT is not of diagnostic value at present.

Lateral geniculate bodies. Isolated lesions of the lateral geniculate body are rare. The blood supply of this region is from the choroidal and thalamogeniculate arteries, so that infarction usually involves the optic tract in addition. Thalamic, third ventricular and pineal region tumours occasionally involve the lateral geniculate body.

Optic radiations. Specific lesions of the optic radiations without other neurological deficit are uncommon. Their blood supply is from perforating branches of the anterior and posterior choroidal and lenticulostriate arteries anteriorly, while the periventricular portions are supplied by deep branches of the middle cerebral artery and, more medially and posteriorly, of the posterior cerebral artery. Infarction is therefore often associated with more widespread neurological deficit (Fig. 4.33).

Vascular disease. The Japanese workers referred to previously divided the optic radiations into three segments. The optic peduncle, running from the lateral geniculate body to the internal capsule, was affected in five of 32 cases, in one of which there

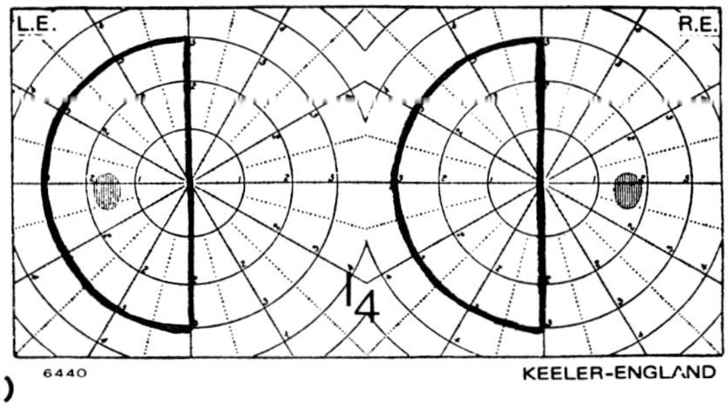

(a)

Fig. 4.34 Thalamic glioma. At the age of 21, this patient suddenly developed a right homonymous hemianopia (a) and a right facial weakness. CT (b,c) showed an enhancing lesion in the left medial temporal/thalamic region, which at angiography was markedly hypervascular, being interpreted as an inoperable arteriovenous malformation.

Some months later, with only slight clinical deterioration (right hemisensory disturbance), the nature of the tumour was evident (d, e): it was larger, partly as the result of cyst formation (arrow); there was contralateral hydrocephalus and presumed dilated draining veins were seen (small arrows).

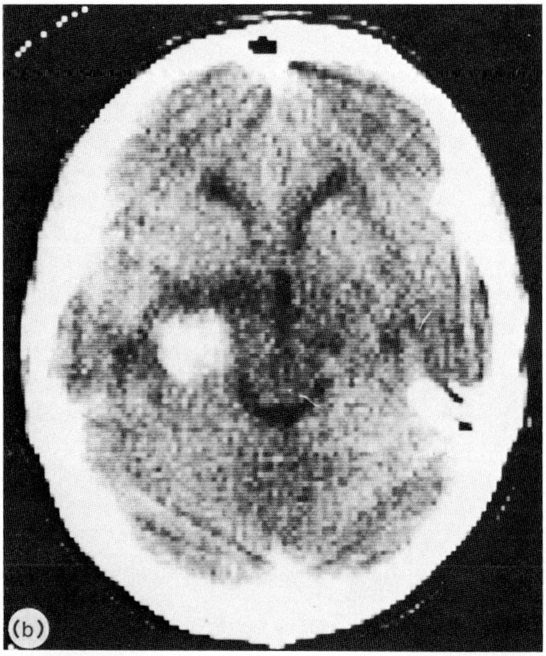

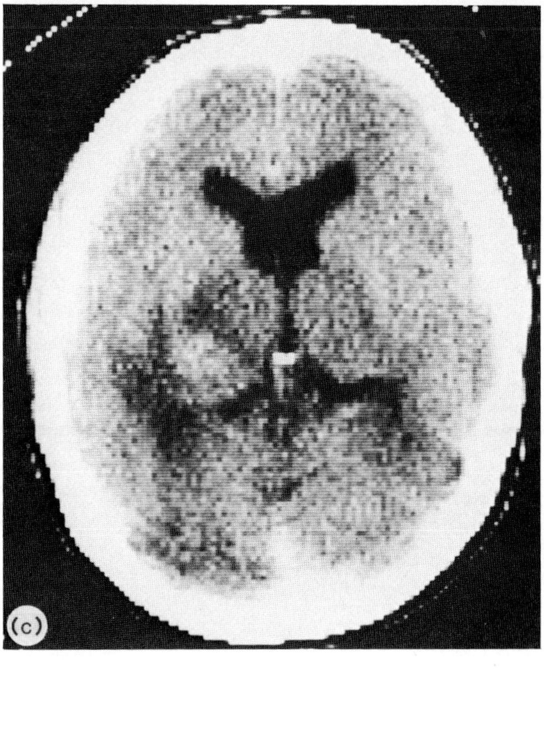

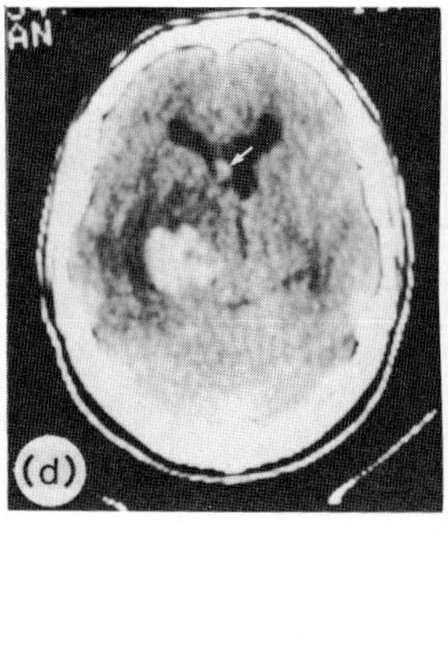

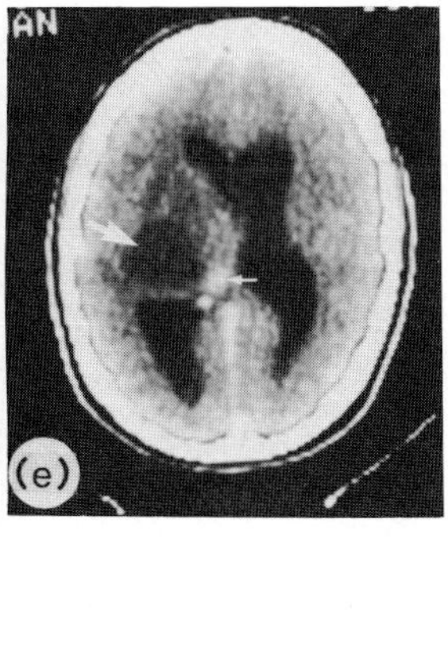

was a thalamic haemorrhage (Fig. 4.34). The middle section was further divided into Meyer's loop (passing around the temporal horn) and the more medial portion; the former was involved in two patients (one with a temporal tumour (Figs. 4.35, 4.36) and one who had had temporal lobe surgery), both of whom had upper quadrantic field defects, and the latter in 15 patients. In all remaining cases without a specified aetiology, cerebral infarction was the presumed cause. Radü and Moseley (1978) reviewed 35 patients with proven carotid artery occlusion. There was CT evidence of cerebral infarction in 27. Homonymous hemianopia was present in three of five patients with generalized ischaemic damage to the affected cerebral hemisphere (i.e. including the posterior cerebral artery territory), in two of three with cortical infarcts apparently confined to the middle cerebral artery distribution, and in one of four with capsular infarction. Homonymous hemianopia was invariably associated with a severe hemiparesis, although more than half the patients in this series had at most a mild paresis. Field defects were absent in the 16 patients with no CT evidence of infarction or with damage confined to the anterior cerebral artery territory. It seems likely that infarction in the middle cerebral territory produces hemianopic defects by involvement of the visual fibres either in the internal capsule, or in their periventricular segments (Fig. 4.37).

Tumours. The periventricular segments of the optic radiation may also be involved by tumours arising within the ventricles, particularly malignant ependymomas, which tend to infiltrate the subependymal tissues.

Demyelination. Schilder's disease (sudanophilic or diffuse cerebral sclerosis) is a form of demyelination (a disputed entity which some pathologists class with the leukodystrophies) in which the white matter of the occipital lobes, including the optic radiations, is particularly affected. Loss of neural tissue may lead to focal enlargement of the occipital horns of the lateral ventricles – a true hydrocephalus ex vacuo. An x-linked recessive form of sudanophilic leukodystrophy occurs in young boys; it is associated with adrenal cortical atrophy, and is therefore known as adrenoleukodystrophy (Fig. 4.38) (see also pp.278–9).

4.10 OCCIPITAL CORTEX

The cortex of the occipital lobe is particularly sensitive to ischaemic injury, a feature it shares with the frontal cortex and the hippocampus. It has been estimated that cerebrovascular disease and cerebral tumours are each responsible for about 40% of cases of homonymous hemianopia (Trobe *et al.*, 1973). However, in cases in which the field defect is an isolated clinical

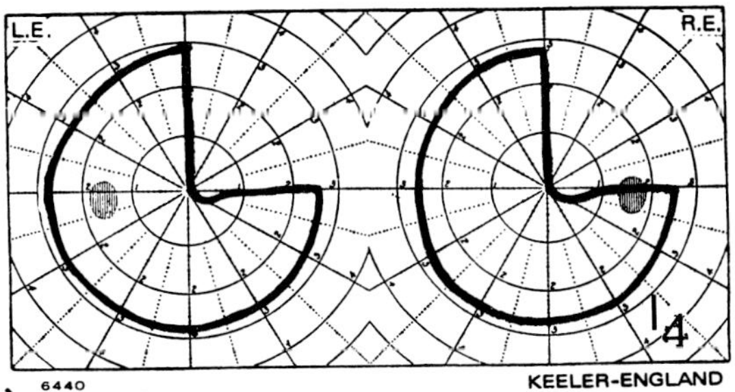

(a)

Fig. 4.35 Temporal glioma. This 65-year old man with a left parietotemporal syndrome had a provisional diagnosis of cerebrovascular disease. He was dysphasic and had a right superior quadrantanopia (a). However, CT (b-d, after intravenous contrast medium) showed a very large temporal tumour, extending up to the thalamus, and causing marked uncal herniation (small arrows). There was extensive central necrosis.

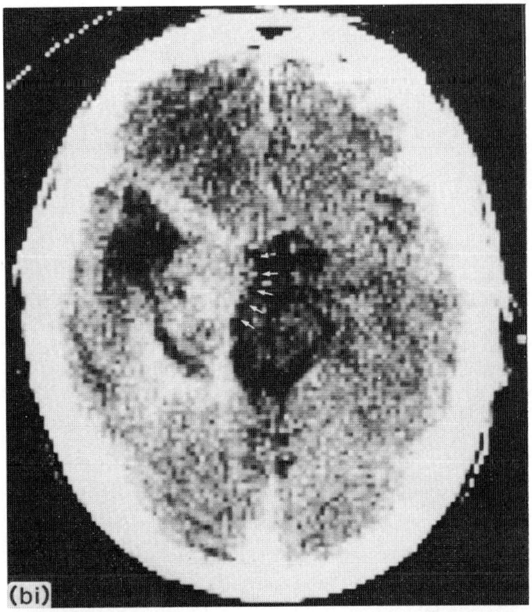

(bi)

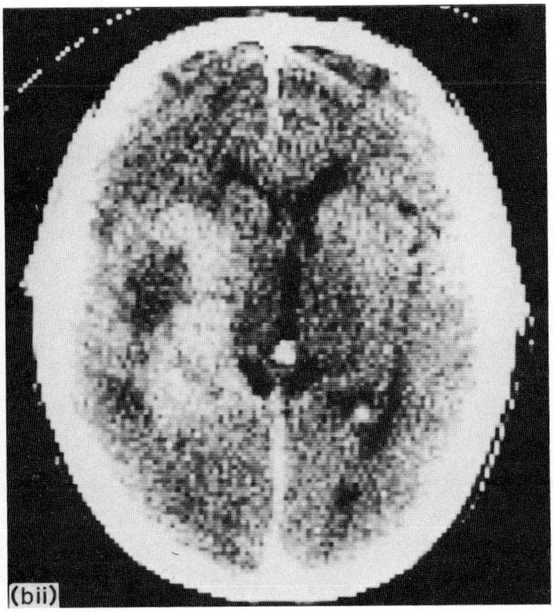

(bii)

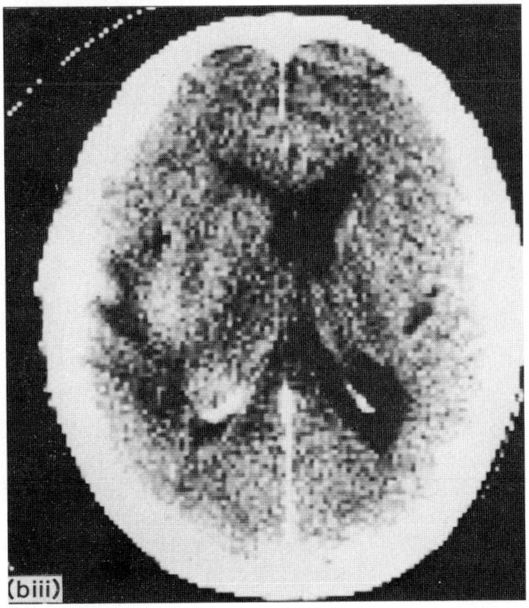

(biii)

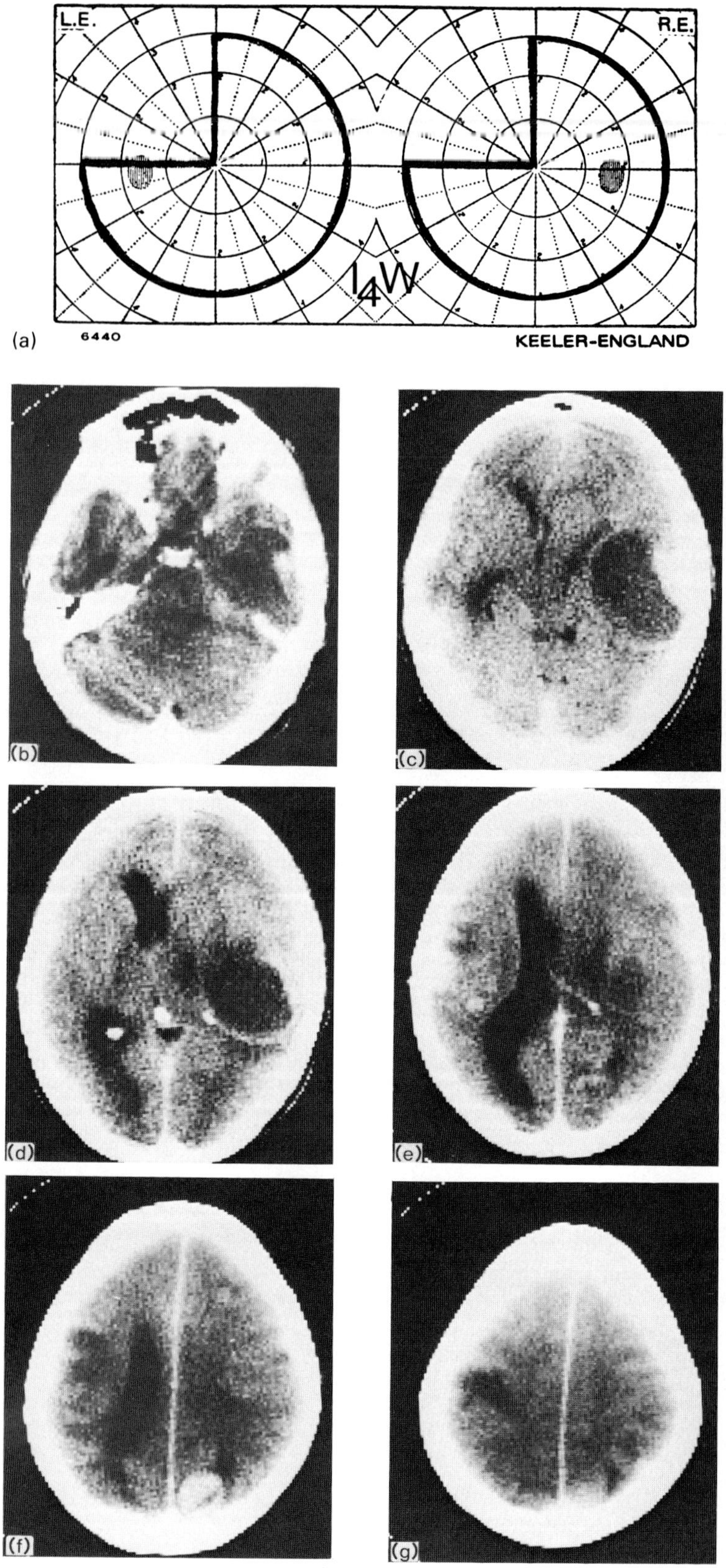

Fig. 4.36 Cerebral metastases. A melanoma had been removed from the back of this 48-year old man several years previously. When he presented with headaches, he was noted to have an odd affect and a left superior quadrantanopia (a). The chest radiograph showed four coin lesions. CT (b–g after intravenous contrast medium) demonstrated multiple metastases. The large, cystic, right temporal lesion is presumably responsible for the field defect, while the high right parieto-occipital nodule lies above the visual cortex (P+2).

Fig. 4.37 Middle cerebral artery territory infarct. A 58-year old man gave a history of right-sided weakness, progressing to hemiplegia, over nine months. He had had two epileptic seizures. Examination showed a complete right homonymous hemianopia (a) and dysphasia. Despite the progressive history, CT shows a very large region of low attenuation, affecting most of the middle cerebral artery territory (b,c); the left lateral ventricle is dilated. The coronal reconstruction (d) passes through the thalamus, of which a small portion (? supplied by the recurrent artery of Huebner) is preserved (small arrow), as is the parasagittal area supplied by the anterior cerebral artery (upper arrow).

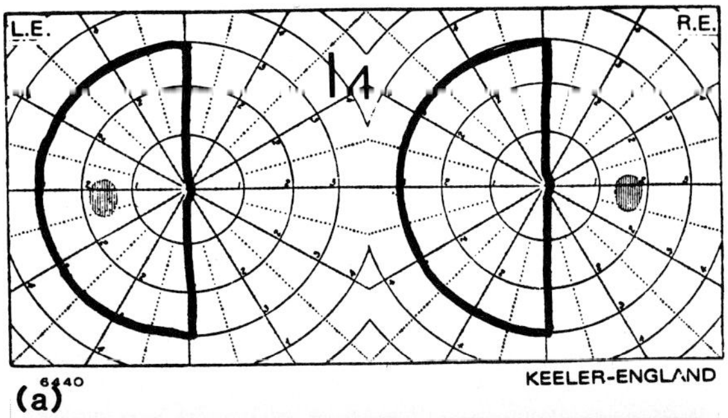

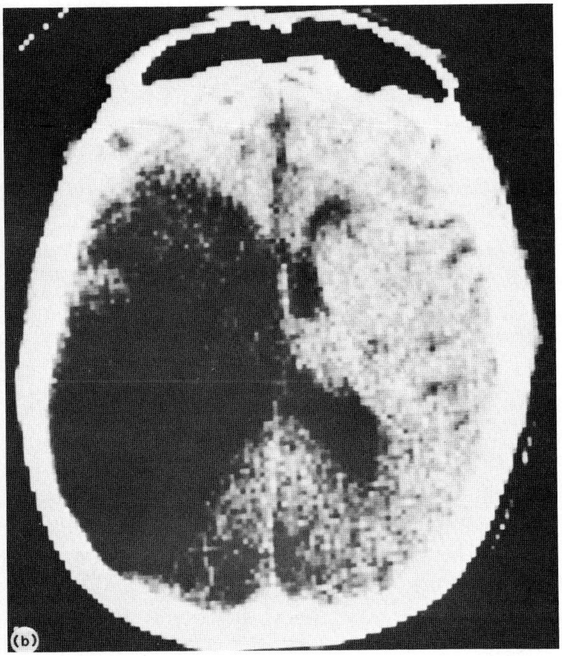

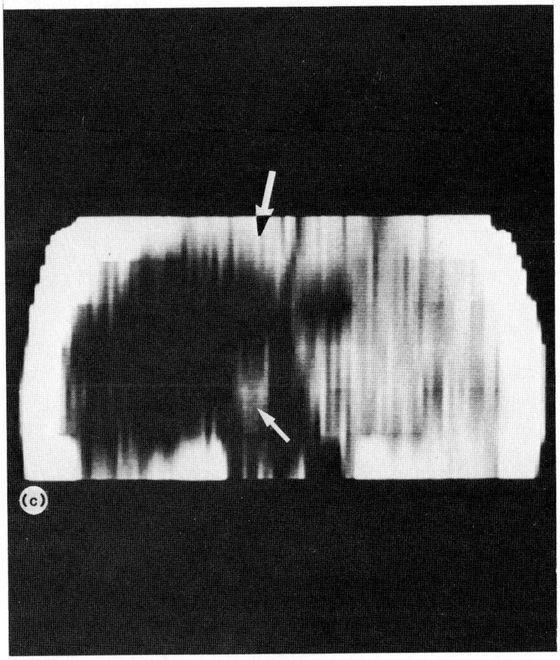

Fig. 4.38 Adrenoleukodystrophy. A boy aged 7 with a gradual deterioration of intellectual performance, found to have markedly reduced visual acuity in both eyes. (a) There is low attenuation in the white matter of both occipital lobes, extending into the posterior parietal regions. The cortex is involved to a lesser extent, and bilateral frontal lesions are also present. (b) After intravenous contrast medium, there is enhancement *adjacent* to the areas of low attenuation.

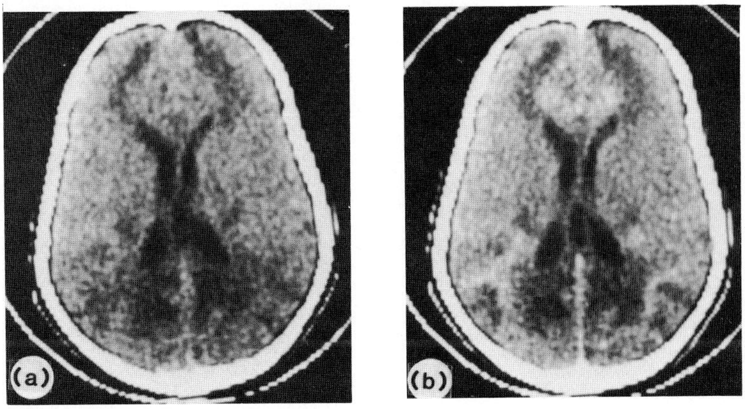

abnormality, the proportion due to vascular disease rises to about 90% (Smith, 1962). Infarction in the posterior cerebral artery territory or in the watershed region between the territories of the middle and posterior cerebral arteries is the commonest cause of cortical visual loss.

CT offers a unique opportunity to correlate clinical defects with cerebral damage *in vivo*. This was carried out in patients with visual loss by McCauley and Ross Russell (1977). Their studies concerned patients with cerebral infarction and closer clinico-anatomical correlation would be expected in this group than in those patients with cerebral tumours where tumour mass, cerebral oedema and vascular disturbances would be compounded. They found that variations in head position rendered it difficult to determine the location of the visual cortex, which is dependent on angulation of the head, the configuration of the tentorium, itself very variable, and other imponderables. Sectioning of cadaver brains in the plane used at CT showed that the calcarine fissure usually lay in the section which also passed through the pineal gland. Since the latter can usually be identified with ease at CT, they numbered the 13 mm sections relative to the pineal. P was the section in which the gland was clearly seen, P+1 and P−1 the adjacent higher and lower sections, etc. Identifying an area of infarction by abnormally low attenuation values and comparing the findings with the visual field defects, they obtained the results shown in Table 4.5.

There were also four patients with bilateral homonymous hemianopias, who all showed bilateral occipital infarcts. Two of this group of patients also had disorders of higher visual function such as prosopagnosia, dyslexia, dysgraphia and visual agnosia.

In four patients, including one with a complete hemianopia (but with macular sparing) there was no evidence of infarction. Two of these patients had small paracentral scotomas, and it was presumed that they had infarcts near the macular area, which were too small to be identified at CT. There were apparently silent contralateral occipital lesions in two patients, although in one of these the presumed infarct was in the P+3 section, and therefore probably in the parastriate area.

Table 4.5 CT findings in patients with field defects due to cerebral infarction (after McAuley and Ross Russell, 1977).

Field defect	*Section(s) showing low attenuation*					
	P−2	*P−1*	*P*	*P+1*	*P+2*	*None*
Upper quadrant (5)	1	4	4	1	0	0
Lower quadrant (6)	0	0	1	3	2	1
Hemianopia (5)	0	3	4	4	2	1
Homonymous scotoma (4)	0	1	1	1	0	2

Fig. 4.39 Occipital infarction (acute). A 69-year old man suffered repeated attacks of right cerebral ischaemia for more than two years, leaving him with a residual left hemiparesis and mild dementia. Ten days before this CT study he had another attack, after which he was found to have a complete left homonymous hemianopia (a). CT was carried out (b) before and (c) after intravenous contrast medium. The low attenuation, mature right frontal infarct (arrow) which had been present two years previously, showed no enhancement. However, an acute right occipital infarct, barely visible on the preinjection scans, showed marked enhancement, involving the whole occipital lobe, including the occipital pole (small arrows).

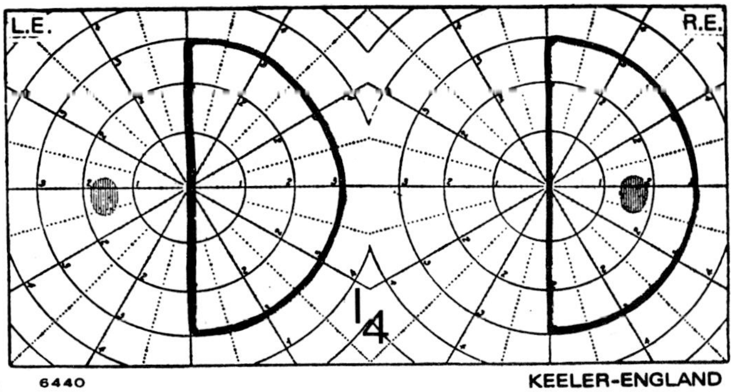

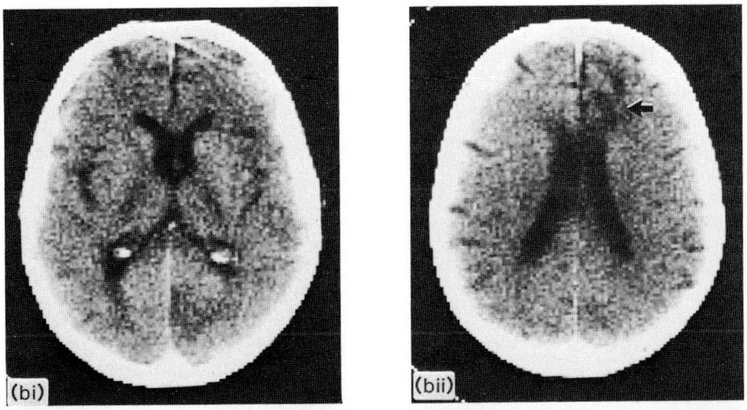

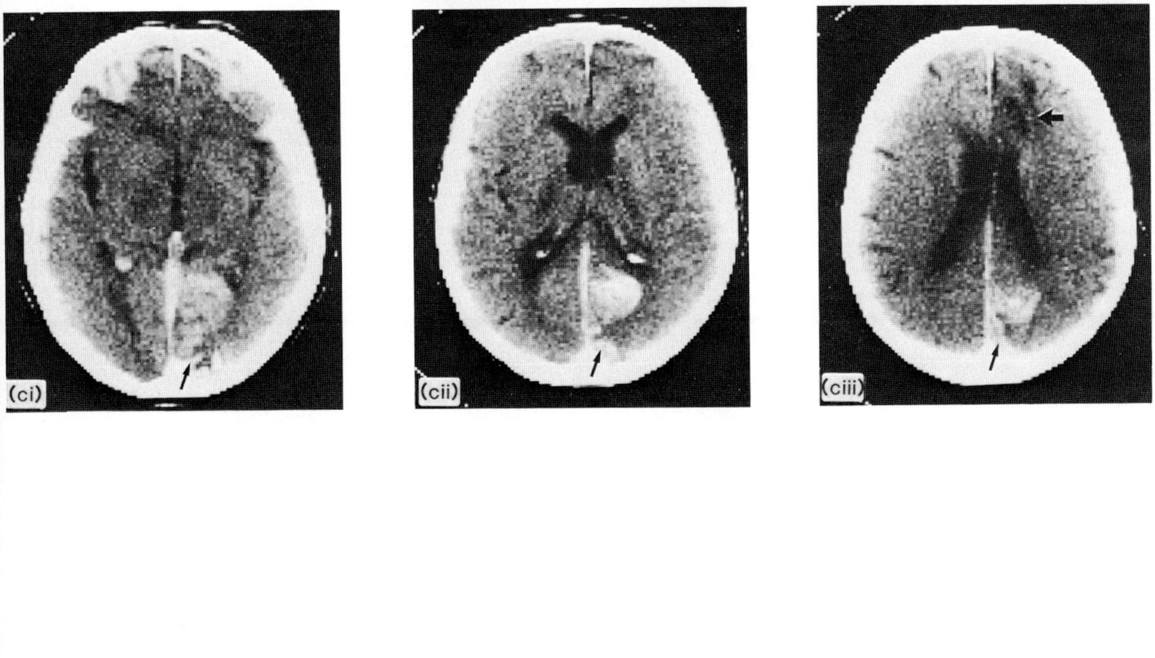

Five patients had lesions which appeared to involve the optic radiation. One patient with an upper quadrantic scotoma had a posterior temporal lesion and correlation with the classical anatomy of the visual pathways was impossible.

A marked difference between the patients with superior and inferior quadrantic defects was noted with regard to macular sparing. Of the five patients with upper field defects, only one showed macular sparing, while there was at least partial sparing in every one of seven patients with exclusively lower field defects. In three of the five patients with complete hemianopia the macula was spared; one of these had a normal CT scan.

Lastly, the mean number of sections on which an infarct could be identified was as follows: complete hemianopia 3.5; upper quadrantanopia 2.0; lower quadrantanopia 1.2.

This study has been discussed in some detail because it appears to be unique in its relationship of field defects to CT data; some of the results could be predicted, others are of considerable interest. It should be noted that the authors conclude that 'occipital infarcts causing isolated visual field defects involve more than just primary visual cortex as several cases clearly involved the para- and even peristriate areas, together with the posterior optic radiations. This is to be expected from the distribution of the posterior cerebral artery.'

Classical infarction of the posterior cerebral artery territory as a result of thromboembolism affects the medial surface of the occipital lobe, often sparing the occipital pole, supplied by branches of the middle cerebral artery (Figs. 4.39 and 4.40).

Ross Russell (1978) has also described the clinical and CT findings in a group of patients in which generalized cerebral ischaemia caused by hypotension or extensive extracranial disease gave rise to lesions affecting the border-zone or watershed areas of the anterior/middle and middle/posterior cerebral artery territories. These patients presented with visual or visuospatial symptoms (Fig. 4.41); they had normal central acuity but three out of five showed difficulty in initiating appropriate eye movements, although ocular movements were full. There was often considerable clinical recovery.

CT in these patients showed bilateral, symmetrical parieto-occipital lesions, i.e. affecting the zone lateral to the occipital cortex, and extending forwards in a paramedian position, corresponding to the anterior/middle cerebral artery watershed zone (Fig. 4.42).

Not dissimilar findings were described by Pearlman *et al.* (1979) in a case of 'central colour blindness' with a congruous superior altitudinal field defect and normal acuity. CT showed infarction of the lingual gyri, occipitotemporal gyri and adjacent areas on both sides.

Tumours, abscesses and other inflammatory conditions, can also affect the occipital lobes (Figs. 4.43, 4.44 and 4.45), but full

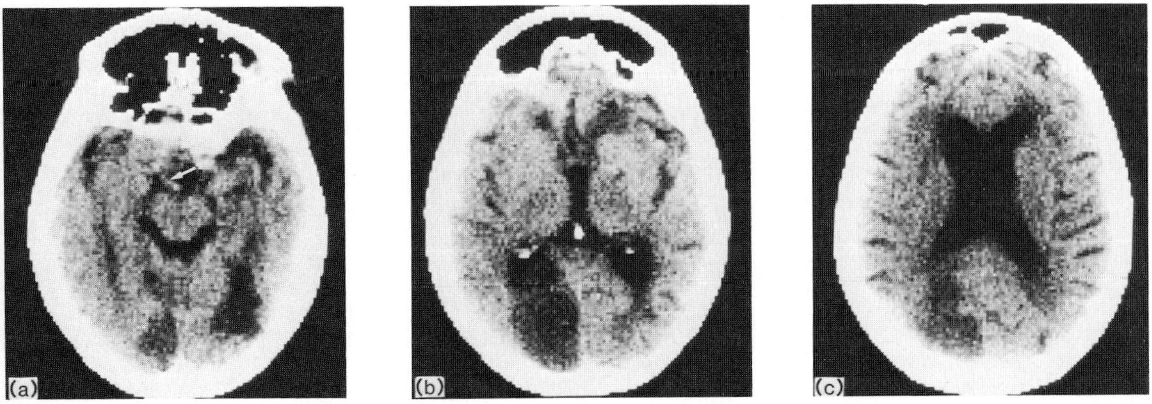

Fig. 4.40 Mature occipital infarct. This 83-year old woman presented with a history of 'blurred vision' for three weeks. An initial clinical diagnosis of temporal arteritis was not substantiated. She had a complete right homonymous hemianopia, and CT showed low attenuation, in the left occipital lobe, typical of an infarct in the posterior cerebral artery territory, extending above and below the pineal (a = P–2; b = P; c = P+2). There was also widespread cerebral and brainstem atrophy (note the wide basal cisterns) with focal ventricular dilatation in the right temporal region. The basilar artery (arrow) was prominent. Ill-defined areas of low attenuation around the lateral ventricles are of the type seen in hypertensives.

discussion of these cerebral disorders is beyond the scope of this book.

4.11 DISORDERS OF HIGHER CEREBRAL FUNCTION

Information from area 17 (striate cortex) projects to area 18, (parastriate area) and this projects in turn to area 19, and also via the splenium of the corpus callosum to corresponding points in the contralateral hemisphere. Information is processed towards more sophisticated perceptual interpretation in the parietal and temporal lobes. The dominant parietal lobe (usually left) is important in visual analysis and higher defects may thus be recognized despite the integrity of the primary visual pathways.

Dominant parietal lesions	*Non-dominant*
Alexia – inability to read	Constructional apraxia
Object agnosia – failure to name objects	Visual spatial abnormalities
Prosopagnosia – failure to recognize faces	

Isolated defects of cognitive function or, in some cases with bilateral disease, complex perceptual problems may be seen. Patients with dyslexia without dysgraphia have a disconnection syndrome when information from the right cortex is unable to reach the visual integration area in the left cortex. This produces the inability to read, but writing is normal and field testing shows a right homonymous hemianopia. Bilateral parieto-occipital disease may produce total visual loss with denial of blindness (Anton's syndrome).

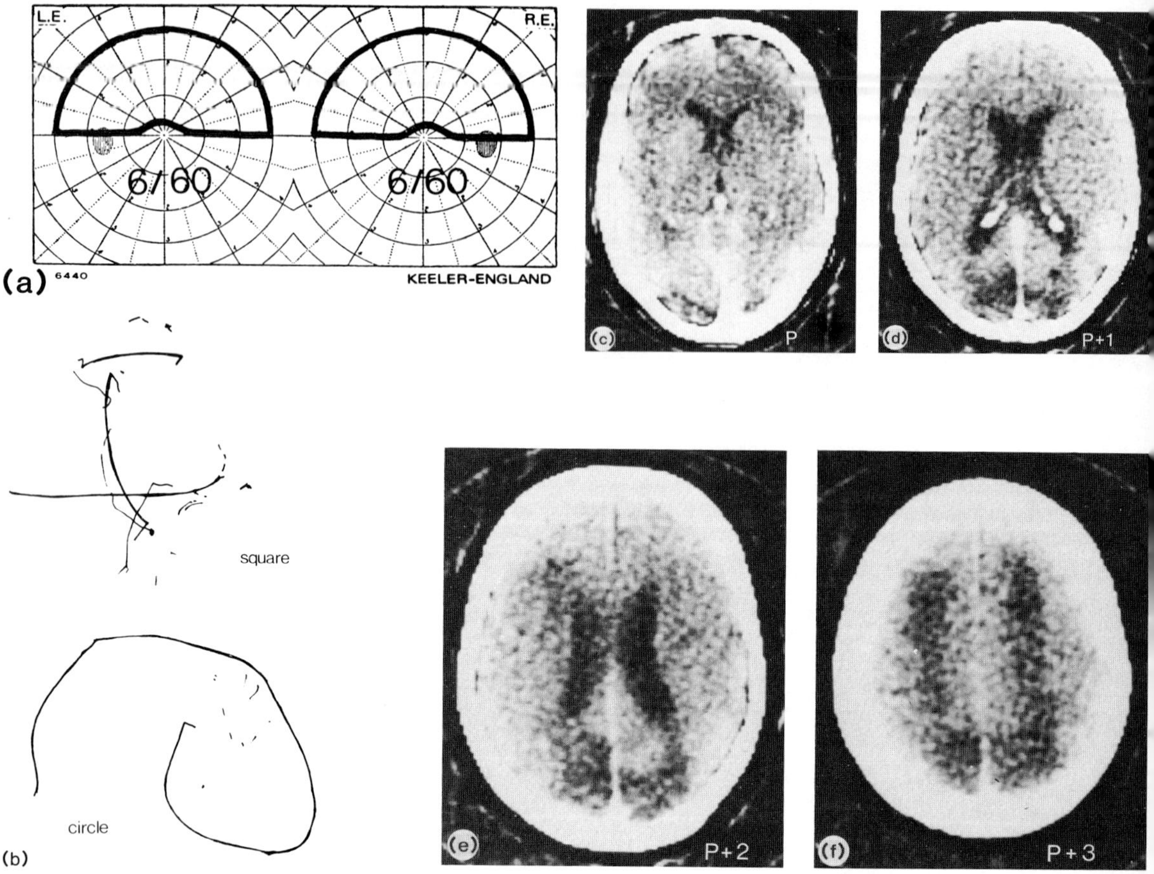

Fig. 4.41 Cerebral infarction producing visual disorientation. A 57-year old woman survived a respiratory arrest due to viral encephalitis, but subsequently developed severe visual disorientation. She showed bilateral inferior altitudinal defects which grossly impaired acuity (a). She had visual disorientation, with constructional apraxia and could not read or write (b). Upgaze and convergence were limited, saccades were slow and optokinetic nystagmus was reduced in all directions. VERs were virtually absent above the inion. CT (c–g) demonstrated extensive areas of low attenuation extending upwards from the P+1 level in the occipital region, involving the cortex and the centrum semiovale.

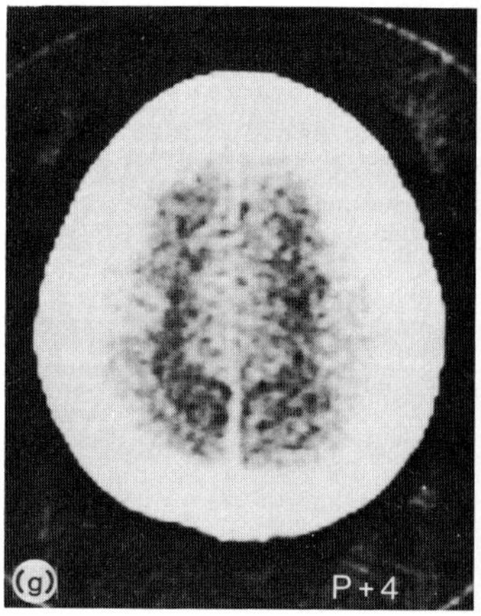

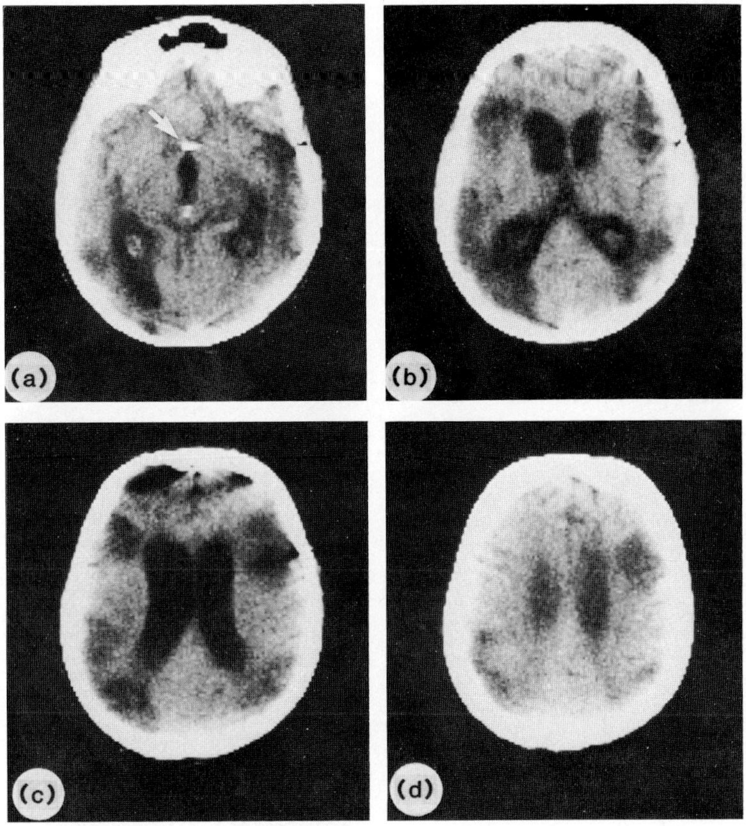

Fig. 4.42 *'Watershed' infarction.* Severe cerebral damage following peroperative hypotension. There is hydrocephalus (secondary to subarachnoid haemorrhage – note a clip on the anterior communicating artery – arrow), and wedge-shaped areas of low attenuation are seen in both cerebral hemispheres. They are predominantly anterolateral in the watershed area between anterior and middle cerebral arteries, and posterolateral, at the middle and posterior cerebral artery territory interface. The bulk of the territory supplied by each of the major cerebral arteries is intact.

Patients with parieto-occipital cerebral disease are occasionally referred to the ophthalmologist for visual assessment. Central acuity must be established before the true nature of the visual disturbance can be determined. Snellen testing is reduced because of word agnosia; certain techniques can be employed:

1. The use of single letters for distant or near visual testing.
2. Tests of colour vision.
3. Simple tests of perception and recognition.
4. Asking the patient to write in small letters.

We see two or three patients a year in whom complex visuo-perceptual disorders are present, but not appreciated. CT offers a major advance in anatomical localization. Some of the commoner phenomena are included in Table 4.6. In severe cases, a combination of these features may be present.

Fig. 4.43 Occipital haematoma with resolution. A 49-year old woman presented with a sudden onset of a left hemianopia (a, solid line) with macular and some upper quadrant sparing. CT (b) showed an acute intracerebral haematoma in the right parietal region. Some months later, when the visual fields were normal (a, broken line), there was still a large posthaemorrhagic cavity, with underlying ventricular dilation (c–e). This residual lesion clearly lies outside the visual cortex, indicating that the field defect was an indirect pressure phenomenon. (Previously published in 'Computerized tomographic scanning (EMI Scan) in neuro-ophthalmology' by Sanders, M.D. and Gawler, J. *Trans. Ophthal. Soc. U.K.* **XCV** Part II, 1975).

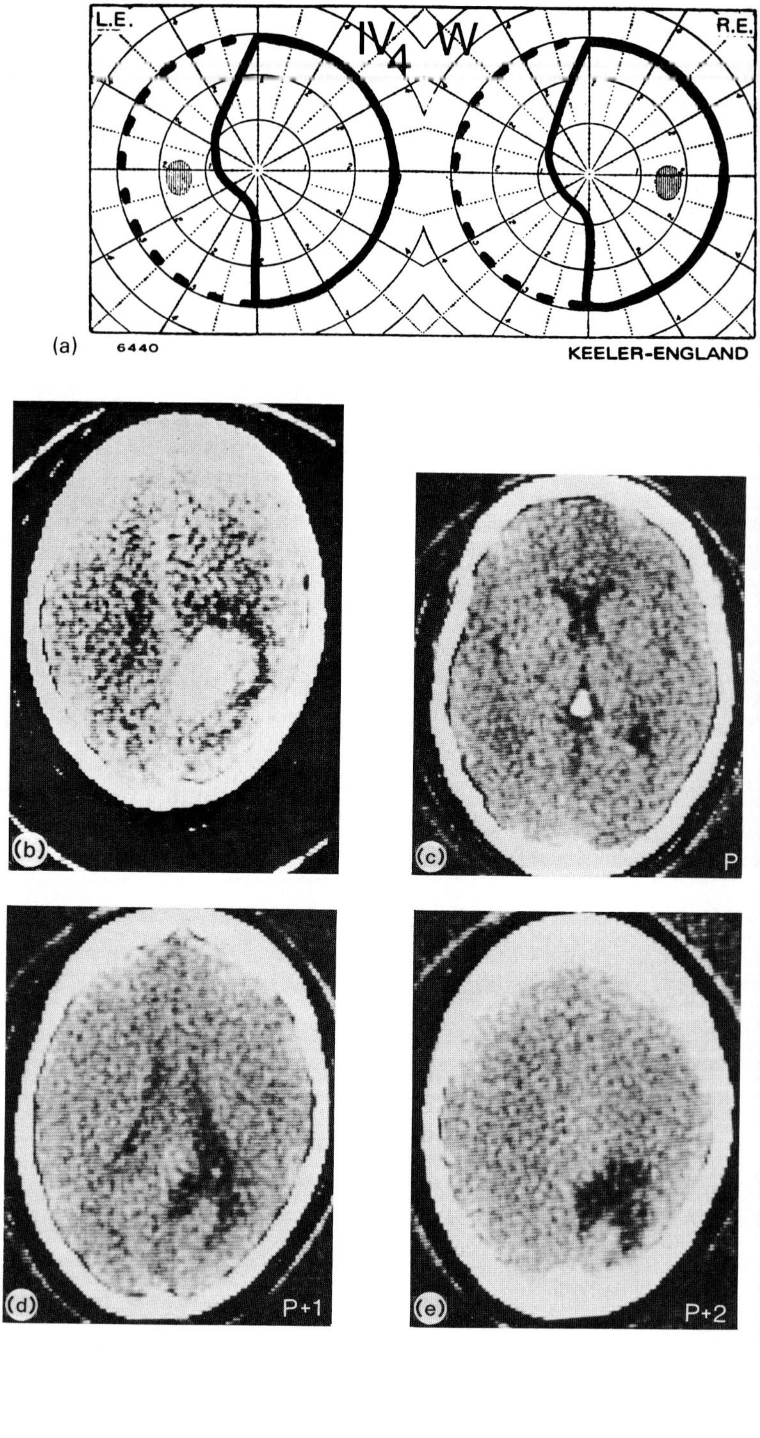

Fig. 4.44 Occipital glioma. Right parieto-occipital headache was the presenting symptom in this 63-year old woman, but examination showed a left homonymous hemianopia with relative sparing of the superior quadrant (a). There was no papilloedema. CT (b,c, after intravenous contrast medium), showed a right occipital tumour, probably cystic. The markedly irregular cyst wall and extensive cerebral oedema indicate its malignant nature. The mass effect is least marked in the infrapineal sections, explaining the incomplete superior component of the hemianopia.

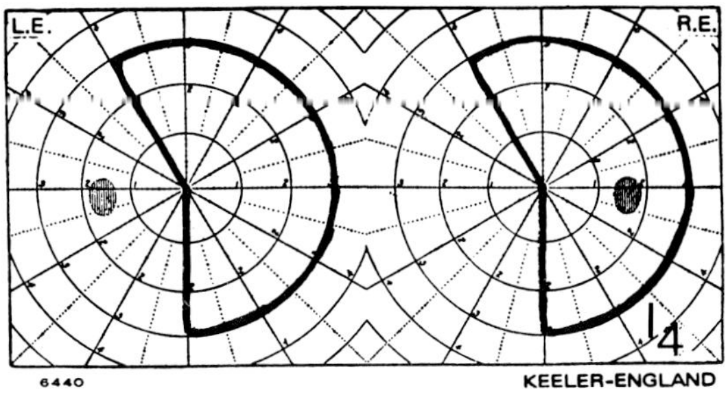

(a)

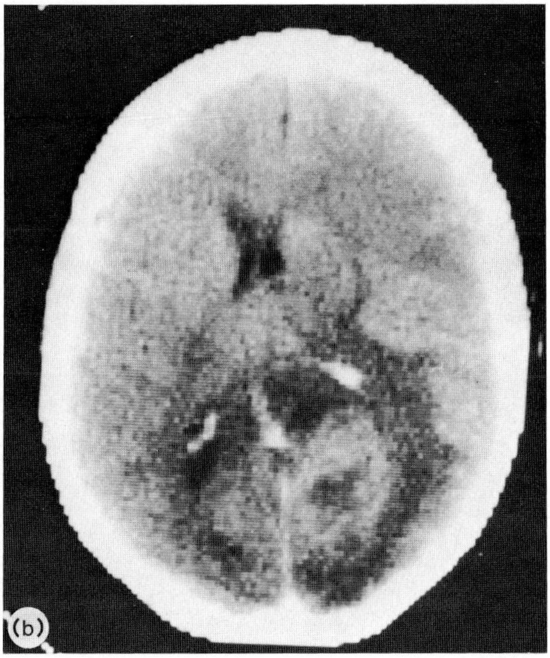

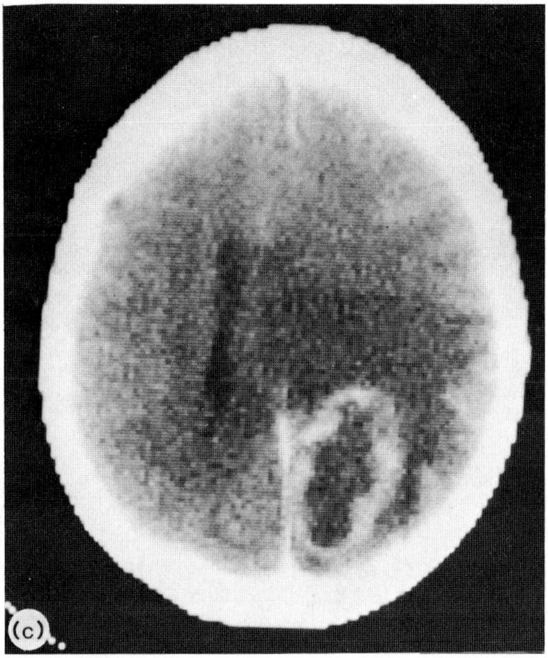

Table 4.6 Anatomical correlations in disorders of higher visual function.

Defect	*Location at CT*	*Visual field loss*
Dyslexia without dysgraphia (Fig. 4.46)	L occipital cortex and corpus callosum	R homonymous hemianopia
Prosopagnosia (Fig. 4.47)	R (or frequently bilateral) inferior occipital and temporal	L homonymous hemianopia
Visuospatial abnormalities (Figs. 4.48 and 4.49)	Usually R parieto-occipital	Inferior altitudinal if present
Visual perseveration (Fig. 4.50)	R inferior temporal	L superior quadrantanopia

Fig. 4.45 Occipital metastases. Complete loss of vision occurred over several days in a 67-year old man previously operated upon for a malignant melanoma. CT (a) showed areas of mixed attenuation, including streaks suggestive of haemorrhage (arrows) in both occipital lobes. After intravenous contrast medium (b), the full extent of the tumours was shown. Note that on the right the haemorrhagic area appears to lie in the centre of the lesion.

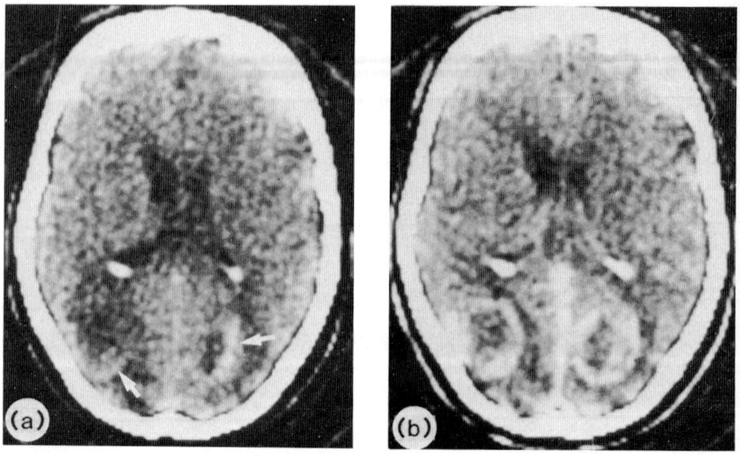

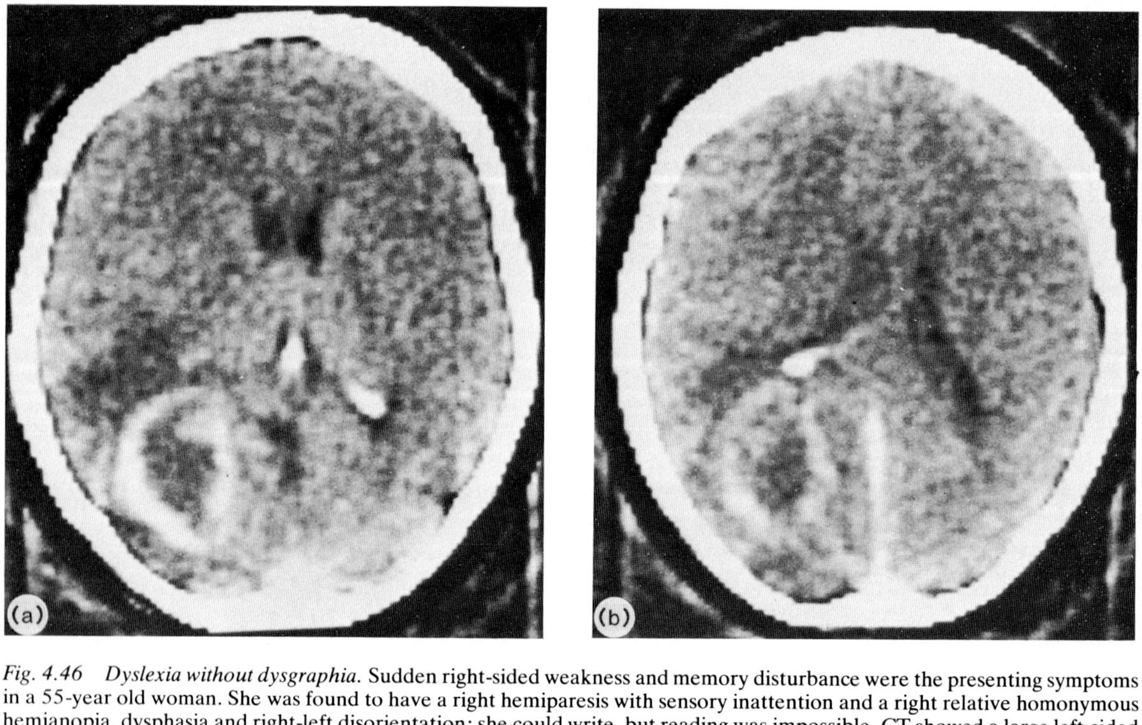

Fig. 4.46 Dyslexia without dysgraphia. Sudden right-sided weakness and memory disturbance were the presenting symptoms in a 55-year old woman. She was found to have a right hemiparesis with sensory inattention and a right relative homonymous hemianopia, dysphasia and right-left disorientation; she could write, but reading was impossible. CT showed a large left-sided lesion of mixed attenuation, with irregular ring enhancement typical of a malignant tumour. It is mainly temporo-occipital (as indicated by *elevation* of the choroid plexus), but may involve the inferior parietal lobe. It lies in the white matter but there is no evidence of involvement of the corpus callosum; the overlying cerebral cortex appears relatively intact.

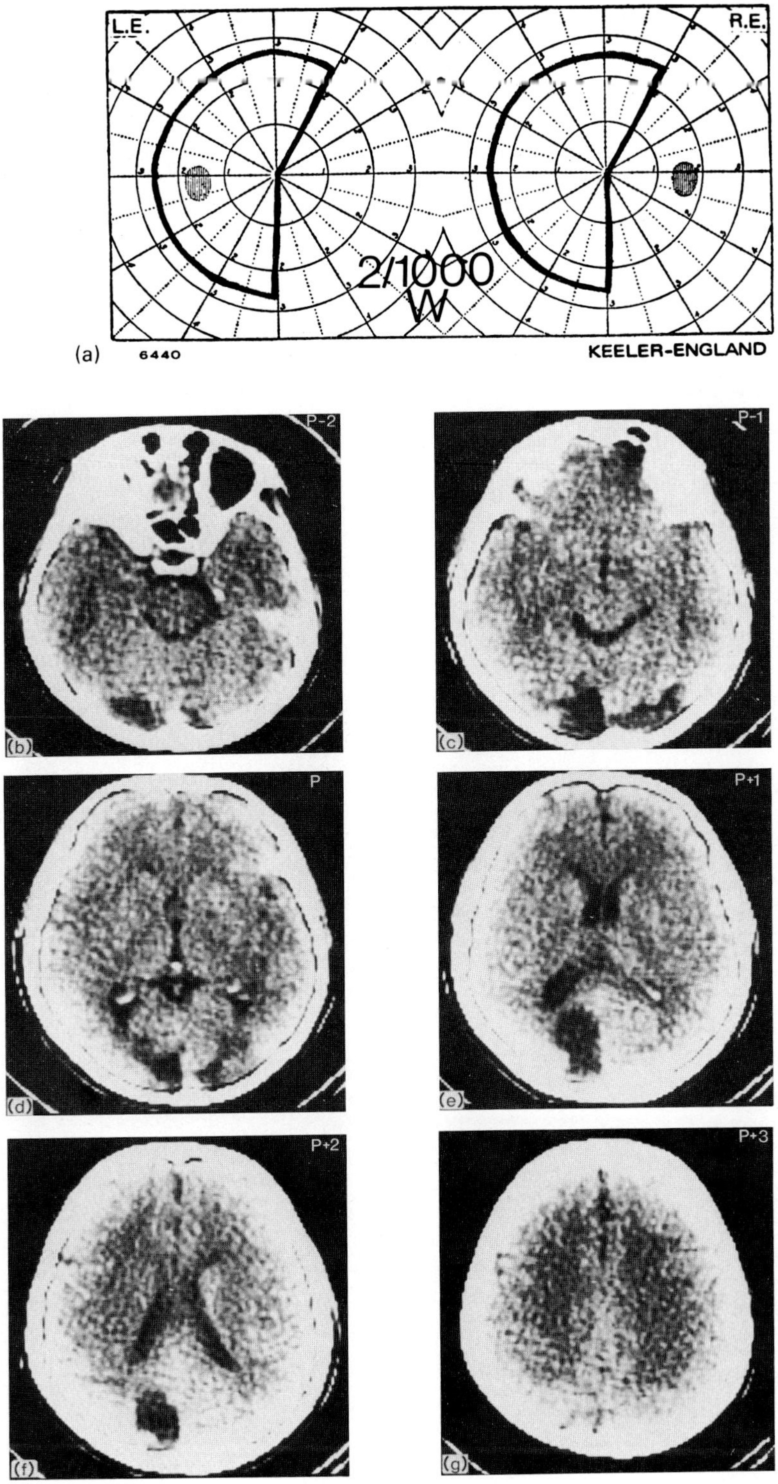

Fig. 4.47 Prosopagnosia with bilateral occipital lobe infarcts. A 49-year old man collapsed in the shower, after which he was unable to see. Over two years his vision improved, but he was unable to read or to recognize people. He was aware of difficulty seeing on the right. Examination showed 6/36 and N48 vision bilaterally. Colour vision was normal, but there was a right homonymous hemianopia with some sparing of the upper field (a). He had prosopagnosia and psychometry revealed a memory defect. CT (b–g) showed low attenuation defects in both occipital lobes, extending from P−2 to P on the right: the anticipated sparing of the left lower visual cortex is not confirmed.

Fig. 4.48 Parieto-occipital glioma causing visual hallucinations. A 57-year old woman presented with headaches and a history of formed visual hallucinations consisting of 'lots of legs moving on a television screen' in the lower left visual field. When first seen she had no visual field defect, but subsequently developed a left inferior quadrantanopia (a). CT (b–e, after intravenous contrast medium) revealed a rounded, inhomogeneous right parieto-occipital tumour, which surgery showed to be a highly malignant glioma.

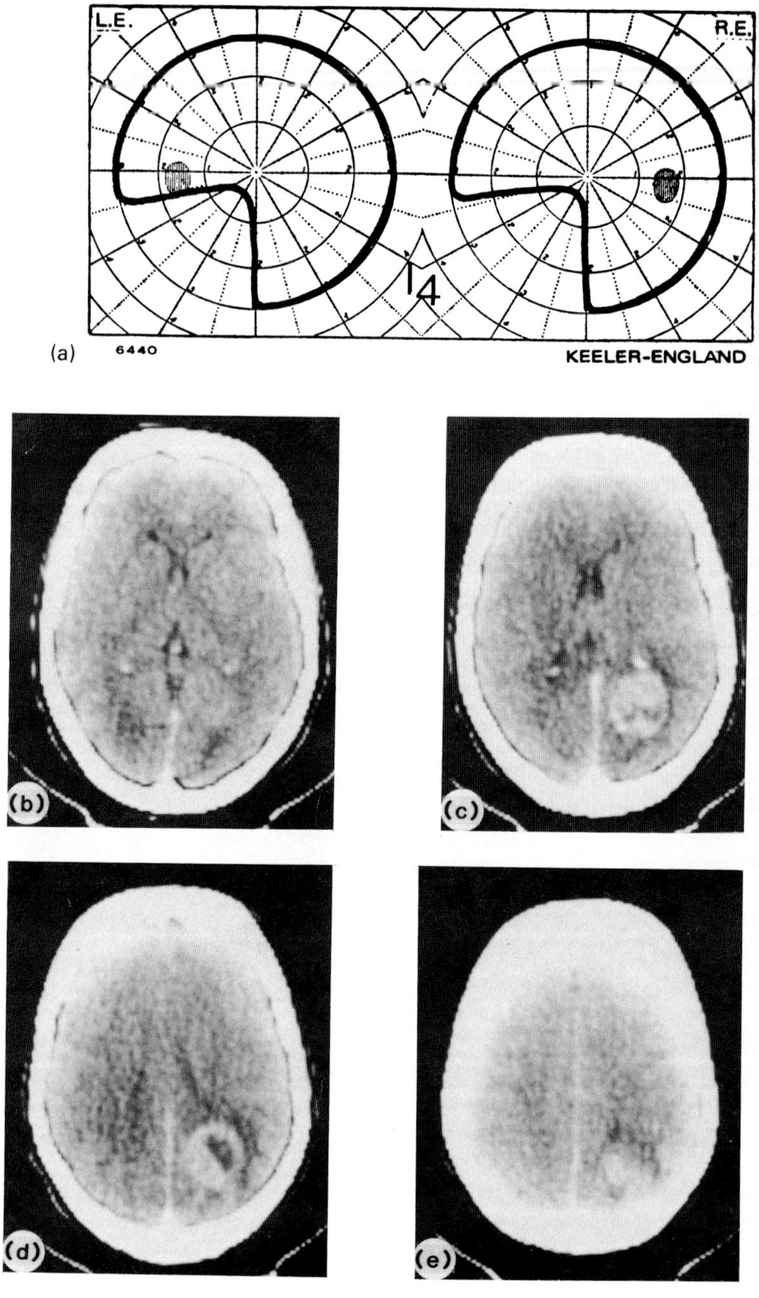

Fig. 4.49 Meningioma causing visual disorientation. A 60-year old man showed global dementia, with left visual inattention and inability to recognize objects and to judge distances or directions. He was found to have a left homonymous hemianopia, with sparing of the temporal crescent (a). CT (b, axial section; c, d, coronal and sagittal reconstructions, after intravenous contrast medium) revealed a typical dense, rounded meningioma in the right occipital region, which was shown to be supplied by the occipital artery (e, arrows), with a somewhat atypical tumour blush (f, open arrow).

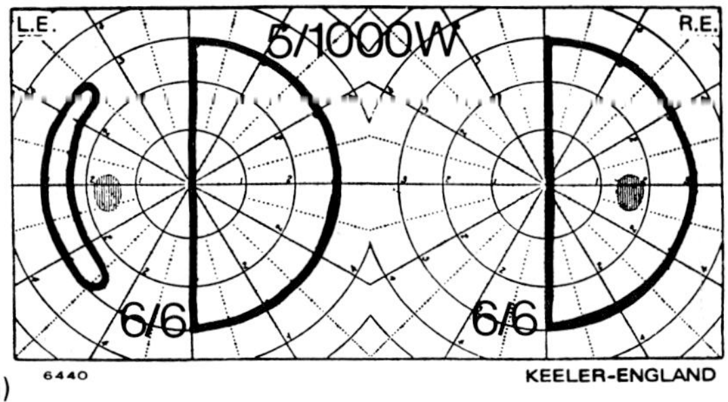

(a)

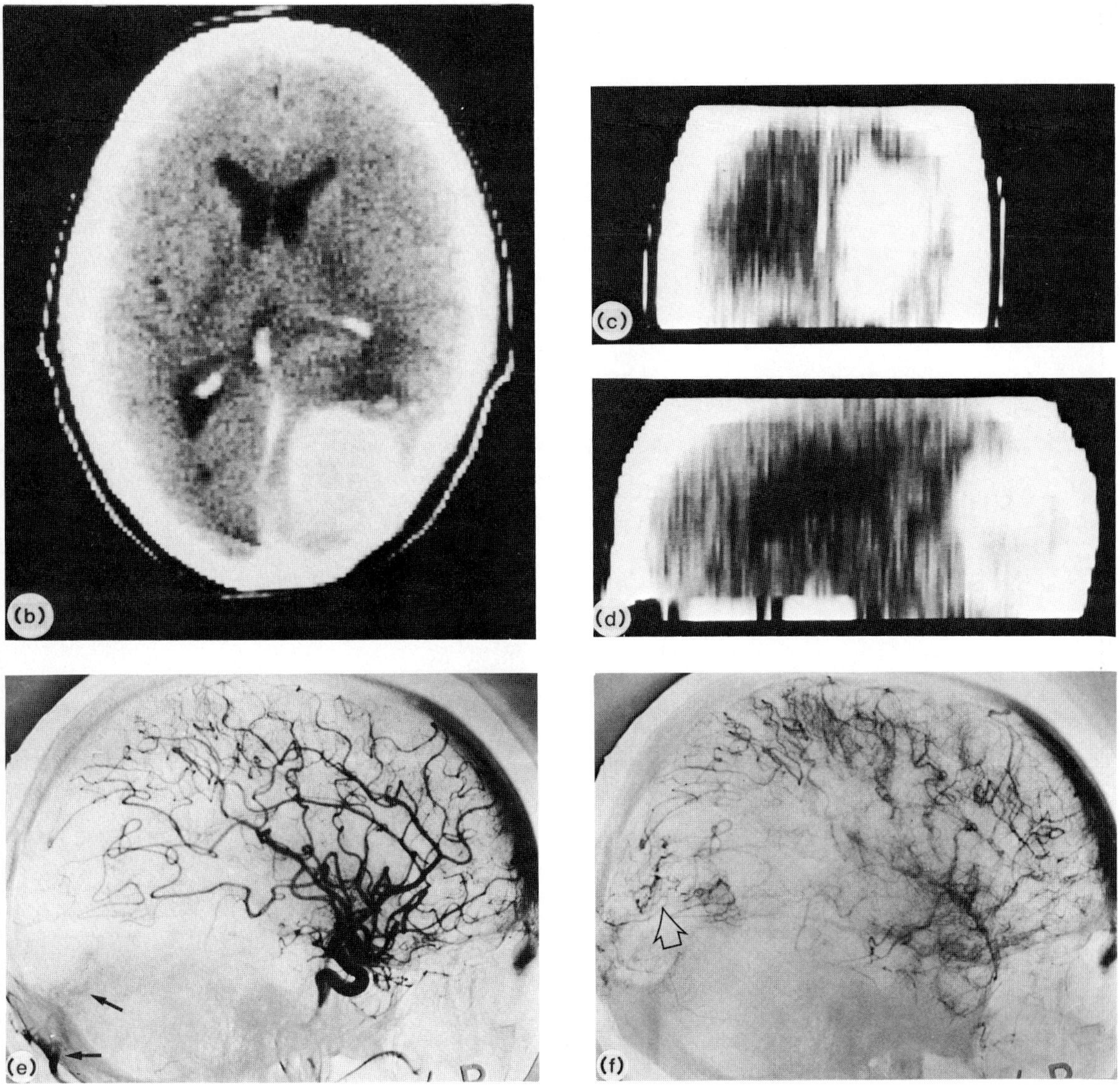

Fig. 4.50 Visual perseveration and hallucinations. A right temporoparietal meningioma had been removed 12 years previously when the patient was aged 45, leaving her with a left superior quadrantic defect. The left eye was subsequently operated upon for glaucoma. Ten days before the CT study she experienced sudden darkening of vision, after which she noted visual perseveration in the left field, distortion of the right side of faces, (metamorphopsia) and frequent visual hallucinations, also on the left. Mild visual disorientation also occurred in the succeeding days. Vision was 6/12 on the right and hand movements on the left; there was a homonymous hemianopia (a). The right disc was pale and there was mild left hemiparesis. The visual phenomena and psychometric testing (b – bicycle and cube) indicated a right temporo-occipital lesion, which was shown by CT (c) to be a large postoperative or ischaemic defect rather than a recurrence of the tumour.

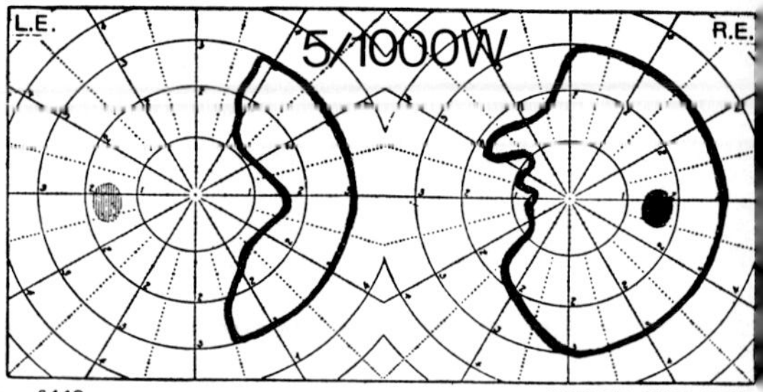

(a)

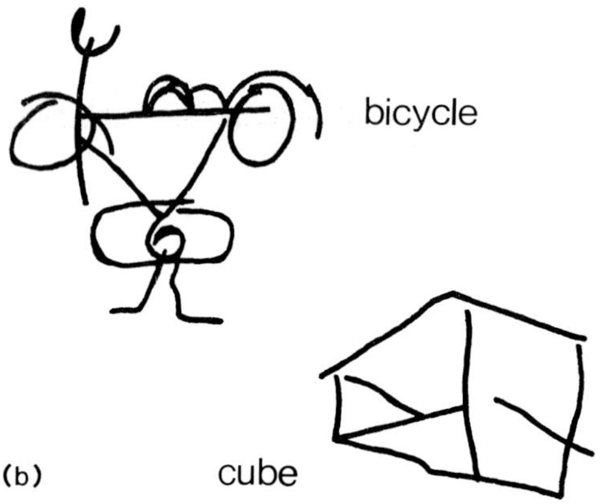

(b)

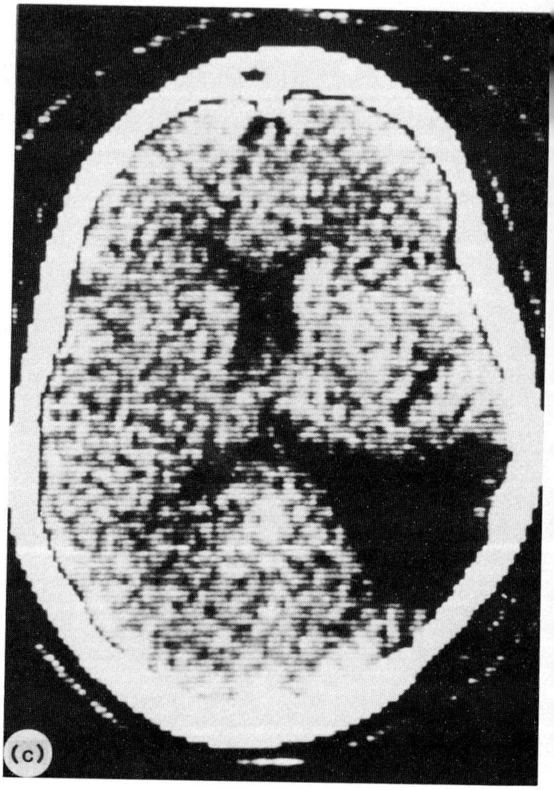
(c)

REFERENCES

Bell, R.A. and Thompson, H.S. (1979), Optic tract lesions and relative afferent pupillary defects. In: *Topics in Neuro-Ophthalmology* (Ed. H.S. Thompson), Williams & Wilkins, Baltimore, pp.164–6.

Decker, R.E., Mardayat, M., Marc, J. and Rasool, A. (1979), Neurosarcoidosis with computerized tomographic visualization and transphenoidal excision of a supra- and intrasellar granuloma. *J. Neurosurg.*, **50**, 814–18.

Fitz, C.R., Wortzman, G., Harwood-Nash, D.C., Holgate, R.C. Barry, J.F. and Boldt, D.W. (1978), Computed tomography in craniopharyngiomas. *Radiology*, **127**, 687–91.

Foley, K.M. and Posner, J.B. (1975), Does pseudotumour cerebri cause the empty sella syndrome?, *Neurology*, **25**, 565–9.

Kan, S. and Matsubayashi, T. (1978), CT in homonymous hemianopia. *Neuroradiology*, **16**, 299–301.

Lin, S.R., Bryson, M.M., Gobien, R.P., Fitz, C.R. and Lee, Y.Y. (1978), Radiologic findings of hamartoma of the tuber cinereum and hypothalamus. *Radiology*, **127**, 697–703.

McAuley, D.L.F. and Ross Russell, R.W. (1977), Vascular disease of the visual radiations and cortex. In: *First European Seminar on Computerised Axial Tomography in Clinical Practice* (eds. G.H. Du Boulay and I.F. Moseley), Springer, Berlin, pp.243–8.

Moseley, I.F., Sanders, M.D., Karoutas, G. and Radü, E.W. (1979), CT scan in neuro-ophthalmology. In: *Topics in Neuro-Ophthalmology.* (ed. H.S. Thompson), Williams and Wilkins, Baltimore, pp.302–17.

Naidich, T.P., Pinto, R.S., Kushner, M.J., Lin, D.P., Kricheff, I.I., Leeds, N.E. and Chase, N.E. (1976), Evaluation of sella and parasellar masses by computed tomography. *Radiology*, **120**, 91–99.

Osher, R.M., Corbett, J.J., Schatz, N.J., Savino, P.J. and Orr, L.S. (1978), Neuro-ophthalmological complications of enlargement of the third ventricle. *Br. J. Ophthal.*, **62**, 536–42.

Oxenhandler, D.C. and Sayers, M.P. (1978), The dilemma of childhood optic gliomas. *J. Neurosurg.*, **48**, 34–47.

Pearlman, A.L., Birch, J. and Meadows, J.C. (1979), Cerebral colour blindness: an acquired defect in hue discrimination. *Ann. Neurol.*, **5**, 253–61.

Radü, E.W. and Moseley, I.F. (1978) Carotid artery occlusion and computed tomography. A clinico-radiological study. *Neuroradiology*, **17**, 7–12.

Ross Russell, R.W. (1978), Border-zone infarction and its effects on vision. *Rev. Oto-Neuro-Ophthal.*, **50**, 27–28.

Sanders, M.D. and Falconer, M.A. (1964), Optic nerve compression by an intracanalicular meningioma. *Br. J. Ophthal.*, **48**, 13–18.

Sanders, M.D. and Moseley, I.F. (1979), CT scanning in neuro-ophthalmology: optic nerve compression. In: *Topics in Neuro-Ophthalmology*, (ed. H.S. Thompson) Williams and Wilkins, Baltimore, pp.318–35.

Smith, J.L. (1962), Homonymous hemianopia. *Am. J. Ophthal.*, **54**, 616–22.

Takeuchi, J., Handa, H. and Nagata, I. (1978), Suprasellar germinoma. *J. Neurosurg.*, **49**, 41–48.

Tibbs, P.A., Challa, V. and Mortara, R.H. (1978), Isolated histiocytosis X of the hypothalamus. *J. Neurosurg.*, **49**, 929–34.

Trobe, J.D., Lorber, M.L. and Schlezinger, N.S. (1973), Isolated homonymous hemianopia, *Archs Ophthal.*, **89**, 377–81.

Weisberg, L.A. (1977), Pituitary apoplexy, *Am. J. Med.*, **63**, 109–15.

5 · Optic nerve disease

This chapter deals with the role of CT in optic disc and optic nerve disease. Optic disc swelling is a general term describing the morphological appearances of the optic disc, which may be due to congenital abnormalities or a wide variety of local disease processes. These local conditions have to be distinguished from papilloedema due to raised intracranial pressure where investigation and therapy is of immediate importance. Discussion of these subjects is followed by a review of optic nerve tumours.

5.1 PAPILLOEDEMA

Clinical features

The advent of CT has removed for the clinician the difficult decision whether to investigate with potentially hazardous techniques a patient suspected of having a brain tumour. Although large intracranial tumours may be present without papilloedema, the optic disc has remained an important clinical indicator of the level of the cerebrospinal fluid (CSF) pressure. Patients may present with bilateral papilloedema and have a normal CT while suffering from a wide range of conditions often lumped together under the term 'benign intracranial hypertension', but spinal cord tumours, malignant infiltration of the subarachnoid space, high CSF protein and arteriovenous malformations of the meninges should all be excluded.

The term 'papilloedema' is properly reserved for conditions producing raised intracranial pressure.

The clinical appearance of papilloedema is determined by a number of variable factors which include:

1. The shape and size of the disc prior to swelling.
2. The degree, duration and fluctuation of the elevation of CSF pressure.
3. The relationship between the intraocular pressure, CSF pressure and the blood pressure, affecting optic disc perfusion.

Considering these variables it is possible to categorise five stages of papilloedema.

1. Early papilloedema. The disc margin and the nerve fibre pattern are often blurred and the nerve fibres appear thickened. Venous pulsation is usually absent; no haemorrhages or

cotton wool spots are seen. Fluorescein angiography shows dilated superficial vessels and peripapillary leakage into the retina.

2. Fully developed papilloedema. Perfusion of the disc is reduced so that numerous infarcts or haemorrhages are present and marked dilatation of the superficial peripapillary plexus is seen on fluorescein angiography.
3. Chronic papilloedema. There is moderate disc and nerve fibre swelling, with occasional haemorrhages or cotton wool spots. Marked dilatation of the superficial capillary plexus is seen on angiography, with residual leakage.
4. Vintage papilloedema. Haemorrhages or infarcts are absent, but punctate bright opacities due to neural degeneration are seen within the disc, and occasionally opticociliary shunt vessels are present.
5. Atrophic papilloedema. The end result of untreated papilloedema produces severe loss of neurones with concomitant visual loss and optic disc pallor.

CT in papilloedema

Early CT studies of the orbit demonstrated changes in the size and form of the 'optic nerve' in patients with papilloedema. Swelling of the optic nerve is restricted by intraneural septa and any apparent increase in diameter is due to dilatation of the subarachnoid space between the nerve and the dura mater, with possibly some thickening of the dura and arachnoid mater. The patency of this space was confirmed radiologically by Manelfe *et al.* (1978), who described one case in which metrizamide, a water-soluble iodinated contrast medium injected into the spinal subarachnoid space, circulated into the optic nerve sheaths. CT studies showed expanded 'nerves' of high attenuation with a central filling defect representing the optic nerve. On a repeat scan some days later the nerves appeared of normal attenuation (Fig. 5.1).

Enhancement of the optic nerve sheaths can be seen after intrathecal metrizamide in a concentration giving an iodine level of 170 mg/ml. In a series reported by Fox *et al.* (1979), five patients showed very slight increases (3–5 EMI units), though one patient with cerebrospinal fluid rhinorrhoea showed an increase in attentuation coefficients of 15 EMI units. It is possible that this patient had benign intracranial hypertension giving rise to the leakage of fluid and also rendering the optic nerve sheaths more patulous. In another case, slight enhancement of the nerve sheath was seen distal to a surgically proven sheath meningioma, removal of which resulted in complete recovery. The authors suggested that the patency of the sheath, as indicated by the passage of the contrast medium, was a favourable prognostic sign. Further experience will be necessary to evaluate the use of intrathecal contrast medium in investigating patients with optic nerve disease. Although none of the patients in this

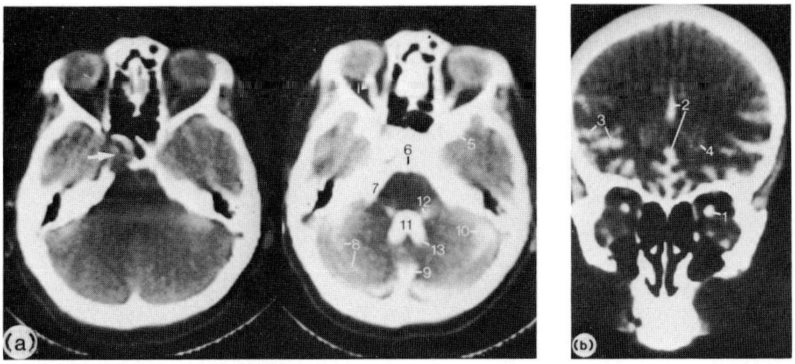

Fig. 5.1 Metrizamide in optic nerve sheaths. Metrizamide CT cisternography carried out for investigation of an eroded sella turcica (arrow). (a) Before and after injection; same axial plane. (b) Coronal section after injection of metrizamide. 1. Optic nerve sheath; 2. interhemispheric fissure; 3. Sylvian fissure; 4. frontal horn of lateral ventricle; 5. subarachnoid space over temporal lobe; 6. pontine cistern; 7. cerebellopontine angle cistern; 8. cerebellar hemispheric sulci; 9. vallecula; 10. lateral cerebellar cistern; 11. fourth ventricle; 12. lateral recess; 13. posterosuperior recess. (Courtesy of Dr V.L. McAllister).

series suffered any ill effects, transient scotomata have been reported (Aubin *et al.*, 1978), so that potential risks have to be evaluated.

The transverse diameter of the optic nerve is extremely difficult to assess at CT. If the CT section is thicker than the optic nerve (taking into account possible tortuosity of the nerve in the plane of section), then partial volume phenomena will tend to decrease its apparent size. However, if the section is thinner than the diameter of the nerve at right angles to the plane of section, there is no guarantee that any individual section passes through its greatest diameter. Measurement of the transverse diameter may be increased by obliqueness of the nerve to the plane of section.

Salvolini and his co-workers (1978) used the neuro-ocular index (NOI: see Chapter 2) to assess the size of the optic nerves. Their results in normal cases indicated a normal variation of up to 50% in the diameter of the midpoint of the nerve as compared with the transverse equatorial diameter of the globe. Although it was their impression that the NOI was increased in patients with papilloedema, less than one quarter of their observations were outside the range they had established as normal. This would certainly be in accordance with our own experience.

In addition to increasing the diameter of the optic nerve sheath, the increased volume of fluid within the sheath gives rise to increased tortuosity. Patients with papilloedema may therefore show apparently enlarged nerves, tortuous nerves or nerves which are both large and abnormally tortuous.

Cabanis *et al.* (1978) claimed that this exaggeration of the normal slight tortuosity of the optic nerves was present in up to 80% of patients with papilloedema. The assessment of the degree of tortuosity is complicated by the observation that some patients without any evidence of optic nerve disease may show definite tortuosity, either horizontally, in the form of lateral angulation of the midportion of the nerve, or vertically (Figs. 5.2 and 5.8). Milder degrees of tortuosity may also be noted in abduction.

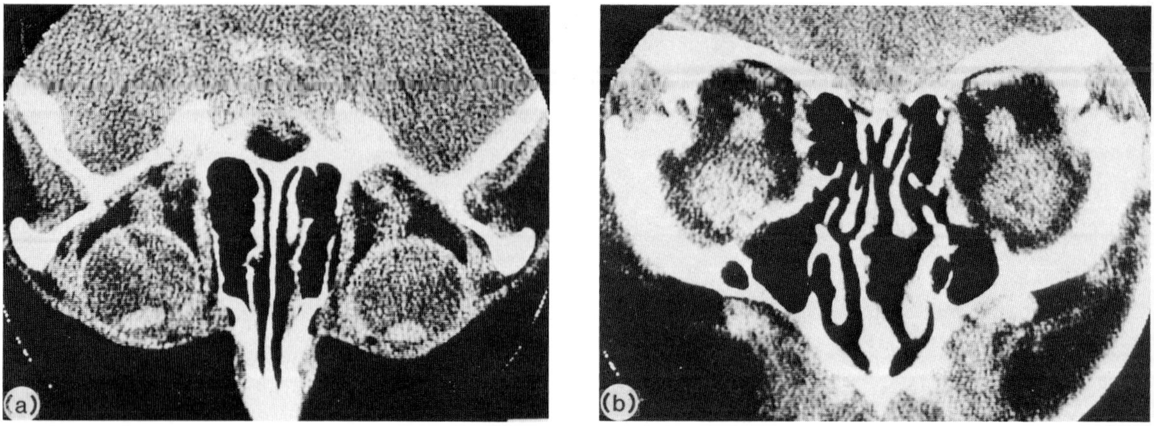

Fig. 5.2 Tortuous optic nerves. This patient suffered an ophthalmic artery occlusion on the right; there was no perception of light in the right eye. Both optic nerves appear abnormally tortuous and angular (a), but are not thickened (b). The orbits are small in anteroposterior diameter (cf Fig. 5.3), and this tortuosity may be explained by a disproportion between the nerves and the orbits.

Increased tortuosity in patients without papilloedema may be the result of a disparity between the length of the nerve and the anteroposterior diameter of the orbit.

Dilatation and/or increased tortuosity of the optic nerves has been observed in obstructive hydrocephalus, in the presence of intracranial mass lesions, in benign intracranial hypertension and in retrobulbar neuritis. Accurate correlation between the optic nerve changes at CT and the degree of papilloedema is not yet available, but the changes are usually confined to patients with long-standing papilloedema. We have, however, seen one patient with distended sheaths approximately ten days after the onset of papilloedema, so that the potential for rapid dilatation would appear to exist (Fig. 5.3).

We have had the opportunity to carry out a CT examination on a patient with bilateral gross papilloedema some days after unilateral incision of the optic nerve sheath. The nerve on the operated side was thought to be of smaller diameter than its fellow. In another case, a young man with presumed benign intracranial hypertension, marked resolution of disc swelling after incision of the nerve sheath was not accompanied by marked decrease in size of the nerves at CT, despite dramatic improvement in the papilloedema (Fig. 5.4).

Bilateral papilloedema

CT examination provides the lynch pin of modern diagnosis of bilateral papilloedema. Patients can be divided immediately into two groups: those in whom CT shows no causative lesion and those in whom it shows a mass lesion and/or hydrocephalus.

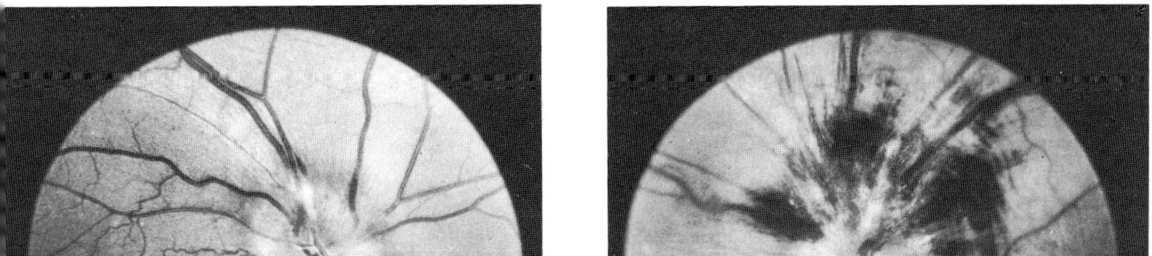

Fig. 5.3 *Acute papilloedema with subdural haematoma.* Shortly after a minor head injury, a 57-year old man developed headaches and retro-ocular pain. Investigations revealed closed angle glaucoma; the optic discs were normal. Bilateral peripheral iridectomy was performed but the headaches persisted. Two weeks after surgery the patient was found to have gross bilateral papilloedema with numerous haemorrhages on the right (a, b) without other neurological abnormalities. CT of the orbits (c–e) showed swollen optic nerves, whose curve was slightly exaggerated, while cranial scans (f) demonstrated a left subdural haematoma (arrows). At surgery, bilateral chronic subdural collections were found. Postoperative recovery was satisfactory, and four months later the discs were flat and the optic nerves appeared normal (g).

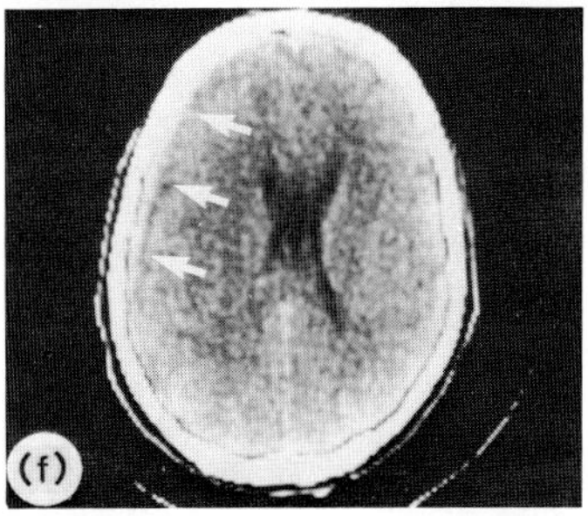

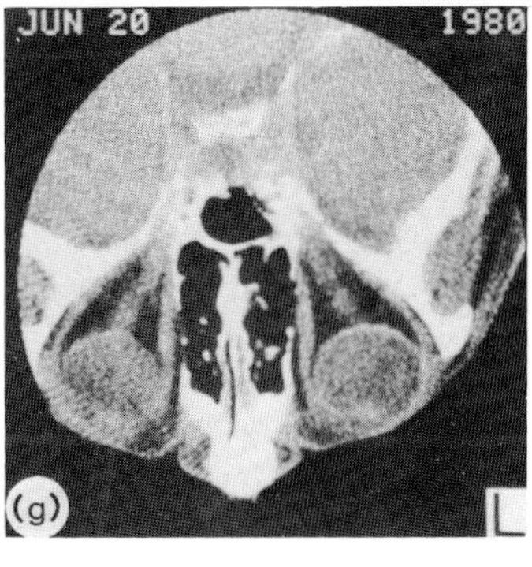

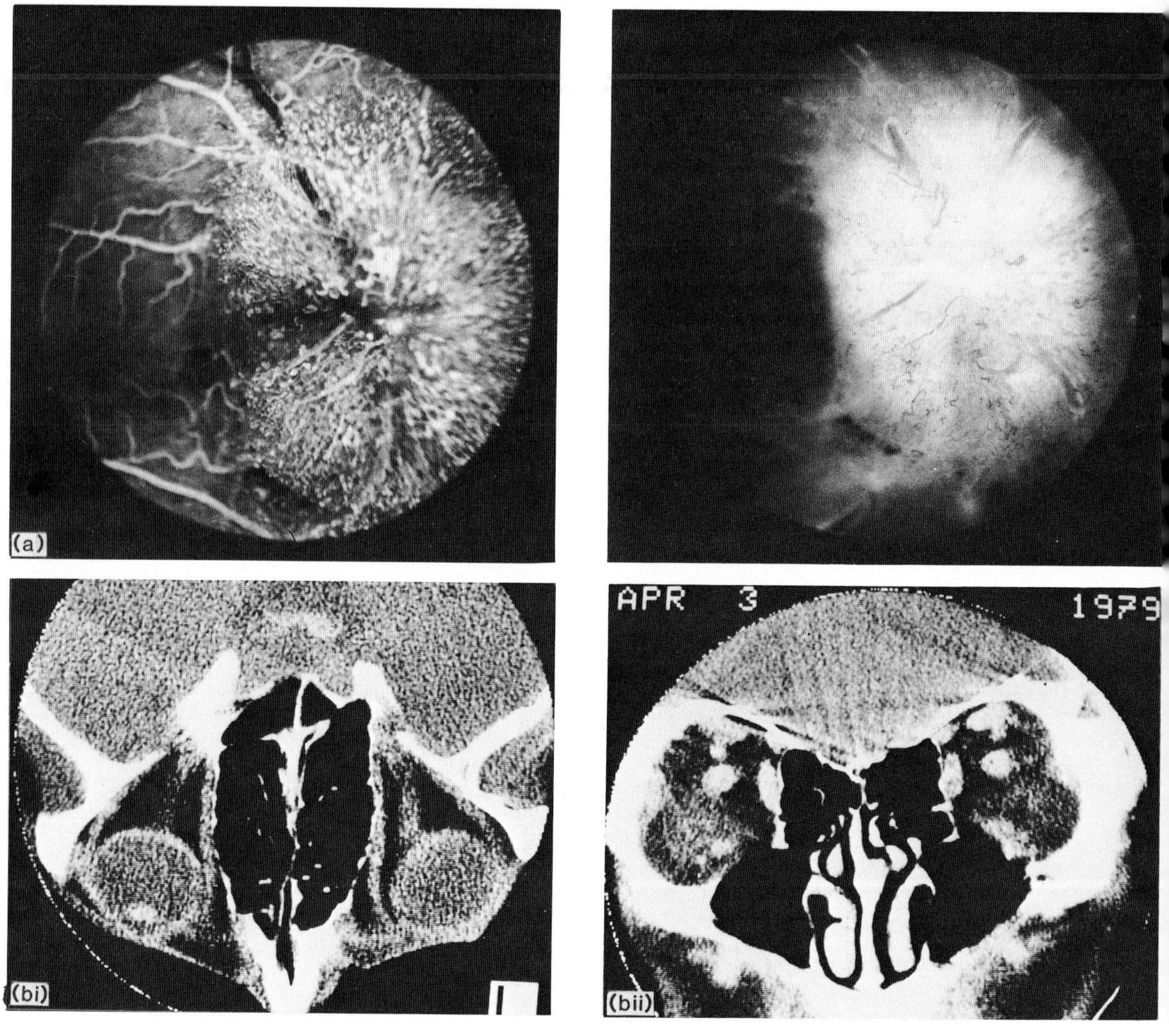

Fig. 5.4 Benign intracranial hypertension with incision of optic nerve sheaths. A 32-year old man complained of obscurations of vision, which increased in frequency to 2–3 times/day. He was found to have gross bilateral papilloedema (a) right eye, venous and late pictures. Acuity was 6/12 on the right and 6/6 on the left; the blind spots were anlarged, and he had a binasal inferior quadrantanopia. CSF pressure was 440 mm water. Steroids had no beneficial effect and it was decided to decompress the optic nerve sheaths, which CT (b) – 3/4/79) had shown to be mildly distended. This was carried out in April and May, 1979, after which he had no further obscurations and the papilloedema improved considerably (c) right and left eyes; late pictures. CT however, showed only a minor reduction in the size of the optic nerves (d). (The cause of the raised CSF pressure was subsequently found to be due to bilateral glomus tumours).

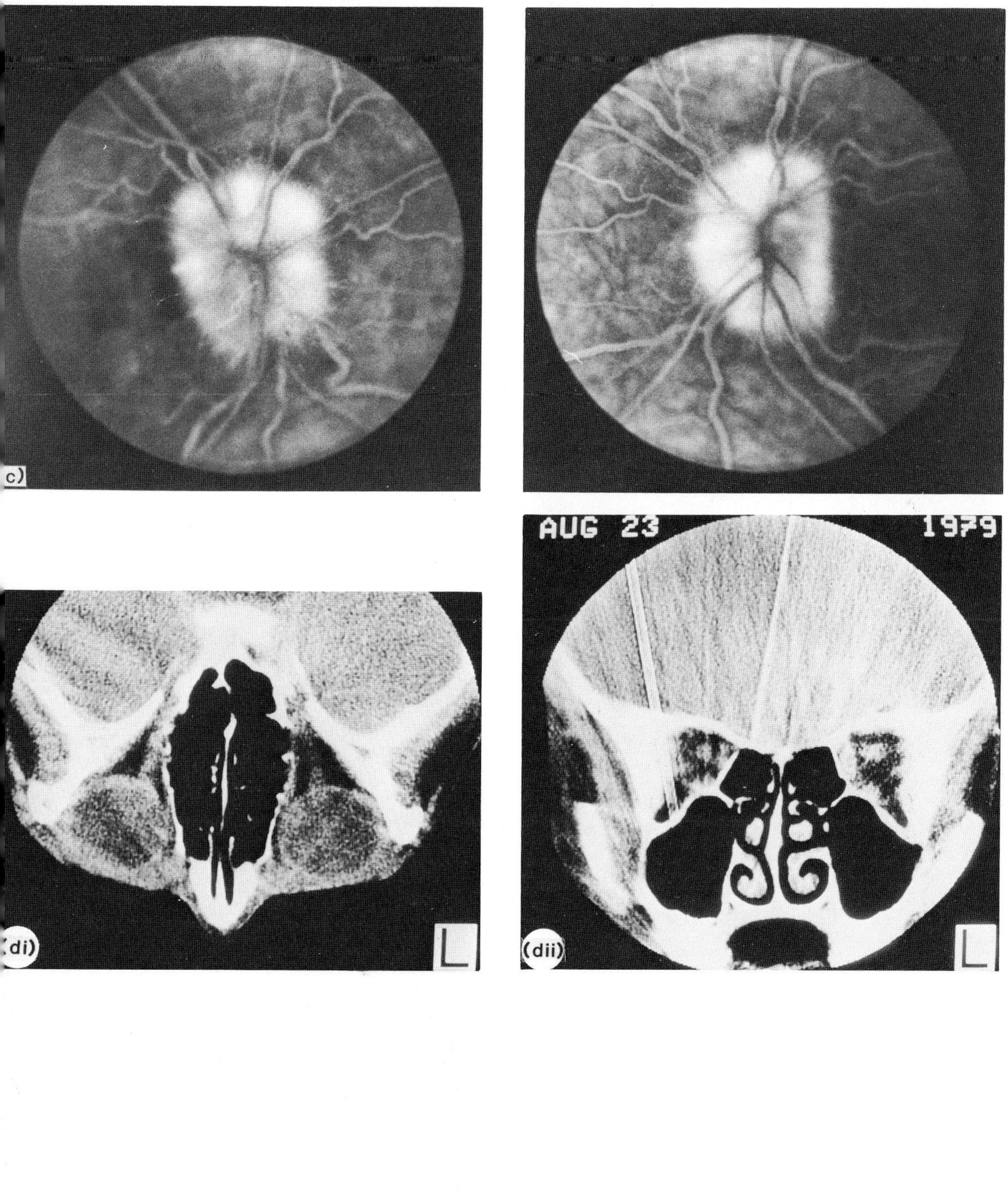
c)
AUG 23
1979
(di)
L
(dii)
L

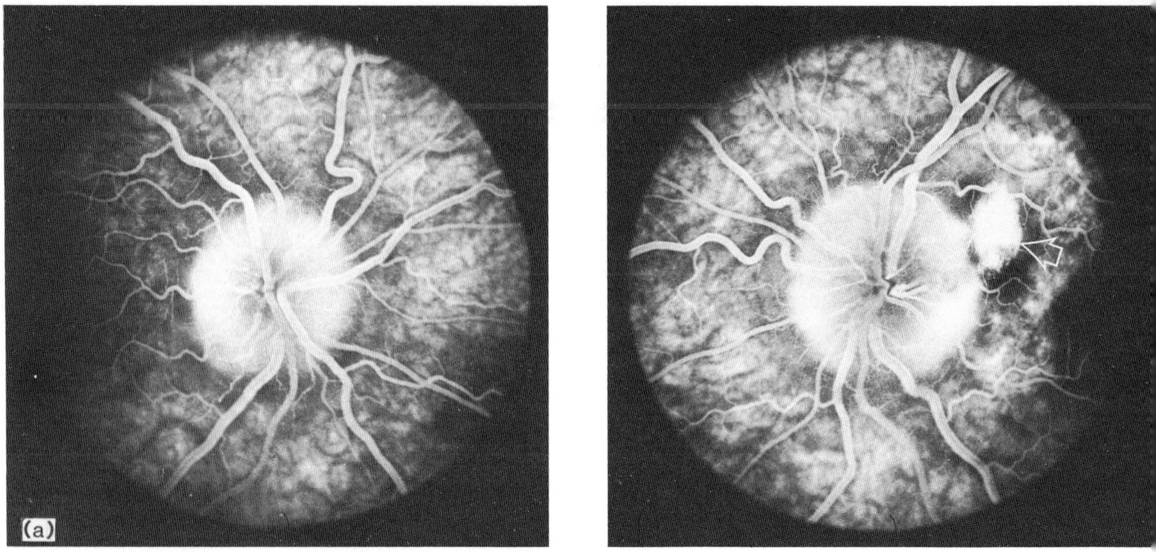

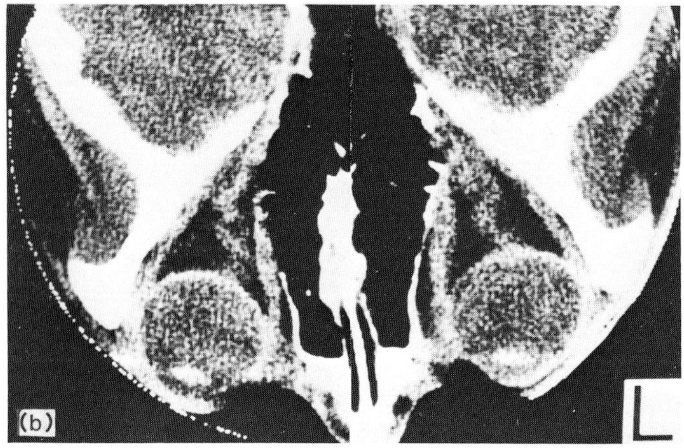

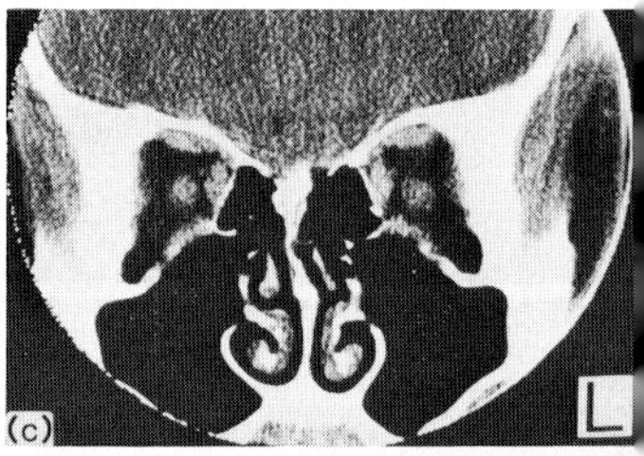

Fig. 5.5 Benign intracranial hypertension. A 15-year old girl presented with menorrhagia sufficient to cause anaemia; she was mildly obese. She also complained of poor vision, and examination revealed normal acuity but extremely constricted fields with enlarged blind spots and bilateral chronic papilloedema (a). (There was also a peripapillary disciform lesion in the left eye – open arrow). CT (b) showed swollen, somewhat tortuous optic nerves, confirmed on coronal sections (c) and lateral ventricles which were small, but within the normal range (d). This latter finding authorized lumbar puncture, at which CSF pressure was 290 mm water.

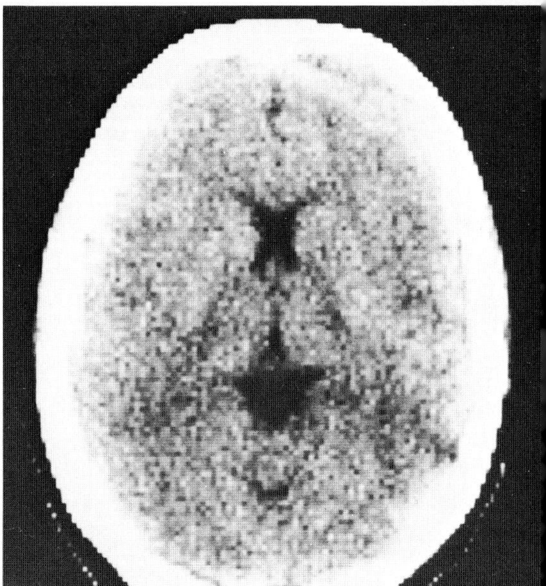

Normal CT

Bilateral papilloedema in the presence of a normal CT study is, in the absence of abnormal physical signs, usually a manifestation of benign intracranial hypertension (pseudotumour cerebri) (Fig. 5.5). This condition typically occurs in obese young females with endocrine or haematological disturbances, and a recent history of drug ingestion is sometimes obtained. The elevated cerebrospinal fluid pressure may persist for years and the main complication of this is visual loss. Recent series suggest an incidence of visual loss of 23% (Johnston and Paterson, 1974). Thus, continued visual assessment is an important factor in follow-up and management.

Several retrospective studies of patients with a final diagnosis of benign intracranial hypertension studied by CT have been described. Huckman *et al.* (1976) applied rigid diagnostic criteria: papilloedema without focal neurological signs and with a battery of normal investigations: cerebrospinal fluid analysis, electroencephalogram, isotope brain scan and carotid angiogram. Of their 17 patients, all female, 15 complained of headache, six of blurred vision, three of menstrual disturbances and one of diplopia. All showed papilloedema and five were thought to be obese. Their CT studies (with and without intravenous contrast medium in every case) were normal. In particular, the lateral ventricles were virtually identical in size with those of an age-matched normal group, and computer analysis of the cerebral attenuation coefficients did not support the suggestion of generalized cerebral oedema.

These findings were confirmed by Weisberg and Nice (1977), who pointed out that the diagnostic yield in those cases with normal sized ventricles and no evidence of mass lesions was not increased by intravenous contrast medium. We would agree with their suggestion that in *patients being investigated for bilateral papilloedema* in whom CT shows no abnormality, contrast medium administration is unnecessary. Similarly, additional radiological studies are not required; the next investigation should be diagnostic lumbar puncture. The necessity of normal cerebrospinal fluid and of the absence of physical signs other than in the eyes, however apparently remote, was underlined by Ridsdale and Moseley (1978), who described a case of spinal cord tumour causing papilloedema in which cranial CT was completely normal.

Thrombosis of cerebral cortical veins or dural venous sinuses provides one of the few examples where the aetiology of benign intracranial hypertension is adequately understood. (Identification of the aetiology, however, should render the term benign intracranial hypertension inappropriate.) Venous occlusion may follow intracranial infections or trauma, or be associated with polycythaemia or dural arteriovenous malformations. CT examination may be normal. The ventricles may be reduced in size in the acute stage, but this may only be determined retrospectively, as the lower limit of ventricular size is difficult to establish. In severely affected cases widespread low attenuation areas of variable extent may be seen in the white matter of one or usually both cerebral hemispheres. When the area of low attenuation is not extensive, the centrum semiovale tends to be most involved; small areas of haemorrhage within this region of low attenuation have been reported (Kingsley *et al*., 1979). Intravenous contrast medium produces little change in mild or chronic cases, but patients with acute disease, typically infective, show widespread superficial enhancement of areas of the brain which before injection appear relatively normal.

Mass lesions and other causes of papilloedema shown by CT
Bilateral papilloedema may be the result of (a) a mass lesion, (b) cerebral swelling, or (c) interference with the cerebrospinal fluid circulation. Cerebral angiomata can give rise to raised intracranial pressure by causing hydrocephalus (obstructive, or communicating, secondary to haemorrhage), generalized cerebral swelling as a consequence of raised cerebral venous pressure, or purely by raising the venous outflow pressure.

Detection of a mass lesion, displacement of normal structures (Fig. 5.6) or enlargement of the ventricular system will indicate the diagnosis and the need for further studies.

The relationship of papilloedema to CT evidence of raised intracranial pressure

The presence of low attenuation areas around the cerebral ventricles in cases of hydrocephalus was noted by Naidich *et al*. (1976). These areas are thought to represent the results of transependymal passage of ventricular fluid, and they are seen more commonly in acute obstructive hydrocephalus (Fig. 6.14). Wilson and Moseley (1977) noted that these 'periventricular lucencies' (PVL) and the size of the lateral ventricles, especially the temporal horns, bore a rather inconstant relationship to the presence of papilloedema.

A systematic analysis of the correlations between clinical factors, including papilloedema, and PVL was attempted by Moseley and Radü (1979). They showed that papilloedema was more common in hydrocephalic patients with PVL than in those without (the difference being significant, but apparently independent of the severity of PVL), and that the temporal horns were dilated much more frequently in patients with papilloedema who showed PVL than in those who did not.

5.2 UNILATERAL DISC OEDEMA

Investigation of unilateral disc oedema may present one of the most difficult problems in clinical neuro-ophthalmology. The

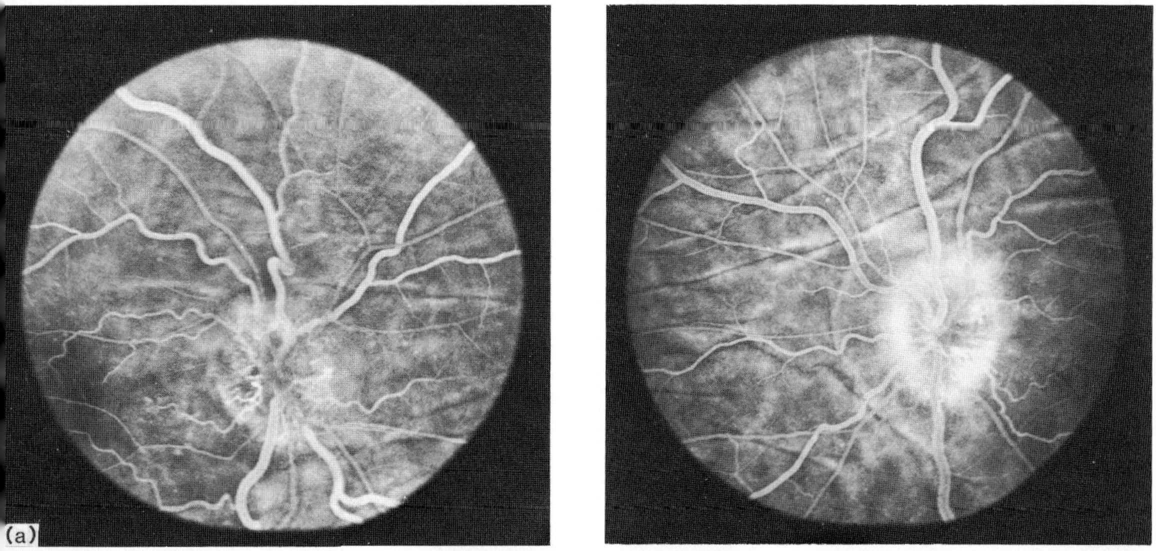

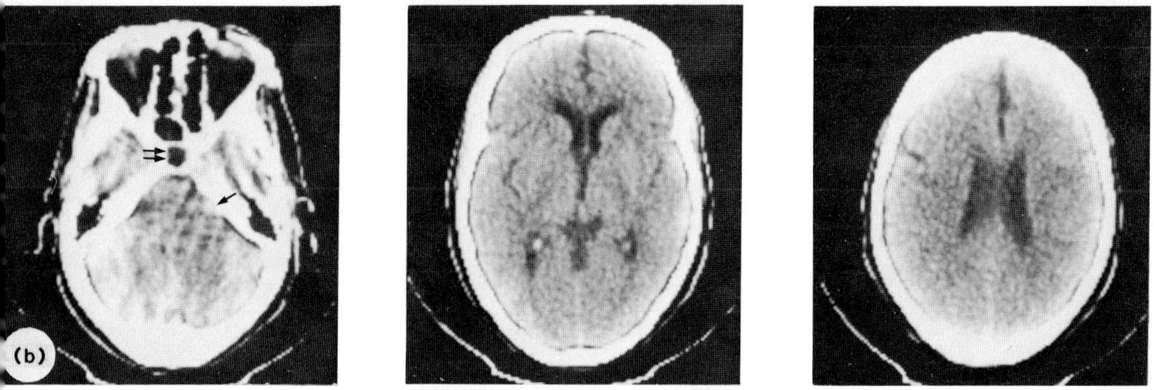

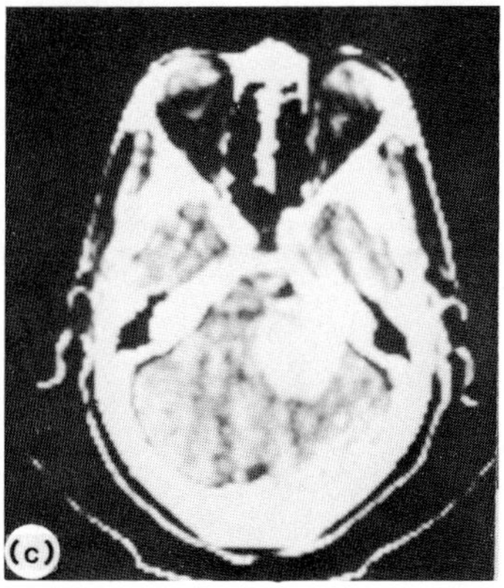

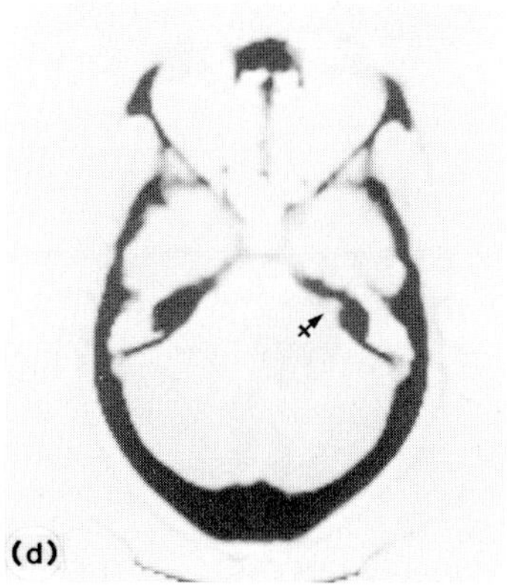

Fig. 5.6 Papilloedema with posterior fossa tumour, without hydrocephalus. A 38-year old man presented with headache and unsteadiness. Examination revealed long-standing papilloedema with opticociliary shunt vessels, choroidal striae and disc leakage on fluorescein angiography (a). In addition he had ataxia and right-sided deafness. CT (b) showed the third and lateral ventricles to be at most minimally enlarged; the temporal horns were not visible. Some fissures and sulci were prominent. The fourth ventricle, however, could not be seen and in the right cerebellopontine angle a small high-attenuation region (arrow) was surrounded by poorly-defined low attenuation. The sellar contents (two arrows) appeared to be of CSF attenuation. After intravenous contrast medium (c) a large cerebellopontine angle mass was seen and it became apparent that the right internal auditory meatus (crossed arrow) was enlarged (d, same section, different window factors). At operation a large acoustic neuroma was removed.

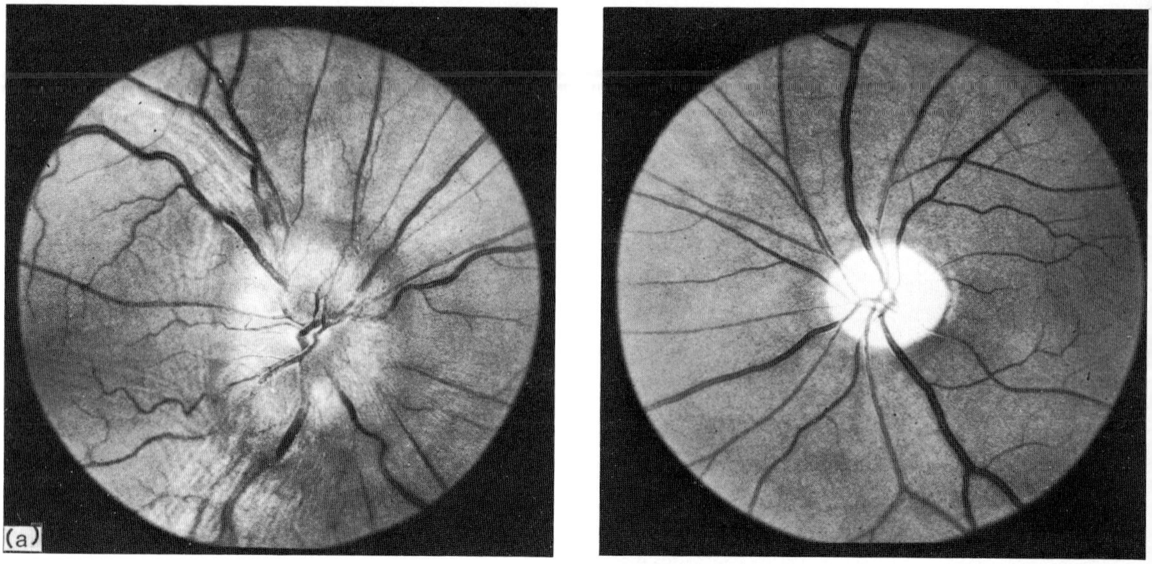

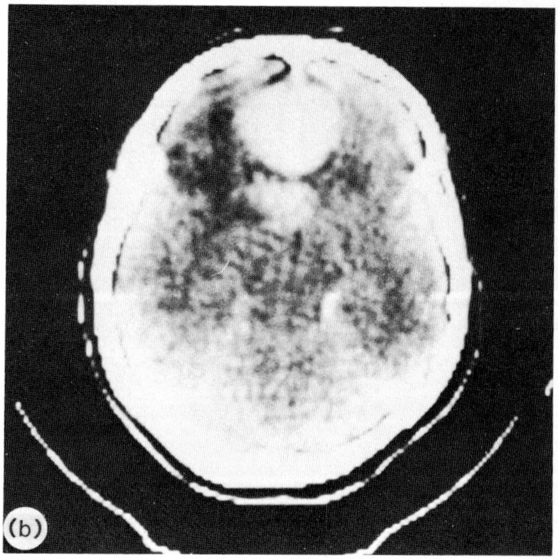

Fig. 5.7 Foster-Kennedy syndrome. A 33-year old woman complained of severe persistent headaches and recent visual loss. Examination revealed advanced optic atrophy on the left and chronic papilloedema on the right. There were no other physical signs. CT revealed a frontal meningioma centrally situated, but extending more to the left side, where there was considerable cerebral oedema. An unusual feature is the bilobular appearance of the tumour.

wide variety of causes may involve extensive investigatory procedures. It is therefore important to eliminate benign congenital lesions, and in a series of patients with pseudopapilloedema, 14% of cases were found to be unilateral (Rosenberg *et al.*, 1979). The most common causes of unilateral disc oedema are local disease of the optic disc, distal optic nerve or sheath. However, orbital disease, orbitocranial processes such as meningioma and granuloma, and raised CSF pressure must be excluded.

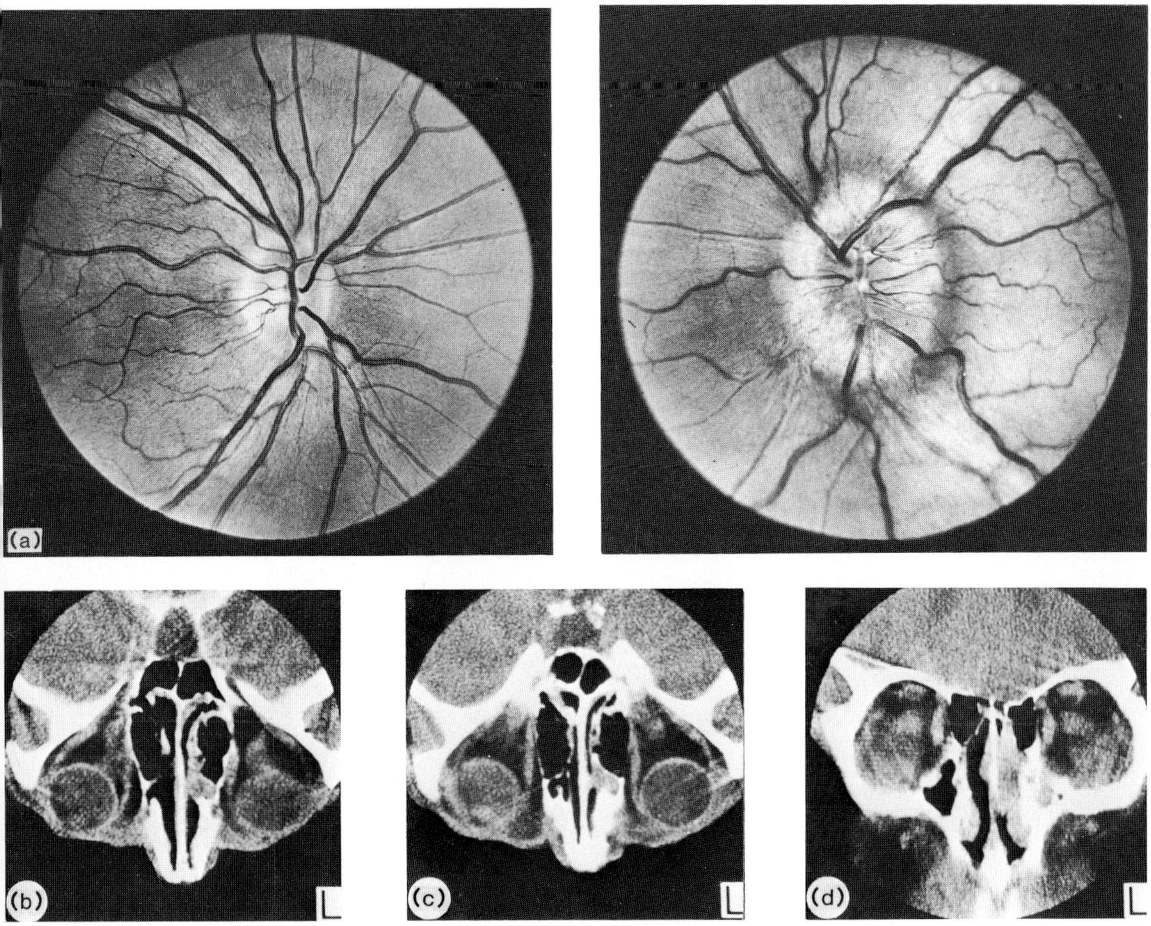

Fig. 5.8 Unilateral papilloedema with bilateral swelling of optic nerves in benign intracranial hypertension. A 34-year old woman with benign intracranial hypertension had papilloedema on the left only (a). CT, however (b,c) showed swollen optic nerves on both sides confirmed by a coronal section (d). Note that, presumably because of exaggerated undulation of the nerves in the vertical plane, neither (b) nor (c) shows either nerve throughout its length. The sella appears empty.

Papilloedema

Unilateral papilloedema may occur with raised intracranial pressure in several different circumstances. Firstly, when a mass lesion compresses the optic nerve or obliterates the nerve sheath on one side, the effects of the raised CSF pressure will not be transmitted to that disc to produce disc oedema and, instead, the disc may be atrophic, with contralateral papilloedema (Foster Kennedy syndrome) (Fig. 5.7). Similarly, one disc may be protected from the effects of raised pressure, but not compressed sufficiently to produce atrophy and this may also indicate a frontal or middle fossa tumour. We have seen a number of

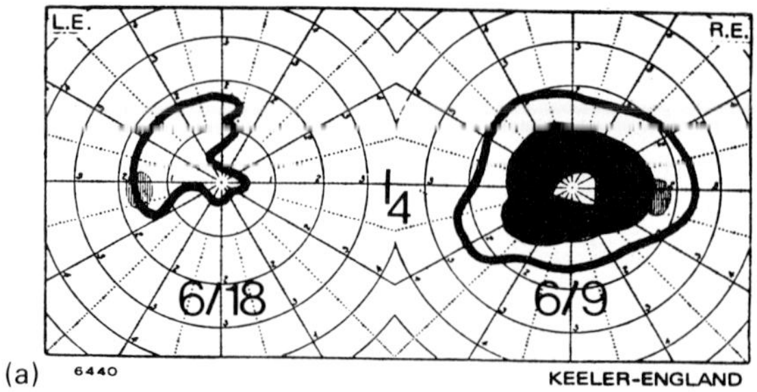

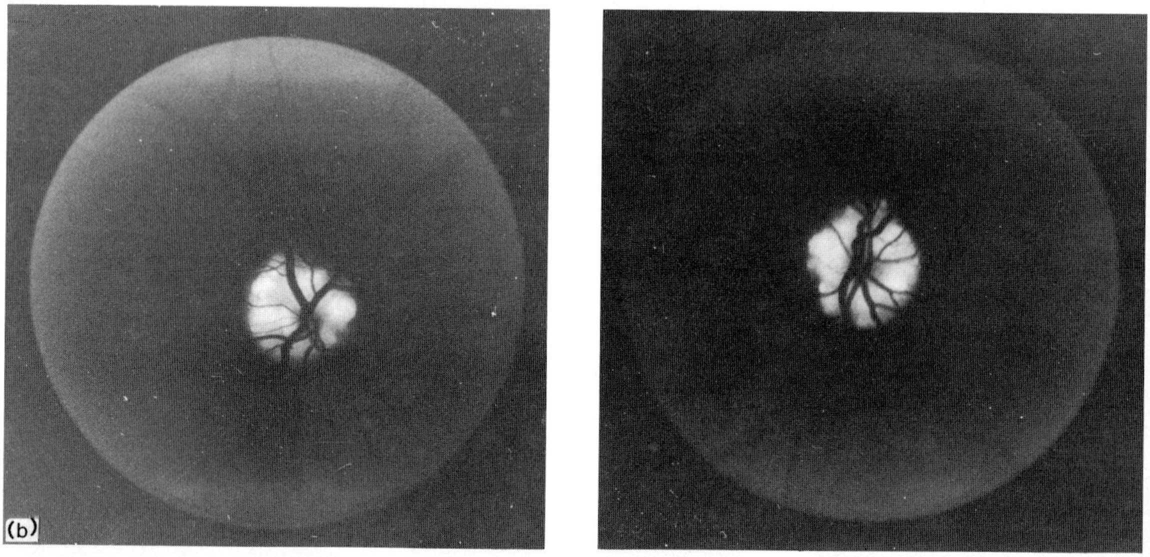

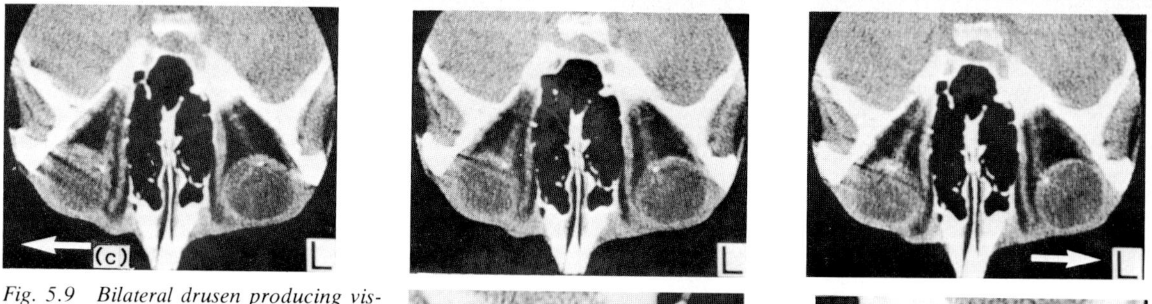

Fig. 5.9 Bilateral drusen producing visual impairment. This 19-year old man has had progressive visual loss in both eyes for many years. Vision at the time of the CT study was 6/9 in the right eye and 6/18 in the left eye, with arcuate defects (a). Examination revealed bilateral drusen with autofluorescence (b). CT confimed the presence of calcification in the nerve heads: (c) centre: in primary position; lateral gaze indicated by arrows; (d) double exposure, showing movement of nerve head and plane of the optic nerves during abduction and adduction (the left moves 7.5 mm, as measured by the computer of the CT scanner).

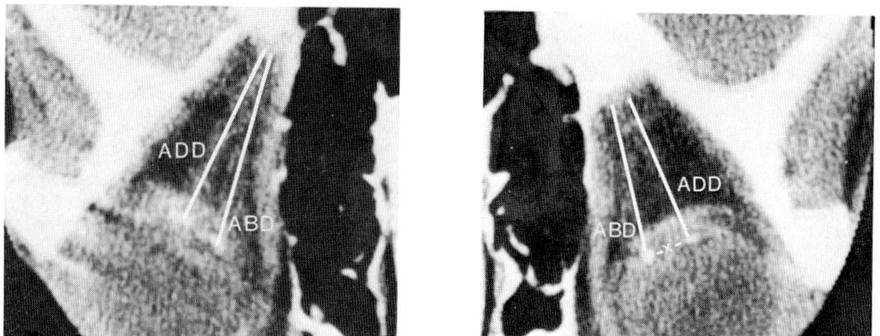

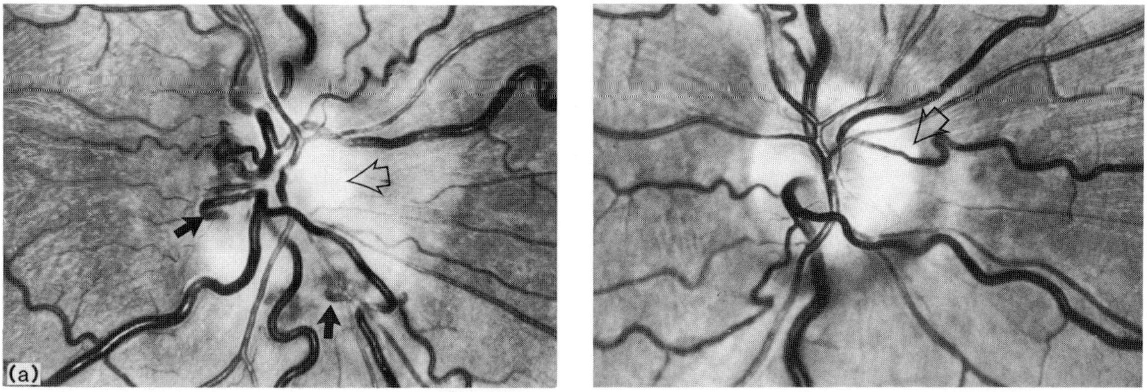

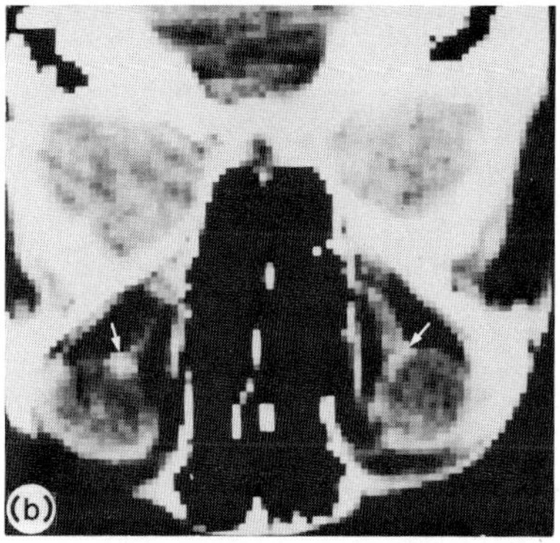

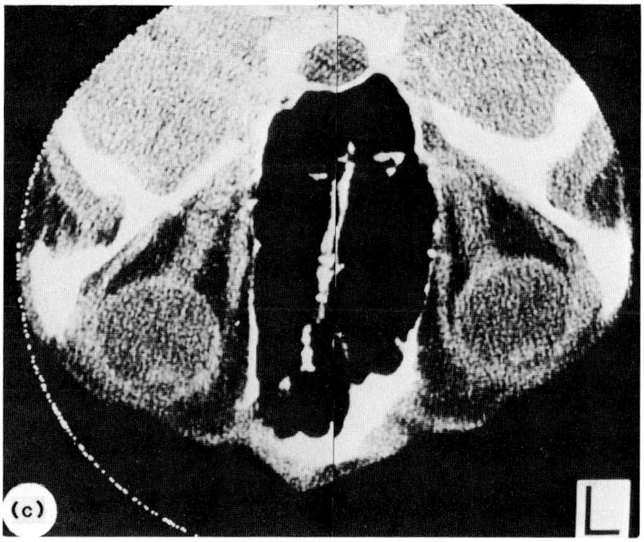

Fig. 5.10 Bilateral drusen with presumed optic nerve sheath meningioma. A 21-year old man had been blind in the right eye since childhood. The left eye was normal. The right optic disc was small and asymmetrical (a). Pale refractile bodies (drusen – open arrow) and many large opticociliary shunt vessels (arrows) were present, while the retinal veins were dilated and tortuous. Multiple drusen were visible on the left (open arrow), but there were no shunt vessels. CT using standard resolution (b) showed densities in both nerve heads, more prominent on the right. They were less obvious on high resolution CT (c, montage of R and L sides), which, however showed both optic nerves to be expanded and slightly dense. Note low attenuation in the sella turcica.

patients with benign intracranial hypertension who presented with unilateral papilloedema (Fig. 5.8) and have attributed this to some defect, possibly congenital, in the patency of the subarachnoid space around the optic nerve on the spared side (Kirkham *et al.*, 1973). Finally, a totally atrophic nerve head does not develop papilloedema, so that any patient with unilateral atrophy who develops raised cerebrospinal fluid pressure will present with unilateral papilloedema.

Congential anomalies of the optic disc

Pseudopapilloedema

The optic disc is variable in size and shape, and when small, with a reduced or absent physiological pit, and with anomalous branching of the retinal arterioles, may resemble papilloedema.

A small full disc, often associated with hypermetropia or astigmatism is the commonest cause of 'pseudopapilloedema' in our experience. The following abnormalities should be considered:

1. Small full discs (with hypermetropia).
2. Large nasal elevation (with myopia).
3. Glial anomalies of the optic disc.
4. Drusen of the disc (i) exposed (ii) buried.
5. Other anomalies, e.g. angiomas, medullated nerve fibres, etc.

Drusen is a term which gives rise to confusion. It is applied to colloid bodies in the pigment epithelium; and to the giant drusen of the optic disc which are seen in tuberous sclerosis. We feel there are advantages in restricting the term to the refractile, lobulated aggregates seen in the disc, which are associated with anomalous vessels and show a propensity for haemorrhage. Such drusen of the disc may remain buried in young children, but tend to emerge during adult life, when confusion with papilloedema may occur. Other ocular abnormalities such as pigmentary retinopathy, angioid streaks or Coats' disease may also be present. Calcification in drusen is found in up to 2% of apparently normal individuals at post-mortem examination, and though the aetiology is unknown, it may represent a form of degeneration of the astrocytes. The calcium deposits may be neither dense nor extensive, but with high resolution CT it is possible to show small, well-defined areas of high attenuation in the region of the nerve head, or just posterior to it, on one or both sides (Fig. 5.9). Standard resolution CT may merely show a rather amorphous area of high attenuation, and since the region of the optic disc may appear of slightly higher attenuation than adjacent sclera in normal subjects, the radiological diagnosis should be made with some caution. CT represents no diagnostic threat to the ophthalmoscope, but in cases of drusen with visual loss a CT scan of the optic nerves may be indicated to exclude the rare bilateral sheath meningioma (Fig. 5.10).

Tilting of the optic disc is a congenital anomaly, found in about 3.5% of normal subjects. The disc appearances are variable, but a 'crescent', due to disparity between the size of the retinal and scleral openings, is visible. There may also be a discrepancy in the elevation of opposite sides of the disc and anomalous retinal vessels may be present. These appearances can mimic papilloedema. Visual field defects (usually an upper altitudinal scotoma) are present in about 50% of cases, probably caused by hypoplasia of nerve fibres (Dorrell, 1978). The CT appearances in a single patient said to have this condition were described by Quevillon *et al.* (1977): 'ectasia' of the inferior nasal quadrants of the globes was reported, although the published images were not striking.

Local causes

The classical clinical features of optic neuritis, ischaemic papillopathy and uveitis are easily diagnosed and represent the majority of cases of unilateral disc oedema. Visual acuity is usually reduced in these conditions and field loss can be demonstrated. Difficulty is experienced with infiltration of the nerve (sarcoid, reticulum cell sarcoma, nasopharyngeal tumours, optic nerve tumours, etc.). The disc swelling may have identical characteristics in all of these conditions, so that particular emphasis must be placed on the history and other aspects of the clinical or ophthalmological examination. Causes of local disc oedema may be classified in the following manner:

1. Inflammatory (a) optic nerve – papillitis;
   (b) ocular – uveitis.
2. Vascular (a) Ischaemic (arterial occlusion, e.g. ischaemic papillopathy);
   (b) congestive (venous occlusion, e.g. central vein occlusion).
3. Primary tumours of the nerve sheath (meningioma or optic nerve glioma).
4. Secondary infiltration by granuloma (e.g. sarcoid) or tumour (carcinoma, lymphoma, leukaemia etc).
5. Ocular hypotony.

5.3 OPTIC NEURITIS

Optic neuritis may be attributable to a wide variety of causes, but sudden central, monocular visual loss with pain on ocular movements is usually due to demyelination of the optic nerves. The commonest cause is multiple sclerosis, but postexanthematous optic neuropathy, which has a better visual prognosis, may also be seen. An early suggestion that plaques of demyelination could be detected by CT within the optic nerves of patients thought to have multiple sclerosis, has not been corroborated by us or by most other groups. Eyerman, Archer and Mayes (1976) apparently detected hyperdense beads or bulges alternating with low density constrictions and isodense swellings of the nerves in retrobulbar neuritis; their report did not include illustrations. The apparent abnormalities detected by some workers may have represented partial volume and other artefacts rather than plaques.

Subsequent work by Mastaglia, Black, Cala and Collins (1977) indicated that the presence of cerebral plaques, seen as white matter low-attenuation lesions (Fig. 5.11) was perhaps more useful for confirming the diagnosis of multiple sclerosis. Lesions were seen in 60% of cases with established disease, 50% of patients with early, probable or latent disease, and in only 14% of patients suspected of having this disease. Thirty per cent of

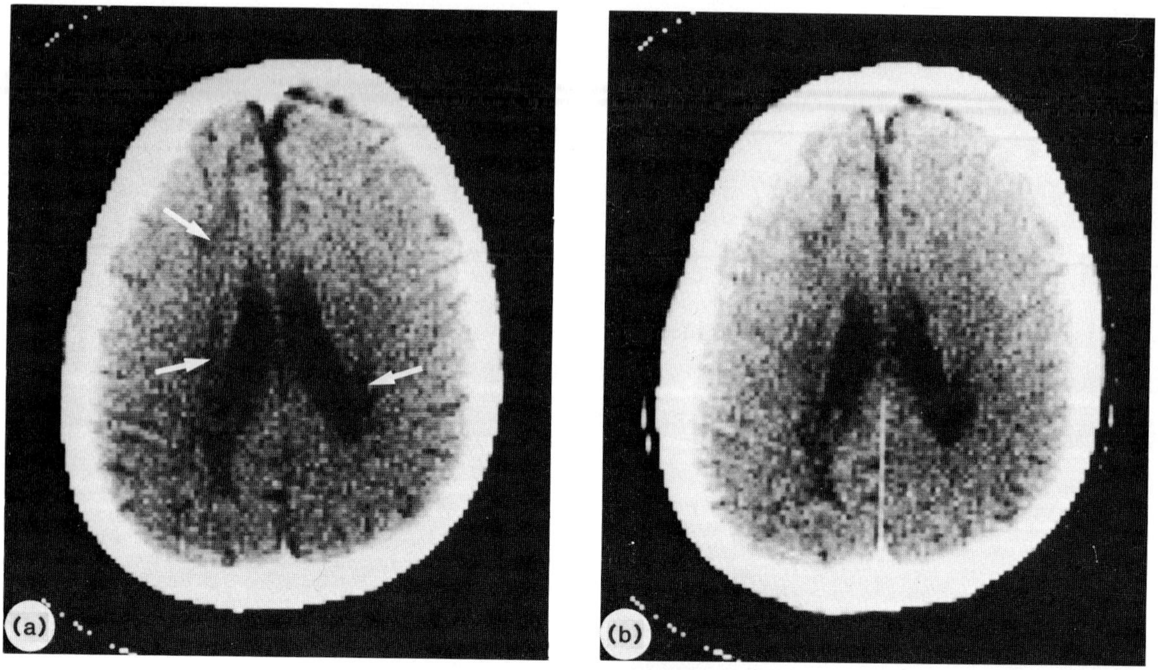

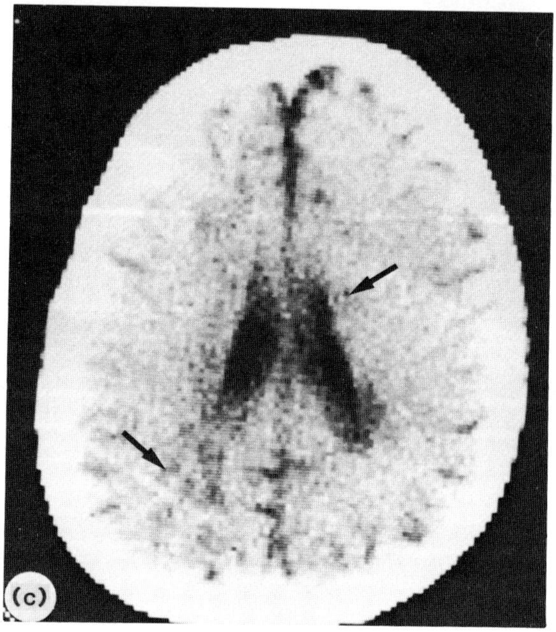

Fig. 5.11 Multiple sclerosis. This 31-year old man developed personality problems one year before the CT study, rapidly followed by lower limb paraesthesia, internuclear ophthalmoplegia and ataxia. Examination showed facial myokymia, ataxia and long tract signs. CSF proteins (39 mg%) included 20% IgG, while visual evoked responses indicated delayed conduction in the right optic nerve. CT (a) showed at least three zones of low attenuation in the deep white matter (arrows). These showed no contrast enhancement (b). The cortical sulci were prominent. After breathing stable xenon for 15 min, (c, same window width and level as a and b) the white matter lesions were more clearly seen and others became evident (arrows).

patients were thought at CT to show 'optic nerve lesions'. Additional neurophysiological evaluation (VER plus somatosensory evoked responses and/or saccadic velocities) increased the positive diagnostic rates in the three groups from 91%, 79% and 42% to 100%, 94% and 57% respectively. Thickening or increased tortuosity of the nerves may be seen in optic neuritis (Fig. 5.12); we have seen one patient in whom a thick nerve assumed normal proportions concurrently with visual improvement (Fig. 5.13).

Salvolini *et al.* (1978) claimed that the nerves may be expanded in Leber's hereditary optic atrophy. This could be explicable either on the basis of neuronal swelling in the acute stage or in relation to the arachnoidal hyperplasia which has been documented in this condition (Fig. 5.19 p. 178). Our limited experience has not confirmed thickening of the nerves, and there may be a need for scans in potential patients from afflicted families to assess the validity of this concept.

5.4 ISCHAEMIC PAPILLOPATHY

This condition may be divided into two clinical groups:

1. Severe infarction of the disc, as seen with giant cell arteritis.
2. Less severe involvement as part of a generalized microvascular disturbance.

Patients in either group may show associated cerebral ischaemia with areas of infarction or cerebral atrophy. Viscosity may play an important part in the events leading up to infarction of the disc, and a few patients have definite polycythaemia rubra vera. Some patients with this latter condition show more or less extensive low attenuation areas in the cerebral white matter, particularly marked in the frontal periventricular and anterior capsular areas. These changes are thought to represent cerebral ischaemia and may be correlated with the findings of reduced cerebral blood flow which we have seen in some patients with ischaemic papillopathy.

5.5 INFLAMMATORY DISC DISEASE AND INFILTRATION

Inflammatory swelling of the disc may rarely occur without associated involvement of the vitreous or anterior uvea, but disc swelling is usually part of the picture of a panuveitis. The disc swelling in inflammatory disease is ill defined and on fluorescein angiography there is minimal dilatation of the superficial peripapillary capillary plexus characteristic of other types of disc swelling, and the presence of concomitant macular oedema is almost pathognomic. CT may show non-specific involvement of the optic nerve or cerebral granulomata of, for example, sarcoid

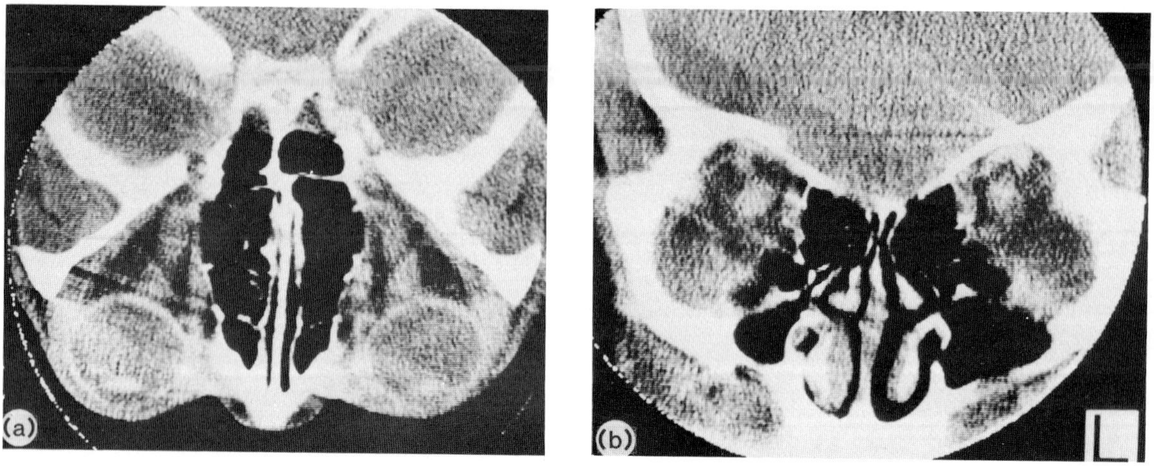

Fig. 5.12 *Optic neuritis.* A 19-year old black West Indian girl gave a history of progressive visual impairment; within four weeks of onset of symptoms she had no perception of light in either eye, with absent pupil responses to light. Eye movements were disconjugate, indicating mesencephalic involvement, and there was sensory disturbance on the left cheek and lips. CSF protein was 65 mg% with 25% IgG. An air encephalogram was normal. CT (a,b) showed optic nerves which appeared slightly swollen and irregular. Within three days of steroid therapy vision improved and two weeks later the patient could walk around the ward. The pupillary light response had returned and the conjugate gaze paresis was less marked.

or tuberculosis. The association of uveitis with cerebral involvement is rare in Reiter's disease, ankylosing spondylitis or other diseases associated with HLA B27. Cerebral involvement may however be seen with Behçet's disease, usually in the form of infarction. We have seen one patient with biopsy-proven cerebral Whipple's disease who showed multiple well-defined areas of low attenuation, affecting both white and grey matter. There was little mass effect; intravenous contrast medium produced considerable enhancement. The association of panuveitis with cerebral involvement by reticulum cell sarcoma or microglioma and the value of cranial CT in this context are illustrated by Fig. 5.18.

5.6 TUMOURS OF THE OPTIC NERVE

Primary neoplasms of the optic nerve are rare; gliomas of the optic nerve, which form about 80% of such tumours, have an incidence approximately 0.5% that of malignant melanoma. Meningiomas form most of the remainder, while fibromas and cysts are exceedingly rare. Secondary tumours of the optic nerve may be the result of direct infiltration from the adjacent paranasal sinuses, or represent spread from the intracranial subarachnoid space. Less commonly they are truly metastatic.

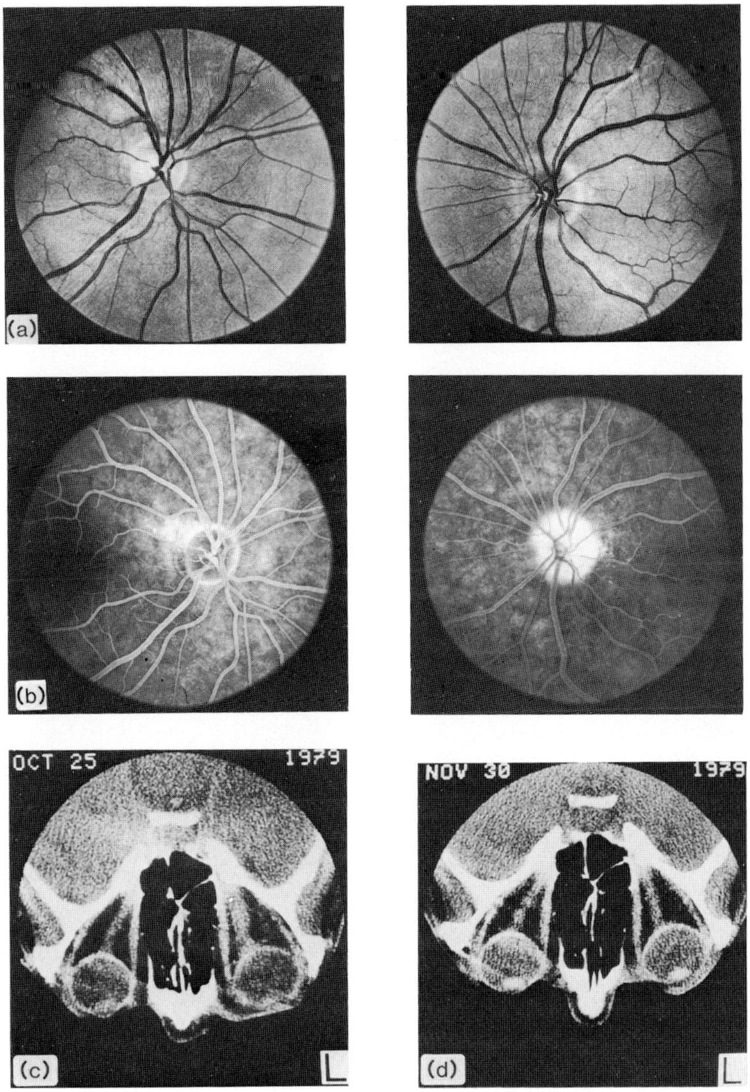

Fig. 5.13 *Optic neuritis*. The vision in the left eye of a 45-year old woman suddenly deteriorated to counting fingers. There was a central scotoma. The left optic disc was swollen (a) and showed leakage at fluorescein angiography (b) NB, left eye on right of page). The left optic nerve was clearly swollen at CT (c) (NOI–L: 25% R: 15%), and was slightly irregular. Systematic steroid therapy produced complete clinical and radiological resolution in one month (NOI – both sides 15%). A further CT scan showed resolution of the nerve swelling (d).

Optic nerve glioma

This tumour usually presents before the age of 10 years, and is much more common in girls than boys. Presenting signs include visual loss, often unilateral, and proptosis. The degree of visual loss and proptosis is extremely variable; it may be rapid, although pain is not usually a feature. Despite marked proptosis, ophthalmoplegia is rare, indicating the intraconal localization of the lesion. The optic disc changes at presentation range from marked disc oedema to atrophy, and are determined by the

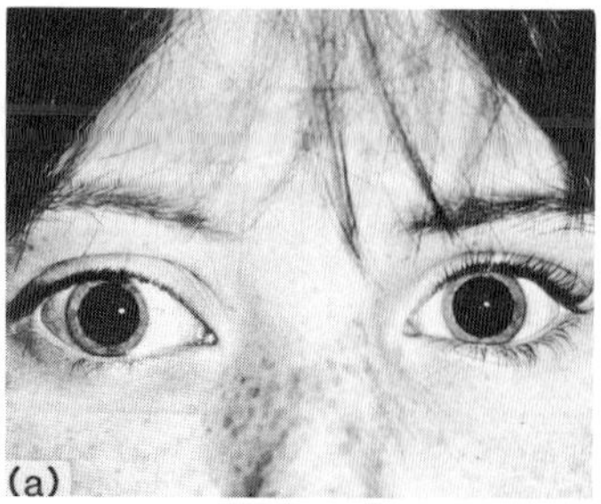

(a)

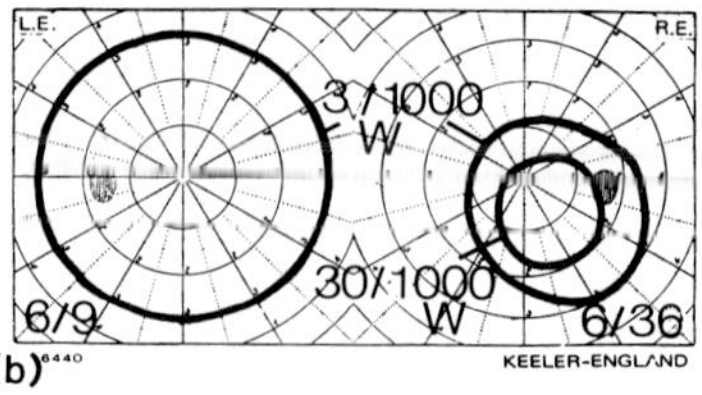

(b)

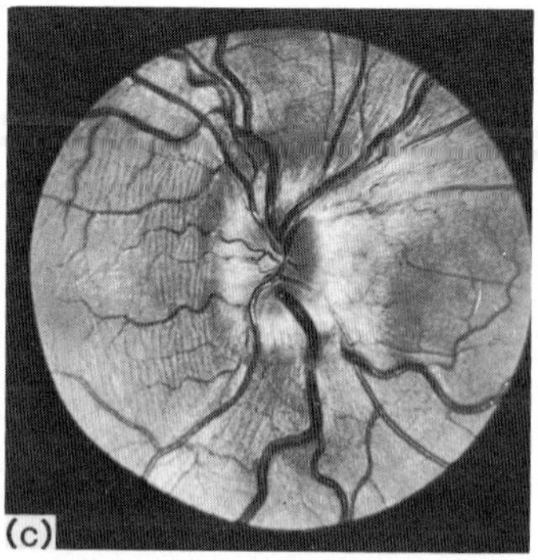

(c)

Fig. 5.14 Optic nerve glioma. A 9-year old girl was noted to have poor vision in the right eye, with mild proptosis (a). Visual acuity was grossly impaired and the right eye field was constricted (b). In 1975 the right disc was swollen with retinal striae and thickened neurones (c) but by 1976 it had become atrophic with loss of nerve fibres; the left eye remained normal (d). Steroids produced some improvement and radiotherapy was also given. CT (d) showed a grossly expanded optic nerve, enlarging the orbit. The right optic canal appeared normal in size. Subsequent scans up to four years later have shown no change, and there is no evidence of intracranial tumour (f). This patient's acuity and field have remained static over five years.

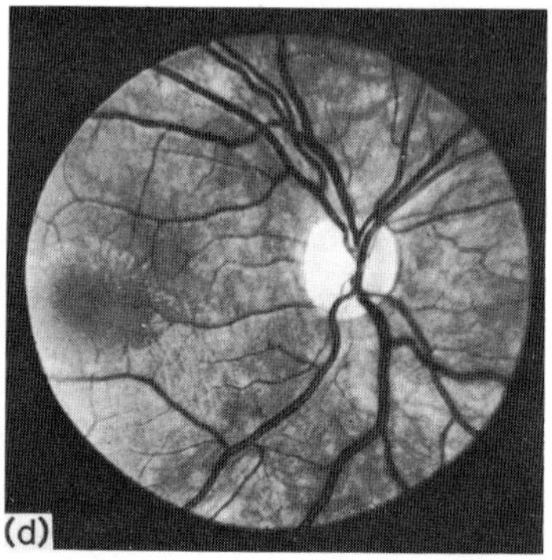

(d)

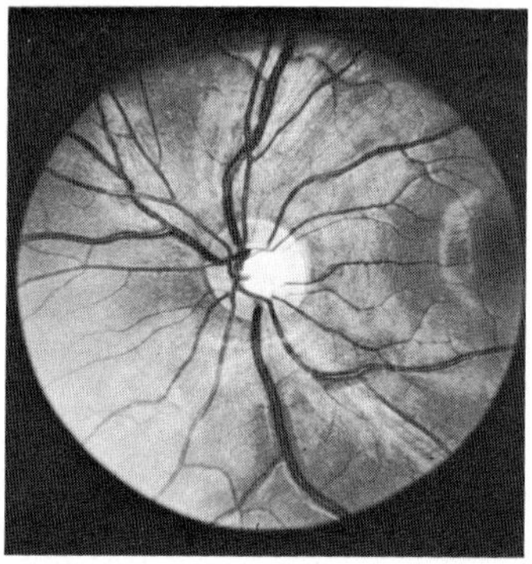

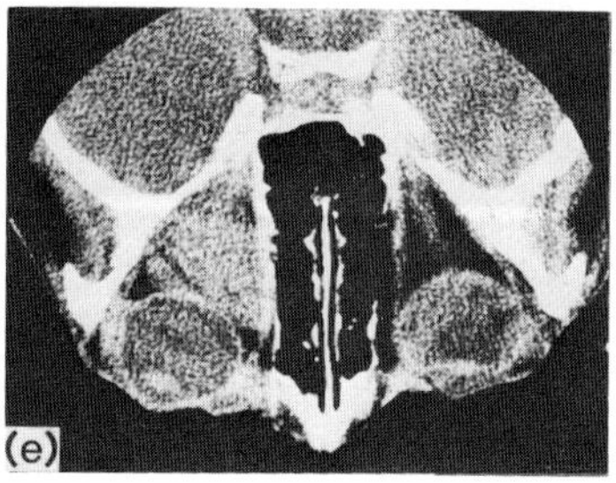

(e)

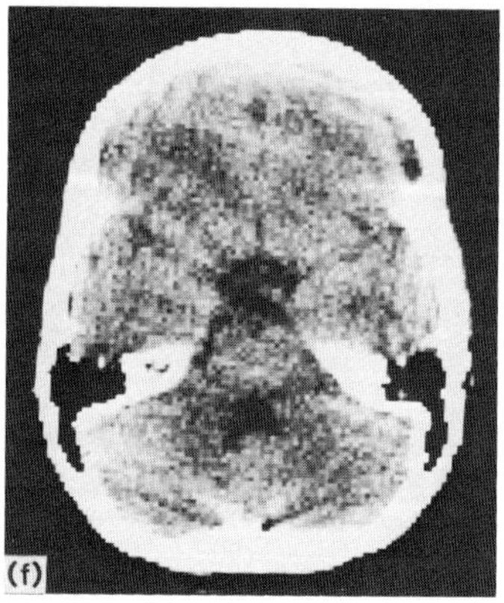

(f)

situation and duration of the tumour. Disc oedema suggests that the tumour involves the distal optic nerve, but progressive damage to neurones produces atrophy, and opticociliary shunt vessels may be the only sign of past disc oedema.

Careful systemic and ocular examination is necessary because of the association with neurofibromatosis. A family history should be sought, as the latter is a dominant condition and examination of the patient and family for café au lait spots is necessary. Five or more café au lait spots with well-defined borders seem necessary for conclusive diagnosis, and plexiform neuroma should also be sought. Endocrine signs of growth abnormality, precocious or retarded puberty, and a history of polyuria or polydipsia are important, as they indicate hypothalamic spread.

Ocular signs include iris neurofibromata, thickened corneal nerves, a predisposition to congenital glaucoma and fundus lesions, often pigmented; occasionally bizarre phacomata may be seen. Pulsation of the globe due to deficiency of the sphenoid neurofibromatosis with phaeochromocytoma and polyglandular syndromes lends further complexity to this fascinating entity.

Optic nerve gliomas are usually benign pilocytic astrocytomas, bone may be difficult to detect clinically, but tonometry shows diagnostic movement of the applanation head. The association of but the pathological appearances form a spectrum, with a few cases having a more malignant course, and although this usually occurs in adults (Hoyt *et al.*, 1973) we have seen one case in a child. The rapid onset of symptoms does not usually indicate malignancy but probably represents ischaemia or metabolic decompensation of the tumour, as evidenced by the mucoid deposition documented pathologically. Debate still arises concerning the ability of these tumours to spread, or whether adjacent neural tissue has a propensity to undergo gliomatous change. Accurate CT observation may assist in the controversy, but for practical purposes the majority of tumours behave in a benign manner, although a few have the potential for a more malignant course. CT provides the best technique for evaluating the extent of the lesion, including possible involvement of the chiasm and hypothalamus. Systemic steroids may improve vision and reduce proptosis and there is some evidence that radiotherapy may reduce the size of some lesions; once again, CT control is helpful. Excision seems of value for cosmetic reasons when the eye is blind and protuberant.

CT characteristics (Fig. 5.14)

By the time a patient with an optic nerve glioma has a CT study there is almost invariably definite and marked expansion of the nerve. In early cases this expansion may be localized, but generally the entire intraorbital portion appears increased in diameter. The expansion is smooth, giving the nerve a bulbous appearance; it may reach 2 cm or more in diameter. The bony walls of the orbit are thin and expanded. When the mass is large, it is often necessary to confirm by means of coronal sections that a normal optic nerve is not being hidden by an extraneural retrobulbar mass.

Optic nerve gliomas have attenuation coefficients similar to or slightly higher than those of normal brain; very occasionally they may show calcification. Increase in attenuation after intravenous contrast media is not a striking feature.

Since in some cases it is desirable to resect the affected nerve for cosmetic reasons (progression being in general very slow), it may be necessary to demonstrate whether the intracanalicular and/or intracranial portions of the nerve are also enlarged. Detection of minor enlargement of the optic canal is possible by CT, but is probably more accurate by conventional hypocycloidal tomography. When enlargement is more marked, increase in transverse diameter of the canal, which appears filled by brain-attenuation soft tissue, is evident. CT is probably the method of choice for detection of enlargement of the intracranial optic nerves and chiasm and intrathecal metrizamide scanning may have a role in this context. It should, however, be noted that Byrd *et al.* (1978) found pneumoencephalography to be more sensitive for intracranial optic nerve involvement. Careful clinical examination and CT screening must be made of the contralateral optic nerve, both at the initial and subsequent follow-up examinations.

Widespread basal arachnoidal hyperplasia, which has been described in association with gliomas generally, is also a well recognized feature of optic nerve gliomas both in biopsy and autopsy specimens (Hogan and Zimmerman, 1962). This is not surprising as the neural tissue of the optic nerve is exposed to more arachnoid tissue than any other part of the central nervous system. Lindenberg *et al.* (1973) emphasized the association of arachnoidal hyperplasia with gliomas, and even speculated that proliferating oligodendrocytes may produce a growth factor. Arachnoidal hyperplasia may be so extensive as to mimic a tumour (Sanders *et al.*, 1965).

Management

Patients with optic nerve glioma should have full orbital and cerebral CT examination at the time of diagnosis, particularly those with neurofibromatosis. CT may show other lesions in the cerebral hemispheres which have failed to declare themselves clinically (Chapter 4). Repeat studies can be dictated by the clinical course, but in view of the possible risk of radiation exposure as few scans should be done as appears practical (one patient at the National Hospital had a documented glioma of the optic chiasm for 40 years).

Optic nerve sheath meningioma

Meningiomas result from proliferation of the meningoendothelial cells of the arachnoid and within the orbit may arise from the periorbita, in the vicinity of the optic canal, or rarely in relation to the muscle cone. The present discussion is confined to those which appear to arise primarily from the optic nerve sheath. Nerve sheath meningiomas represent less than 20% of optic nerve tumours and, unlike optic nerve gliomas, do not present with sudden loss of vision in young females. An association with

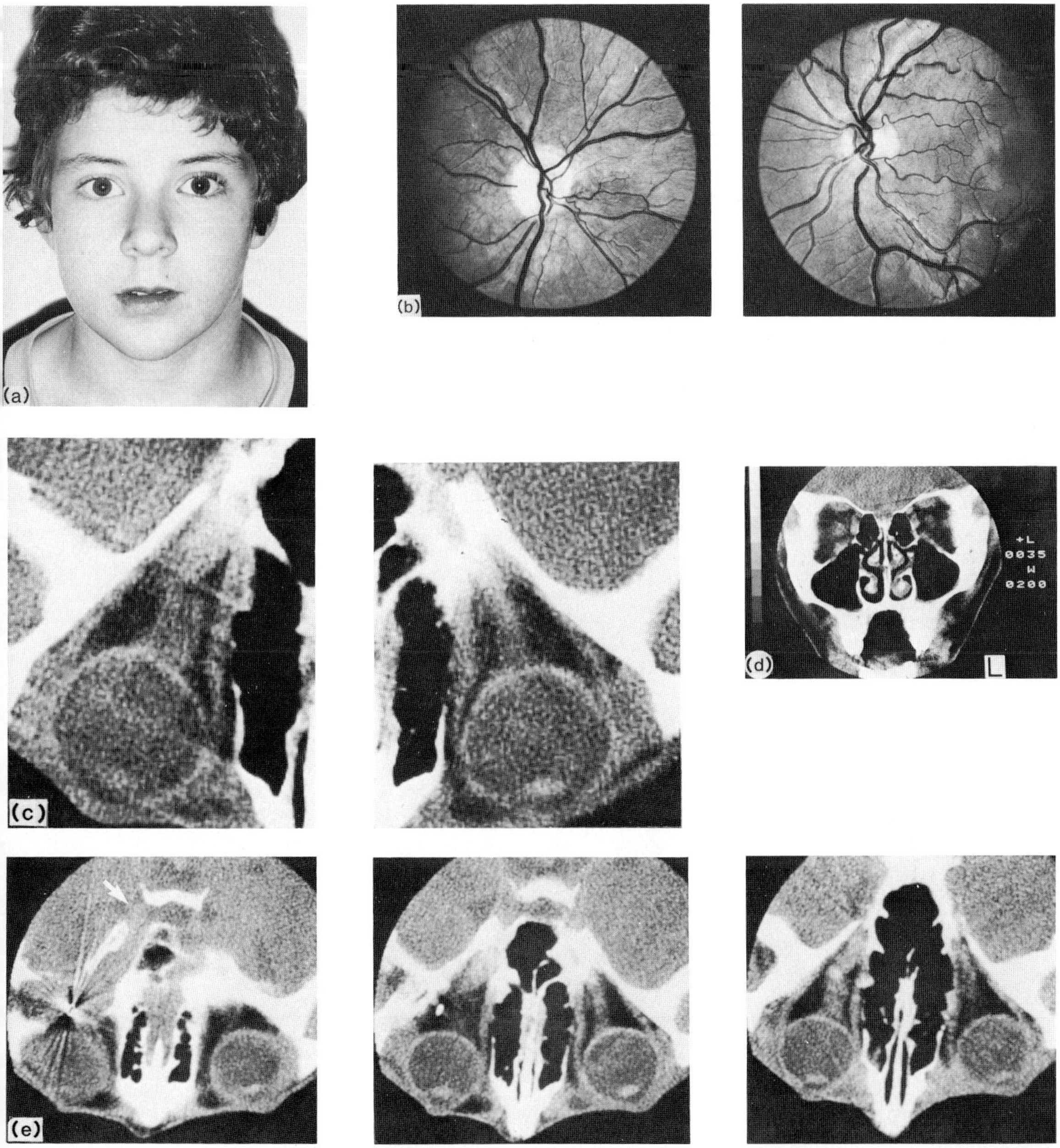

Fig. 5.15 Optic nerve sheath meningioma. This 14-year old boy presented with progressive visual loss in the right eye for several years. There was slight proptosis (a) and he could count fingers in the temporal field. The right optic disc appeared atrophic with loss of neurones (b); the left eye was entirely normal. CT (c) showed a widened, angular optic nerve, with some expansion of the orbital apex; in coronal sections (d), the nerve appeared slightly denser than its fellow. Frontal craniotomy with deroofing of the optic canal revealed a meningioma of the optic nerve sheath, with intracranial extension: six months postoperatively acuity was reduced to hand movements, proptosis was increased and mild ophthalmoplegia persisted. Further scans (e,f) showed little change in the size of the tumour, while demonstration of the intracranial extension (arrow) was unconvincing.

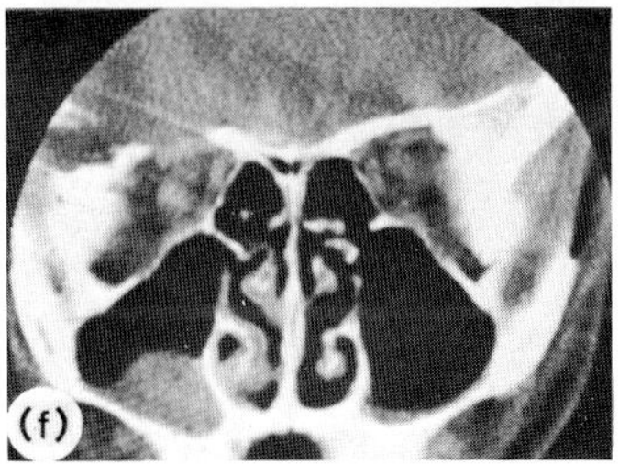

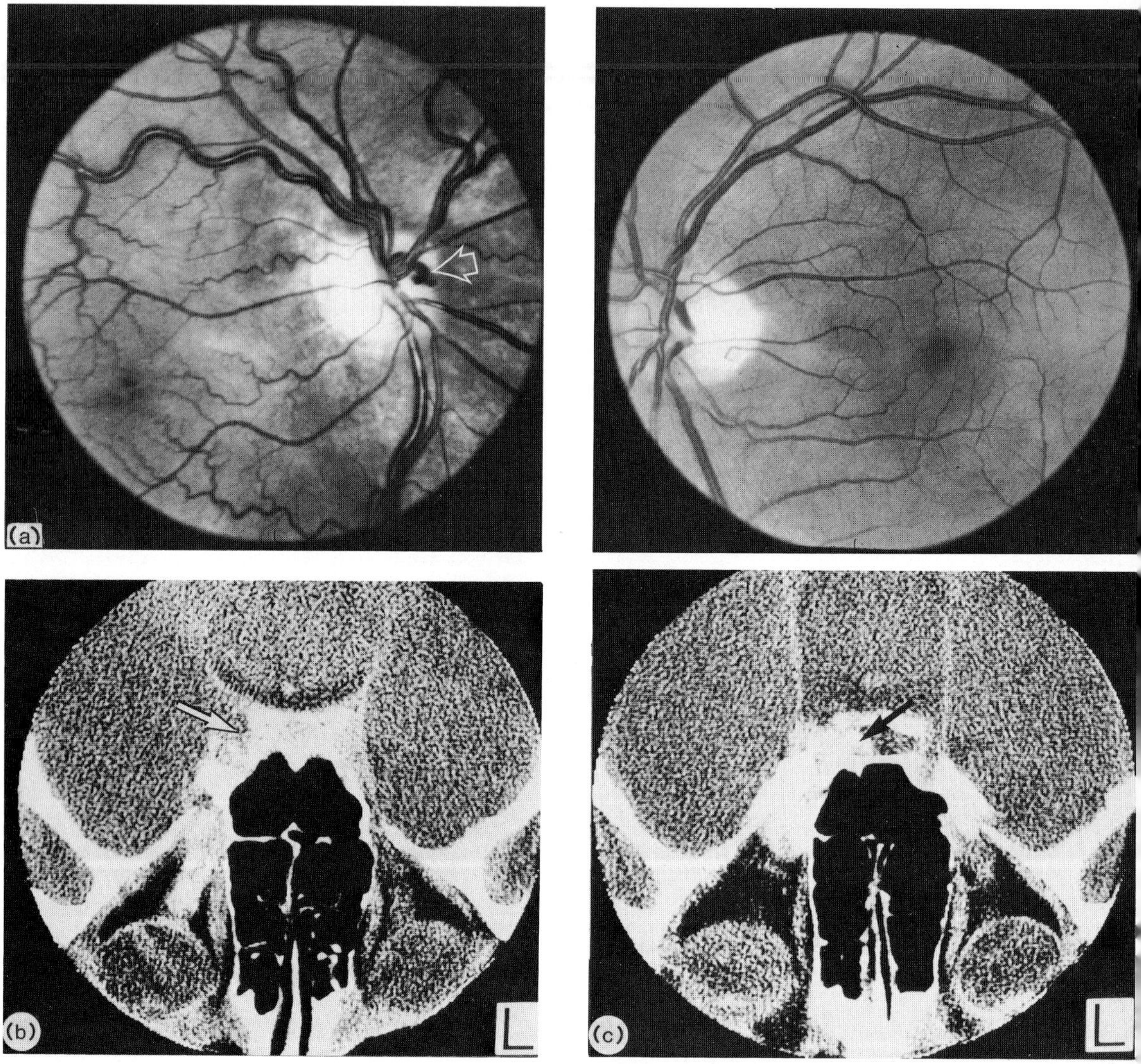

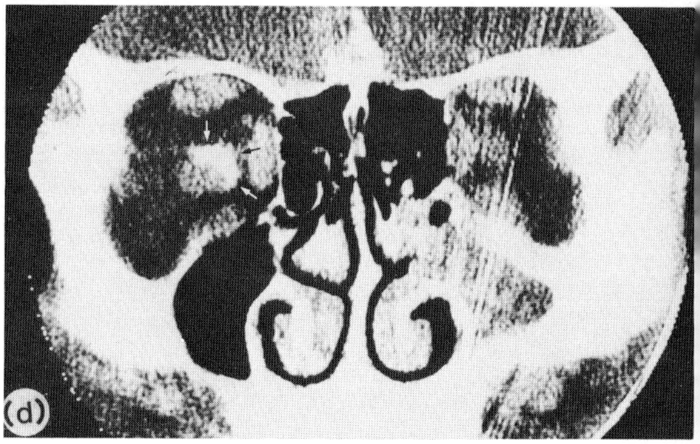

Fig. 5.16 Optic nerve sheath meningioma (presumed). A 34-year old man had been blind in the right eye for 30 years. Examination showed minor perception of light on the right with a reduced pupillary response. There was no proptosis and movements were full. The right disc was atrophic with an opticociliary shunt vessel (open arrow) and the retinal veins were dilated and tortuous with marked loss of retinal neurones (a). The left eye was completely normal, clinically and electrophysiologically. CT showed a densely calcified optic nerve on the right side (b), with calcification extending intracranially and appearing to lie within the sella turcica, almost reaching the midline (c, arrow). Coronal sections (d) confirmed that the calcification was circumferential (small arrows). After intravenous contrast medium, a filling defect was noted in the right cavernous sinus (arrow in b). The left maxillary antrum was opaque. The patient was managed conservatively, and has remained static for four years.

neurofibromatosis has been suggested but our experience has not provided confirmation.

Presentation is usually with progressive visual loss, though some patients present with amaurotic attacks related to ocular position. Fluorescein angiography in these patients shows delayed ocular perfusion during amaurosis with particular delay of the short ciliary system. General neurological examination is usually negative and ocular examination shows reduced acuity and central or arcuate field defects. The optic disc changes are variable and range from florid disc oedema, through chronic disc oedema with shunt vessels, to optic disc pallor alone. The degree of disc swelling is related to the location and duration of the tumour and if opticociliary shunt vessels are present they indicate optic nerve sheath involvement. Disc oedema may be present for many years but subsides as progressive neuronal loss occurs to produce an atrophic disc. Opticocilary shunt vessels indicate past disc oedema, and provide venous return for retinal and optic disc blood via the choroidal system.

This tumour is seen in adults (often men) in the middle decades of life, and a history of poor vision is often present from schooldays, suggesting these are benign lesions. Two patients under the age of 15 years have received surgery at the National Hospital over the past ten years, and only continued observation will indicate whether this surgical intrusion was to their long-term benefit. The more aggressive pattern in some instances in childhood is well documented, though our experience of this is limited.

Bilateral nerve sheath meningiomas rarely occur and CT facilitates this diagnosis. We have seen one case with drusen of the disc and bilateral nerve sheath meningiomas (Fig. 5.10), which poses interesting speculation about their relationship to each other. Diagnosis, however, depends on the clinical picture, as biopsy of the nerve sheath has led to erroneous diagnosis in the past, in relationship to the wide variety of conditions which produce arachnoid hyperplasia and psammoma bodies (*vide infra*).

These tumours tend to spread in a sheath-like fashion along and around the optic nerve, but do not invade it. They may, however, compress the nerve and render it ischaemic, either by infiltration of small blood vessels or by promoting endothelial cell hypertrophy. CT usually shows a nerve which is slightly increased in diameter, sometimes deformed and definitely, often strikingly, increased in attenuation coefficients, showing a further increase after intravenous contrast medium (Fig. 5.15). Calcification is present in some advanced cases and may be seen to involve primarily the periphery of the nerve (Fig. 5.16). The calcification tends to occur in psammoma bodies, and as these are associated with 'benign' tumours, a more benign course may be envisaged, and conservative management recommended.

As in cases of glioma, a careful examination of the size of the optic canal on the affected side must be made. When meningiomas spread through the optic canal, an area of abnormal enhancement after intravenous contrast medium may be evidence of intracranial tumour; it is, however, important not to mistake the normal enhancement of the basal venous sinuses, particularly the cavernous sinus, for intracranial extension of the tumour.

We have seen one case of non-specific granuloma involving the optic nerve which closely mimicked a nerve sheath meningioma (Fig. 6.34). With intravenous contrast medium, however, there was spread of the enhancement around the posterior surface of the globe, a feature we have not observed with optic nerve tumours.

Other optic nerve tumours

Melanomas

Malignant melanoma can very rarely arise from uveal tissues within the anterior portion of the optic nerve. We have seen one such case in the earliest days of orbital CT examination; the studies merely showed a thickened nerve of increased attenuation.

Fibromas

Fibromas and other primary tumours of the optic nerve are documented, but are excessively rare. Lloyd and Ambrose (1977) examined two patients with proven 'cystic hygromas of the optic nerve', but did not describe the CT appearances; their comments suggest that the examinations were regarded as negative.

Metastases (Figs. 5.17 and 5.18)

Metastases, usually from lung or breast primary tumours, may infiltrate the optic disc or optic nerve. When it occurs anteriorly in the nerve, this infiltration produces marked disc oedema with extensive peripapillary changes and CT demonstrates gross thickening of the nerve (Fig. 5.16). Malignant infiltration of the optic nerve is, however, more common in the region of the optic canal, with involvement of the meninges. Patients present with rapid visual loss in one or both eyes. Diagnosis is difficult because fundus examination is usually normal, and CSF examination may also be within normal limits. CT shows no space-occupying lesion, but necropsy reveals infiltration of the optic nerve and the sheaths in the region of the optic canal.

CT demonstration of expansion of the intraorbital optic nerves has been described in two patients known to be suffering from leukaemia, who developed blurred vision, disc oedema and retrobulbar pain (Tourje and Gold, 1977). In both cases the

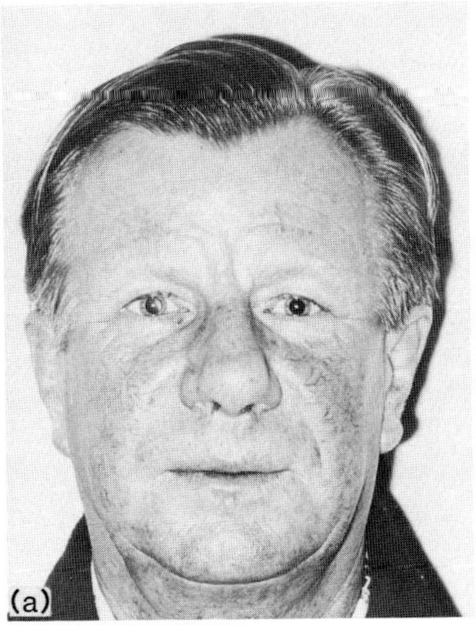

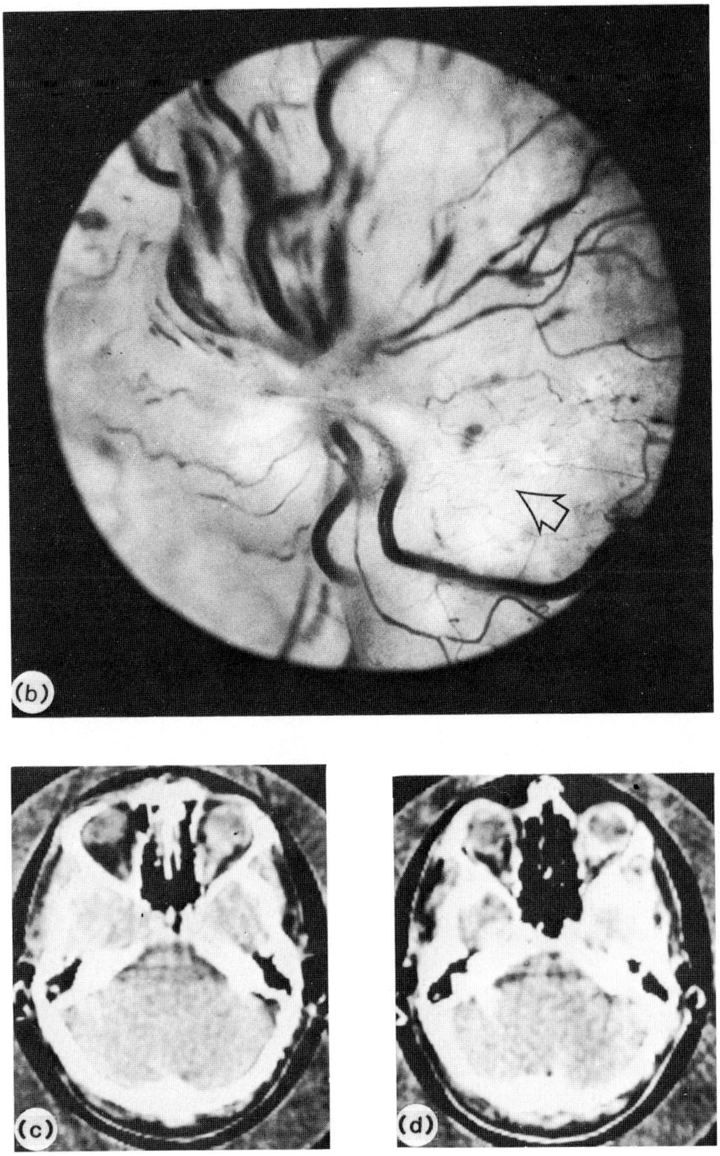

Fig. 5.17 Carcinoma metastatic to optic nerve. Visual loss in the right eye of this 58-year old man progressed to no perception of light in three weeks. There was an abnormal light reflex (a) and fundoscopy showed a grossly swollen optic disc, with elevation of the peripapillary retina (b). Tumour was present in the pigment epithelium and retina (open arrow), confirmed by fluorescein angiography. Dilated veins and superficial haemorrhages were present. CT (c, before and d, after intravenous contrast medium) showed an expanded right optic nerve, with intense enhancement spreading around the posterior surface of the globe. The patient died shortly afterwards with dissemination from a carcinoma of his lung.

clinical changes were unilateral, but in one patient, both nerves were thickened. A follow up study after treatment showed an apparent return to normality in the patient with unilateral changes. A similar picture of a dense, expanded optic nerve (showing no change with intravenous contrast medium), due to leukaemic infiltration, was reported by Price and Danziger (1979) in a patient with slight proptosis.

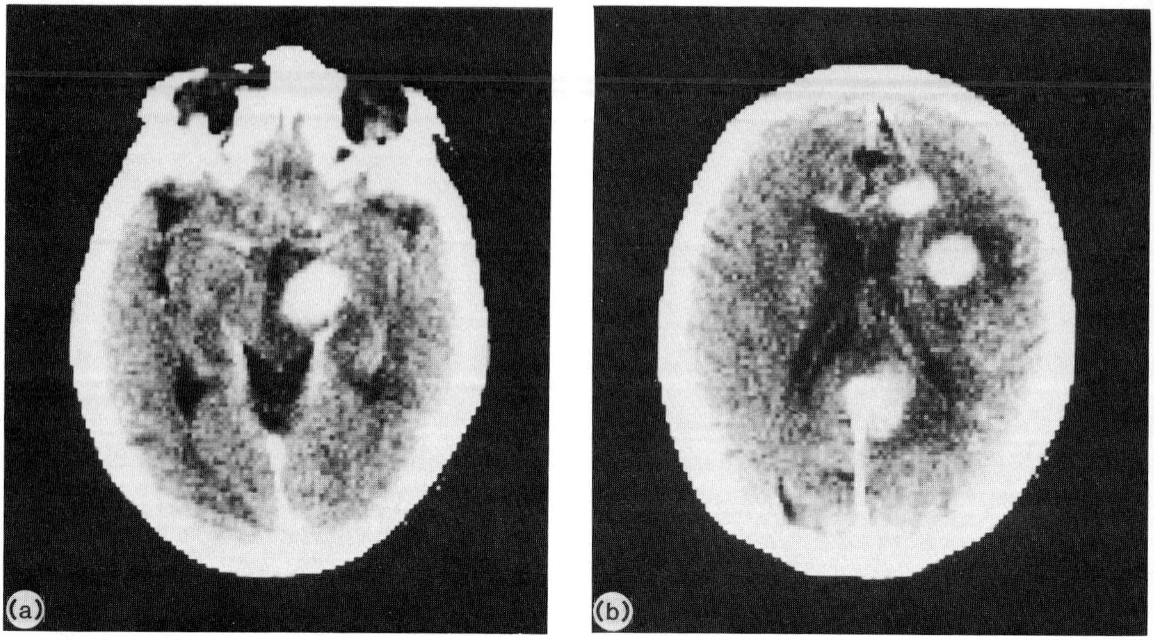

Fig. 5.18 Uveitis and reticulum cell sarcoma (microglioma). The only abnormality on extensive investigation of a 64-year old woman who had suffered bilateral chronic panuveitis for several years was a paraprotein band in the blood. More than one year later she developed a left hemiparesis, when CT (a, b, after intravenous contrast medium) showed multiple rounded, densely enhancing tumours typical of microglioma.

5.7 THE THICK OPTIC NERVE

The facility to evaluate the size of the optic nerve has opened discussion on the pathogenetic mechanisms. Thickening of the optic nerve may be seen in:

1. Papilloedema.
2. Optic neuritis.
3. Granulomatous or neoplastic infiltrative disease.
4. Hereditary optic neuropathy (Leber's disease).
5. Tumours of the nerve or sheath.
6. As a variation of normal.

Whether increase in size of neurones, oligodendroglial cells, fibrous septa, pia, arachnoid or dural hyperplasia are all contributory either individually or collectively, is not yet known.

Arachnoidal hyperplasia of the optic nerve sheaths may be more common than previously appreciated, and may possibly be an underlying common denominator in all these conditions. Arachnoidal hyperplasia is (*de ipso facto*) part of optic nerve meningiomas, but is also well recognized in gliomas, and has

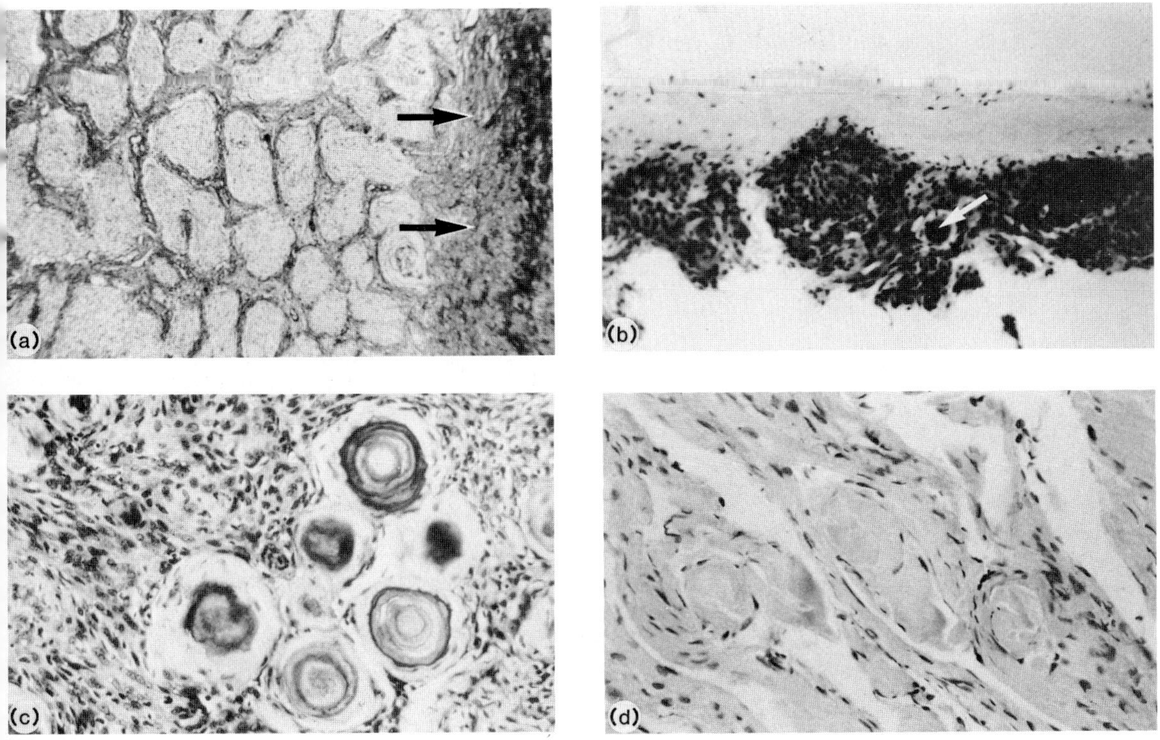

Fig. 5.19 Arachnoid hyperplasia in lesions of the optic nerve. (a) Optic nerve glioma. A dense, superficial layer of hyperplastic arachnoid (arrows) is quite distinct from the well-differentiated tumour. (b) Leber's hereditary optic atrophy. A psammoma body (arrow) lies within the darkely-staining arachnoid. (c) Optic nerve sheath meningioma (patient shown in Fig. 5.15). Massive arachnoid hyperplasia, with numerous calcified psammoma bodies (d) Benign intracranial pressure with chronic papilloedema (patient shown in Fig. 5.4; specimen taken at time of incision of nerve sheath) showing mild hyperplasia of arachnoidal cells. (courtesy of Professor Duchen, Department of Neuropathology, The National Hospital).

been described with optic neuritis, syphilis and Leber's hereditary optic atrophy. In all these conditions psammoma bodies may be seen. In addition we have seen arachnoid hyperplasia in one case of benign intracranial hypertension and papilloedema, in whom the optic nerve sheaths were decompressed, enabling histological examination (Fig. 5.19). Further pathological correlation with CT is therefore of prime importance to our understanding in this sphere. Blind needle biopsy of the nerve sheath has been suggested, with accurate localization facilitated by CT, and success in some patients (Dubois *et al.*, 1979). However, further experience in this technique would seem indicated before widespread use.

5.8 OPTIC ATROPHY

In optic atrophy, the nerve may appear of smaller diameter than

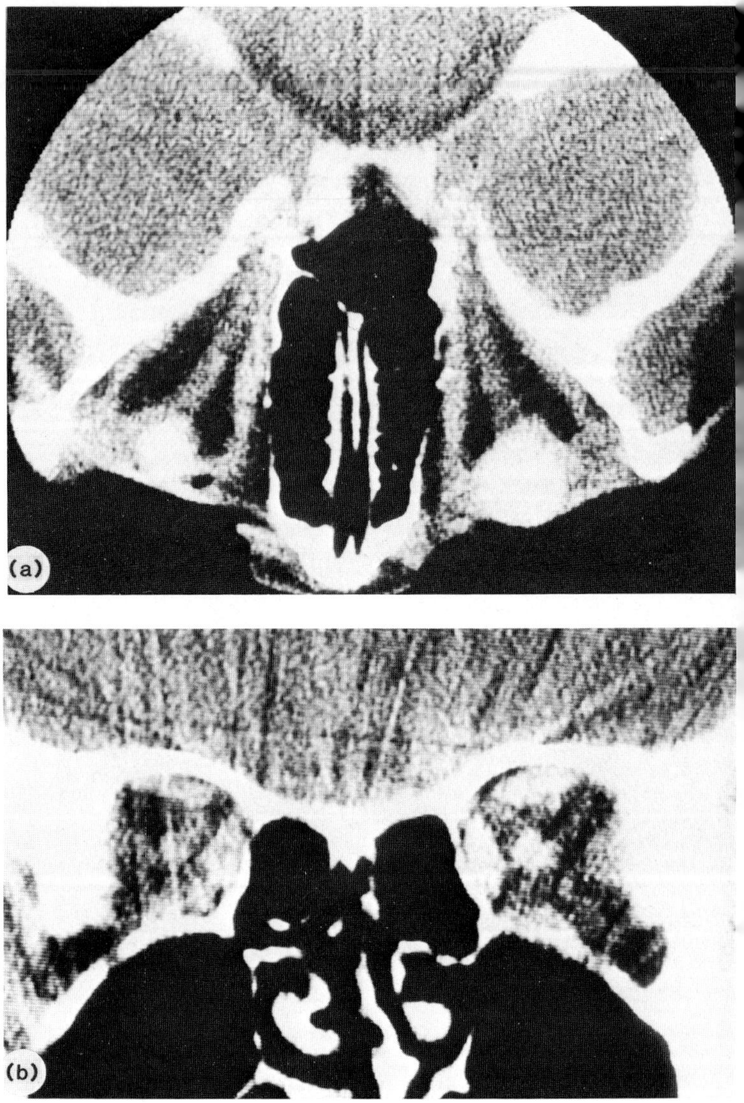

Fig. 5.20 Traumatic optic atrophy. Following criminal assault, it was thought necessary to enucleate both eyes of a 27 year old medical student! Acrylic prostheses were inserted. Subsequent CT (performed to evaluate the possibilities of further surgery) showed the implants, and optic nerves which have *not* obviously wasted.

normal on CT examination, but this change can be very difficult to assess (Fig. 5.20). Expansion of the sheath in papilloedema may be much more obvious than reduction in size as a result of atrophy. Unilateral changes can be more reliably detected by comparison with the healthy side. A normal or, in particular, an expanded nerve at CT in a patient with reduced vision and an atrophic optic disc, is strongly suggestive of a lesion of the optic nerve or the nerve sheath. Optic nerves of small diameter have been shown in optic nerve hypoplasia (Chapter 7).

REFERENCES

Aubin, M.L., Vignaud, J. and Mikol, F. (1978), Scotome transitoire au cours d'une opacification des espaces sous-arachnoidiens des gaines des nerfs optiques par la métrizamide lors d'une tomodensitométrie. *J. Radio. Electrol.*, **59**, 709–10.

Byrd, S.E., Harwood-Nash, D.C., Fitz, C.R., Barry, J.F. and Rogovitz, D.M. (1978), Computed tomography of intraorbital optic nerve gliomas in children. *Radiology*, **129**, 73–8.

Cabanis, E.A., Salvolini, U., Rodallec, A., Menichelli, F., Pasquini, U. and Bonnin, P. (1978), Computed tomography of the optic nerve. Part II: Size and shape modifications in papilloedema. *J. Comput. Assist. Tomogr.*, **2**, 150–5.

Dorrell, D. (1978), The tilted disc. *Br. J. Ophthal.*, **62**, 16–20.

Dubois, P.J., Kennerdell, S., Rosenbaum, A.E., Dekker, A., Johnson, B.R. and Swink, C.A. (1979), Computed tomographic localization for fine needle aspiration biopsy of orbital tumours. *Radiology*, **131**, 149–52.

Eyerman, E.L., Archer, C.R. and Mayes, B. (1976), Multiple sclerosis in brain and optic nerve as seen by standard and high resolution CT. *Neuroradiology*, **12**, 52.

Fox, A.J., Debrun, G., Vinuela, F., Assis, L. and Coates, R. (1979), Intrathecal metrizamide enhancement of the optic nerve sheath. *J. Comput. Assist. Tomogr.*, **3**, 653–6.

Hogan, M.J. and Zimmerman, L.E. (1962). *Ophthalmic Pathology*, 2nd Edn, Saunders, Philadelphia.

Hoyt, W.F., Meshel, L.G., Lessell, S., Schartz, N.J. and Suckling, R.D. (1973), Malignant optic glioma of childhood. *Brain*, **96**, 121–32.

Huckman, M.S., Fox, J.S., Ramsey, R.G. and Penn, R.D. (1976), Computed tomography in the diagnosis of pseudotumor cerebri. *Radiology*, **119**, 593–7.

Johnston, I. and Paterson, A. (1974), Benign intracranial hypertension. 1. Diagnosis and prognosis. *Brain*, **97**, 289–300.

Kingsley, D.P.E.,, Kendall, B.E. and Moseley, I.F. (1978), Superior sagittal sinus thrombosis: an evaluation of the changes demonstrated on computed tomography. *J. Neurol. Neurosurg. Psychiat.*, **41**, 1065–8.

Kirkham, T.H., Sanders, M.D. and Sapp, G.A. (1973), Unilateral papilloedema in benign intracranial hypertension. *Can. J. Ophthal.*, **8**, 533.

Lindenberg, R., Walsh, F.B. and Sacks, J.G. (1973), *Neuropathology of Vision. An Atlas*. Lea and Febiger, Philadelphia.

Lloyd, G.A.S. and Ambrose, J.A.E. (1977) An evaluation of C.A.T. in the diagnosis of orbital space-occupying lesions, In: *First European Seminar on Computerised Axial Tomography in Clinical Practice* (G.H. Du Boulay and I.F. Moseley eds)

Springer, Berlin, pp.154–60.

Manelfe, C., Pasquini, U. and Bank, W.O. (1978), Metrizamide demonstration of the subarachnoid space surrounding the optic nerves. *J. Comput. Assist. Tomogr.*, **2**, 545–7.

Mastaglia, F.M., Black, J.L., Cala, L.A. and Collins, D.W.K. (1977), Evoked potentials, saccadic velocities and computerised tomography in diagnosis of multiple sclerosis. *Br. Med. J.*, **(i)**, 1315–17.

Moseley, I.F. and Radü, E.W. (1979), Factors influencing the development of periventricular lucencies in patients with raised intracranial pressure. *Neuroradiology*, **17**, 65–9.

Naidich, T.P., Epstein, F., Lin, J.P., Kricheff, I.I. and Hochwald, G.M. (1976), Evaluation of pediatric hydrocephalus by computed tomography. *Radiology*, **119**, 337–45.

Price, H.I. and Danziger, A. (1979), The computerised tomographic findings in paediatric orbital tumours. *Clin. Radiol.*, **30**, 435–40.

Quevillon, A., Brouillette, G. and Aube, M. (1977), Syndrome du tilted disc, Tomographie axiale, *Can. J. Ophthal.*, **12**., 216–4.

Ridsale, L. and Moseley, I.F. (1978), Thorocolumbar intraspinal tumours presenting features of raised intracranial pressure. *J. Neurol. Neurosurg. Psychiat.*, **41**, 737–45.

Rosenberg, ,M.A., Savino, P.J. and Glaser, J.S. (1979), A clinical analysis of pseudo-papilloedema. *Archs. Ophthal.*, **97**, 65.

Salvolini, U., Cabanis, E.A., Rodallec, A., Menichelli, F., Pasquini, U. and Iba-Zizen, M.T. (1978), Computed tomography of the optic nerve. Part I: Normal results. *J. Comput. Assist. Tomogr.*, **3**, 141–9.

Sanders, G.S., Allen, R.A. and Straątsma, B.R. (1965), Arachnoidal proliferation of optic nerve simulating extension of intracranial glioma. *Archs. Ophthal.*, **74**, 349–52.

Tourje, E.J. and Gold, L.H.A. (1977), Leukemic infiltration of the optic nerves. Demonstration by computerized tomography. *Comput. Tomogr.*, **1**, 225–8.

Weisberg, L.A. and Nice, C.N. (1977), Computed tomographic evaluation of increased intracranial pressure without localizing signs. *Radiology*, **122**, 133–6.

Wilson, J.L. and Moseley, I.F. (1977), A diagnostic approach to cerebellar lesions. In: *First European Seminar on Computerised Axial Tomography in Clinical Practice* (eds G.H. Du Boulay and I.F. Moseley), Springer, Berlin, pp.123–33.

6 · Disorders of eye movement

This chapter deals with disorders of ocular movements and pupillary disorders. While the neural basis for the control of these structures and their movements is exceedingly complex and still imperfectly understood, some fundamental knowledge facilitates an understanding of the clinical features which result from disturbances at various levels in the brain and provides topographical localization.

6.1 CEREBRAL CONTROL OF OCULAR MOVEMENTS

Conjugate ocular movements have evolved to maintain the fovea of both eyes on the object of interest and the oculovestibular system provides visual stabilization for this, whilst the later phylogenetic addition of the vergence system facilitates a range of focus. Harmonious integration of the ocular motor system demands integrity of the cerebral cortex, the cerebellum, the brainstem and the ocular motor nerves.

Anatomical substrate

One hundred years ago Ferrier discovered the frontal eye fields (Brodman's Area 8) which he proposed as the centre for the initiation and control of voluntary eye movements. However, fast eye movements have also been produced by stimulation of the occipital cortex, cerebellum, superior colliculus, thalamus and brainstem. The corticobulbar pathway is polysynaptic and descends to the contralateral pontine reticular formation. The decussation occurs in the midbrain, and fibres also pass to the collicular region and pretectal area.

Sensory information enters the striate and peristriate cortex and the occipital ocular motor subsystem maintains fixation via a continuous visual feedback system. The emergent pathway encircles the occipital horn of the lateral ventricle to enter the subthalamic region before descending to the superior collicular, mesencephalic and pontine nuclei.

Superior colliculus

A 'dual concept of vision' promulgated in the last decade suggests an important role for the colliculus in subconscious visual perception for 'ambient' or 'noticing' vision, more sophisticated 'focal' or 'examining' vision being reserved for the cortex.

6.2 CEREBRAL LESIONS

Examination of these cerebral pathways is by assessing the ability to generate voluntary saccades (frontal system) to the contralateral side, and the velocity can be assessed clinically by asking the patient to refixate objects in their left and right fields of vision and measured by electro-oculography or infrared techniques. A normal person, in order to pursue a target smoothly to the same side, needs the integrity of the ipsilateral occipital projection and this can be assessed by asking the patient to follow a slowly moving target. Broken up or saccadic pursuit can be seen in a wide variety of conditions ranging from drug toxicity to local cerebral disease. Ipsilateral saccadic pursuit is an important sign of hemisphere disease and may be associated with failure to inhibit the ocular vestibular response to the same side.

Optokinetic nystagmus

Hemisphere function can be assessed by optokinetic stimuli which assess the hemisphere on the side to which a drum is rotating. On rotating the drum to the right a pursuit movement follows the target (R occipital region) and this is followed by a saccade to the left (R frontal region) (Fig. 6.1b). This test is of particular importance in deep parietal lesions and may be defective even when individual saccadic and pursuit movements are clinically normal. Eye movement recordings in deep parietal lesions have shown impaired ipsilateral pursuit, and in particular foveal pursuit (Baloh *et al*., 1980).

Frontal lesions

Acute destructive frontal lesions may show deviation of the eyes to the side of the lesion due to the inability to generate voluntary movements to the opposite side. Gaze to the opposite side may be induced by pursuit or oculovestibular stimuli. Patients with acute frontal lesions are usually severely obtunded and the gaze palsy improves as the patient's general neurological state recovers (Fig. 6.2). Chronic frontal lesions do not produce a similar picture owing to the compensatory ability of the intact frontal hemisphere which is able to generate saccades to each side. Irritative lesions may rarely produce contralateral gaze during the ictal episode.

Occipital lesions

Precise anatomical documentation of the pathway from the parieto-occipital region to the brainstem is lacking, but involvement of the peristriate cortex seems necessary to impair ipsilateral smooth pursuit. Excision of the striate cortex may produce a complete homonymous hemianopia without disturbance of the descending ocular motor pursuit pathway (Weiskrantz *et al.*, 1974).

Deep parietal and thalamic lesions

Saccadic and pursuit movements may be normal, but severe disorganization of optokinetic nystagmus can make a significant

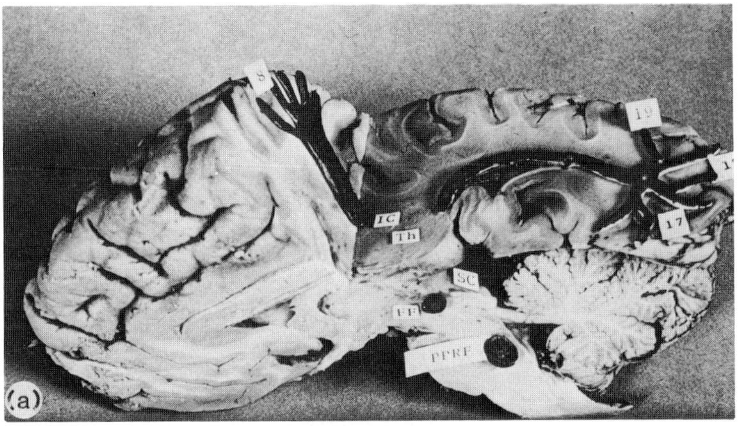

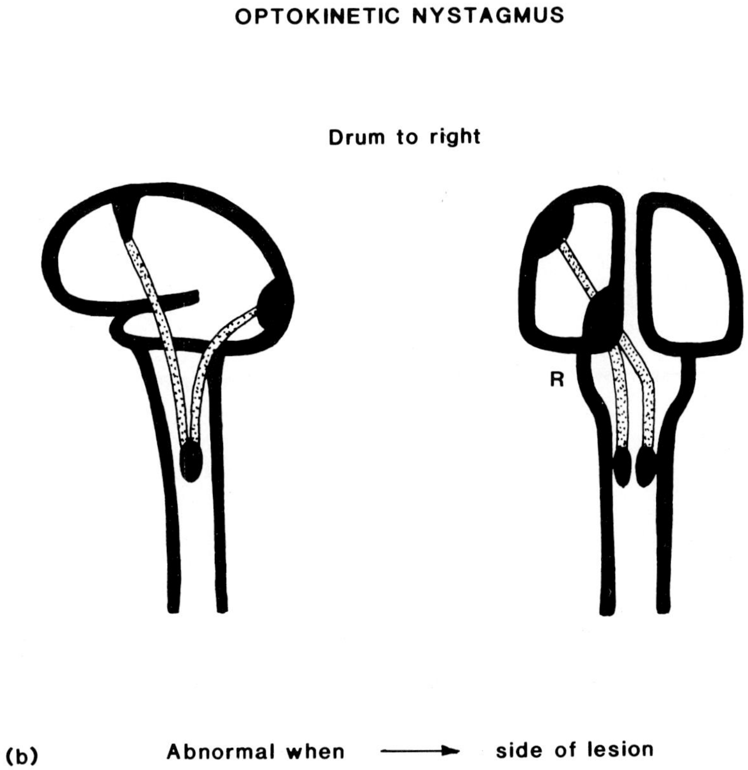

Fig. 6.1 (a) Brain section to show cerebral ocular motor pathways in right hemisphere. The frontal pathway descends from area 8 to the subthalamic region, whilst the occipital pathway projects forwards to the same area. These pathways then descend to the fields of Forel (FF) and pretectal region for the organization of vertical gaze and to the pons (PPRF) for the organization of horizontal gaze. (b) Optokinetic nystagmus for practical purposes is abnormal in cerebral disease when the drum is rotated towards the side of the lesion.

contribution to the diagnosis (Fig. 6.3). Other ocular manifestations of thalamic lesions include paresis of vertical gaze with tonic deviation of the eyes downwards and inwards (Fisher, 1967). It has been suggested that increased intracranial pressure may contribute to this tonic deviation of the eyes, for in one case with a thalamic haemorrhage confirmed by CT, relief of the raised pressure by ventricular shunting produced relief of the ocular signs (Gilner and Avin, 1977).

6.3 CLASSIFICIATION OF SUPRANUCLEAR EYE MOVEMENT DISORDERS (After Daroff)

1. *Gaze palsy or paralysis* (total loss of gaze), can produce:
(a) Saccadic palsy.
(b) Pursuit palsy.
(c) Gaze palsy (both saccades and pursuit palsy).

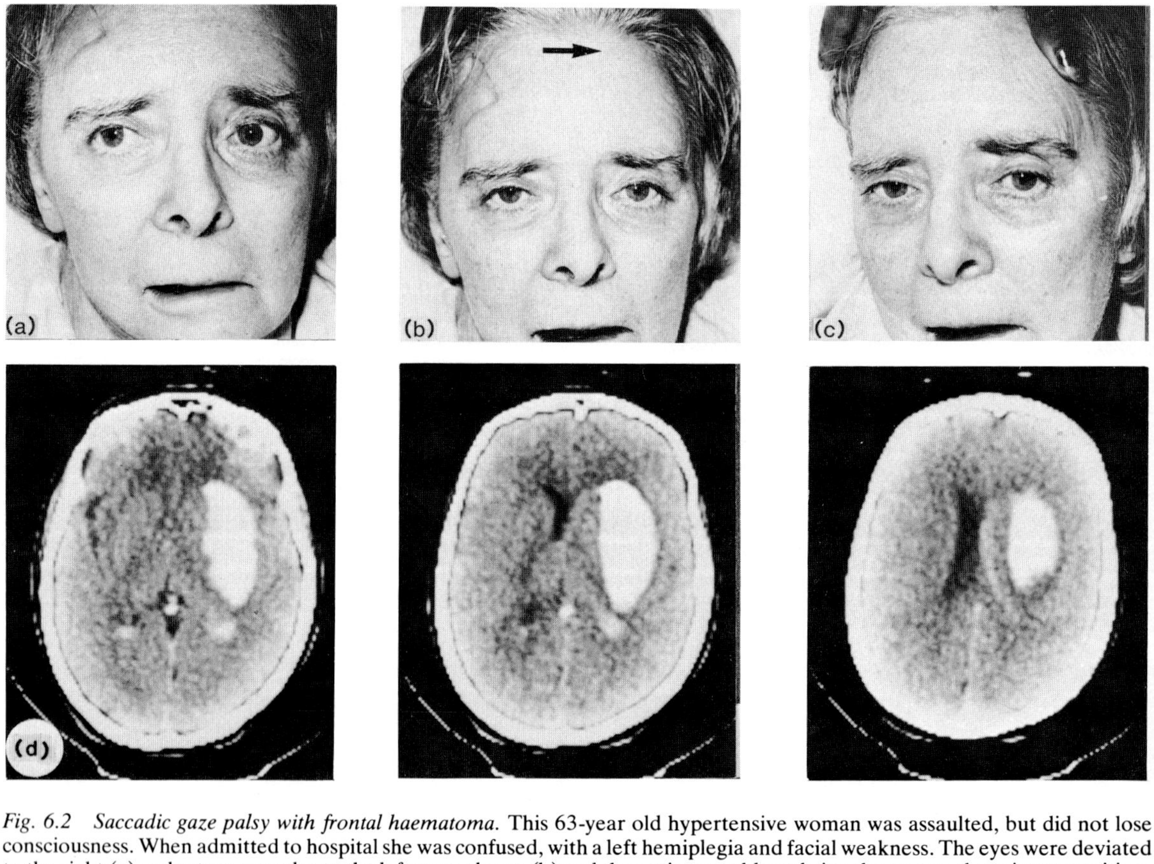

Fig. 6.2 Saccadic gaze palsy with frontal haematoma. This 63-year old hypertensive woman was assaulted, but did not lose consciousness. When admitted to hospital she was confused, with a left hemiplegia and facial weakness. The eyes were deviated to the right (a), voluntary saccades to the left were absent (b) and the patient could not bring the eyes to the primary position; doll's head showed full gaze to the left (c). Optic discs were normal. Radiography showed a fracture of the floor of the left orbit, and CT (d) demonstrated a very large fresh right capsular haematoma, extending into the frontal lobe, with a fine rim of low attenuation, probably indicating clot retraction. There was blood in the right lateral ventricle. Evacuation of the haematoma was followed by rapid improvement, with resumption of straight ahead gaze, and reduced velocity saccades to the left.

Fig. 6.3 Deep parietal lesion with optokinetic nystagmus abnormality. This 30-year old man developed a right hemiplegia, but had no visual symptoms. Examination showed visual acuity of 6/5 in each eye with normal fields, and eye movements were normal to saccadic pursuit and oculovestibular testing. Rotating the optokinetic drum to the left (a) produced deranged movements, whereas rotating the drum to the right was normal. Eye movement recordings confirmed normal saccades, demonstrated impaired pursuit to the left, and abnormal optokinetic nystagmus with the drum rotating to the left (b). Neurological examination showed a right hemiplegia, subtle right sensory signs: two-point discrimination and astereognosis. CT (c) revealed a large area of mixed attenuation around the left trigone, which after intravenous contrast medium (d) was seen to consist of large vessels (arrows) representing an arteriovenous malformation. The great vein of Galen (large arrow) was markedly dilated. There was mild hydrocephalus.

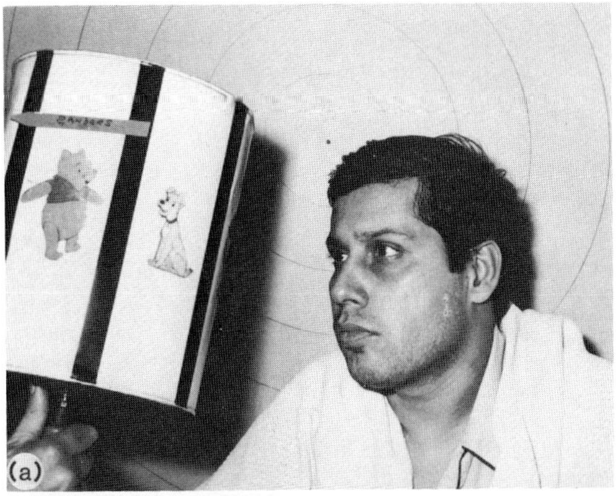

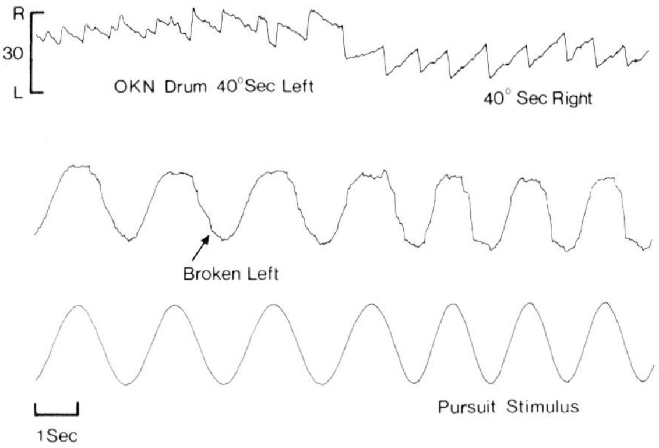

(b)

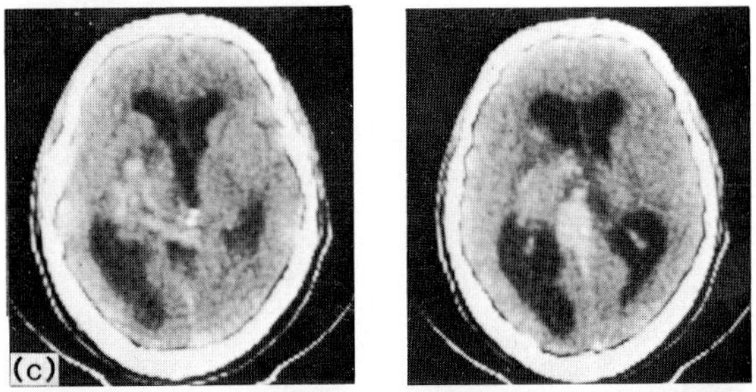

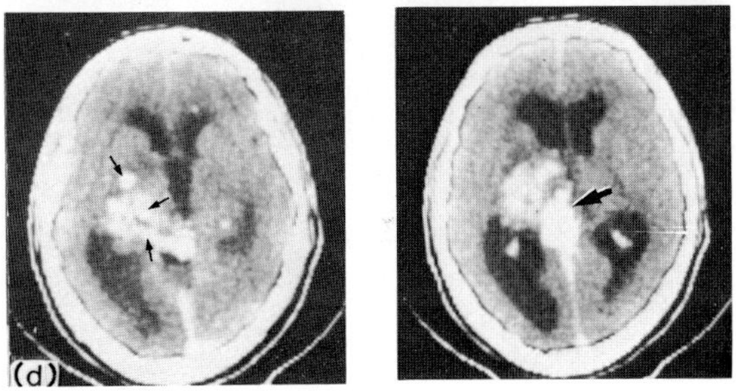

2. *Paresis* (i.e. incomplete or subtotal involvement)
(a) Saccadic (slow saccades; gaze paretic nystagmus; hypometric saccades; inability to maintain eccentric gaze; limited eccentric excursion).
(b) Pursuit paresis (i.e. saccadic pursuit, unidirectional).
(c) Gaze paresis (saccadic and pursuit paresis).

Progressive supranuclear palsy (the Steele-Richardson-Olszewski syndrome)

This degenerative condition involves particularly the neurones in the basal ganglia and midbrain and is characterized by defective saccadic and pursuit function, with intact oculovestibular responses. Vertical movements, particularly downwards, are affected before horizontal, and voluntary before reflex; in late cases, even convergence fails. These eye signs are accompanied by personality change, sudden falls, pseudobulbar palsy, a rigid neck, with characteristic upturning of the head, and some features suggestive of Parkinsonism.

CT shows cerebral atrophy, with enlargement of the ventricles and subarachnoid spaces. The classical feature is atrophy of the midbrain, made evident by prominence of the adjacent cisterns (Fig. 6.4). The changes may be slight and not apparent at routine CT, but visible on pneumoencephalography.

Ophthalmoplegic lipidosis

This lysosomal disease of undetermined aetiology produces a progressive degenerative neurological disease in young children,

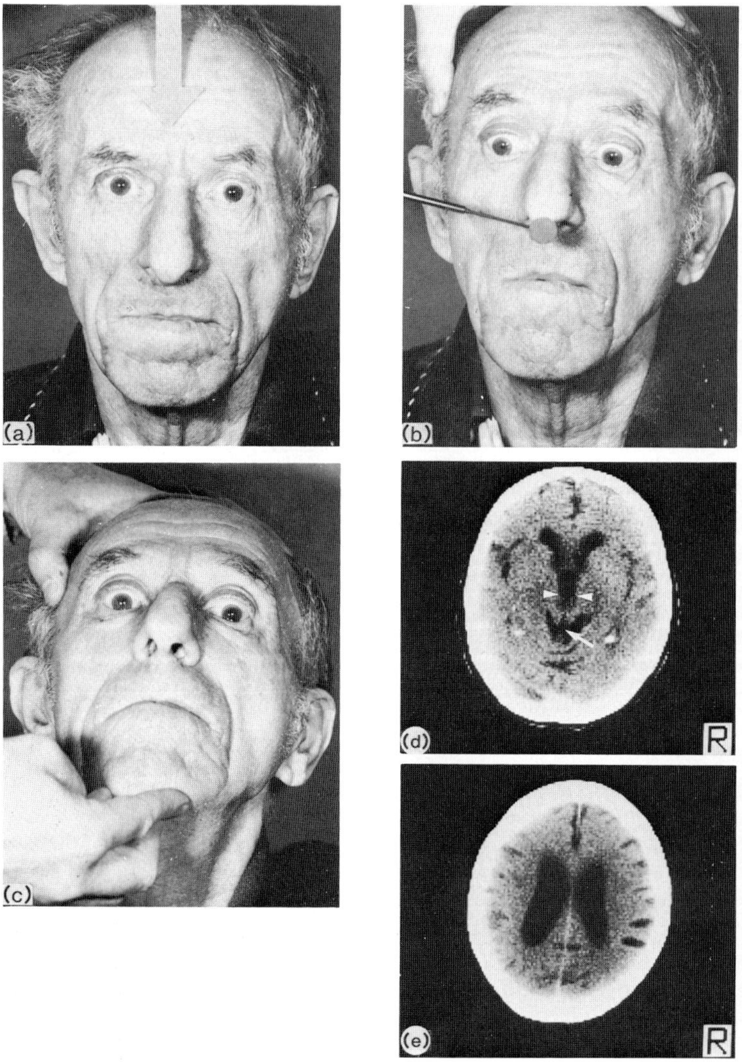

Fig. 6.4 Progressive supranuclear ophthalmoplegia. A 68-year old man gave a history, progressing over four years, of unsteadiness, clumsiness of the hands and memory loss. He had noted an inability to look down. Examination confirmed mild dementia. Vertical gaze, particularly downwards, was markedly restricted; this was most evident on attempted voluntary movement (a), but also on following a downward moving target (b), but doll's head movements showed a full range (c). Convergence was also reduced. Right and left gaze produced mild nystagmus. There was a paucity of facial movements and generalized hypertonia. CT (d, e) showed generalized cerebral atrophy, particularly marked in the tectal region, with widening of the third ventricle (arrowheads) and enlargement of the quadrigeminal cistern (arrow).

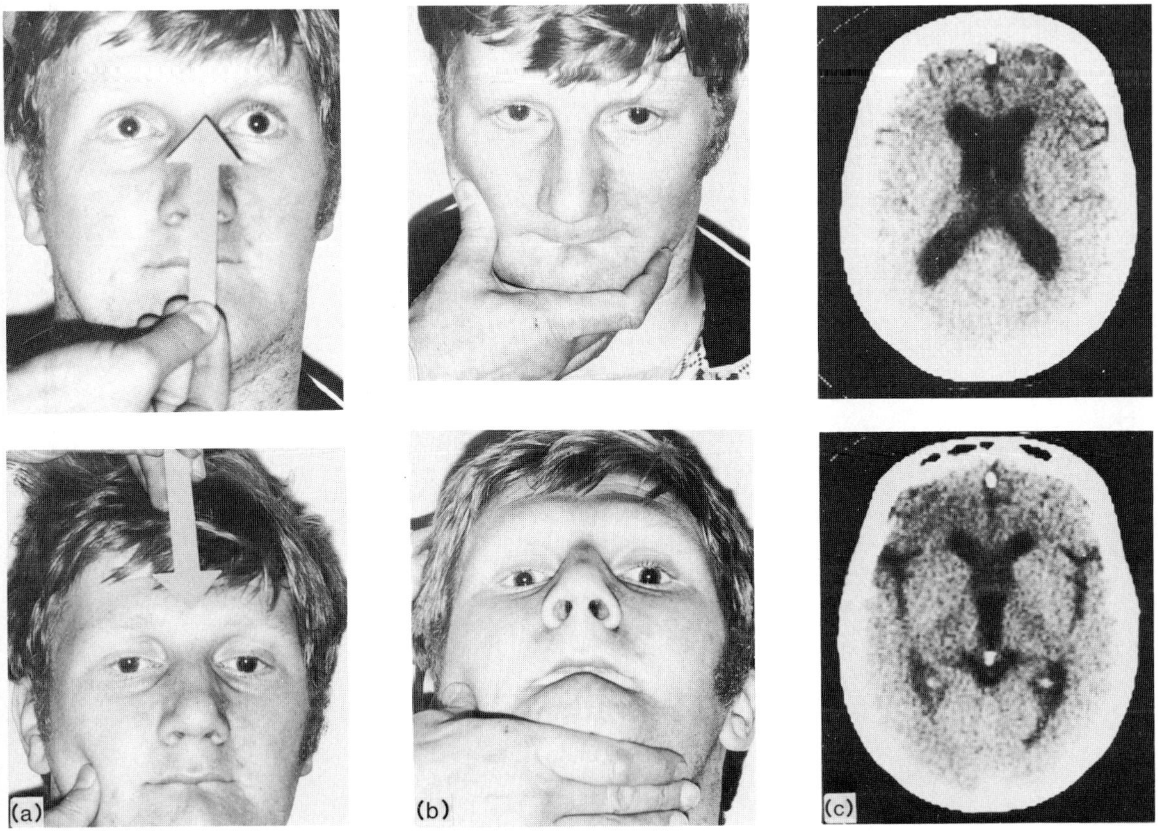

Fig. 6.5 Ophthalmoplegic lipidosis. This young man, who had always been mentally subnormal, developed manic depression and choreoathetoid movements after mumps encephalitis at age 16. His vision was normal but vertical saccades were absent; (a) pursuit was absent for elevation and limited for depression. Doll's head movements were normal (b). He had cerebellar ataxia and dysarthria and the liver and spleen were enlarged. CT (c, carried out at age 21) showed non-specific generalized cerebral atrophy, but bone marrow biopsy showed foamy sea-blue histiocytes with granules, indicative of ophthalmoplegic lipidosis.

with ocular motor abnormalities similar to the Steele-Richardson syndrome seen in adults. Vertical saccades are initially involved, followed by vertical pursuit, and then involvement of the horizontal system. Finally, convergence and the oculovestibular reflexes are deranged. Initial studies suggested this was a late form of Niemann-Pick Disease, with detection of the sea-blue histiocyte (Neville *et al.*, 1973), but intensive study has failed to elucidate the enzymatic abnormality. The first child seen by one of us demonstrated remarkable head thrusts to induce vertical refixation movements similar to those seen in ocular motor apraxia (Sanders and Wybar, 1969). We have examined one case by CT, showing mild atrophic changes only (Fig. 6.5).

6.4 SUPRANUCLEAR OPHTHALMOPLEGIA

Certain diffuse degenerative disorders may induce a progressive disintegration of the cerebral control of ocular movements, with

Fig. 6.6 Olivopontocerebellar degeneration with tapetoretinal changes. This 21-year old man complained of long-standing, progressive ataxia. Vision was reduced to counting fingers. The retinal vessels were attenuated, and at fluorescein angiography (a) there was generalized pigment epithelial atrophy with a peripapillary halo in which choroidal vessels were visible. Large pigment epithelial defects were present peripherally. Saccades were totally absent, and on pursuit there was some preservation of left and downgaze (b). Doll's head movements were also limited. CT (c) revealed signs of cerebellar and pontine atrophy: large cisterns (pontine cistern, arrow; vallecula, crossed arrow), prominent sulci (small arrows) and enlargement of the fourth ventricle.

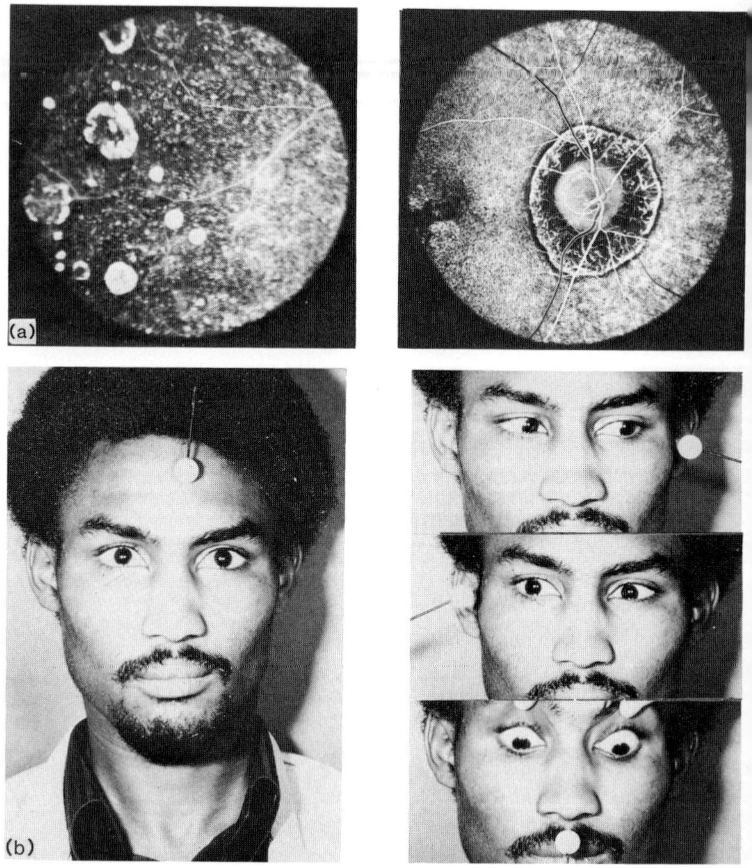

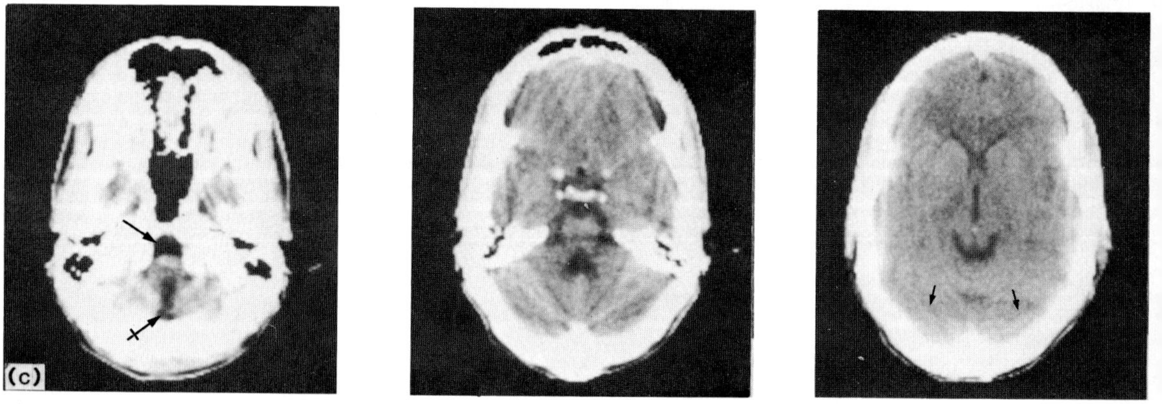

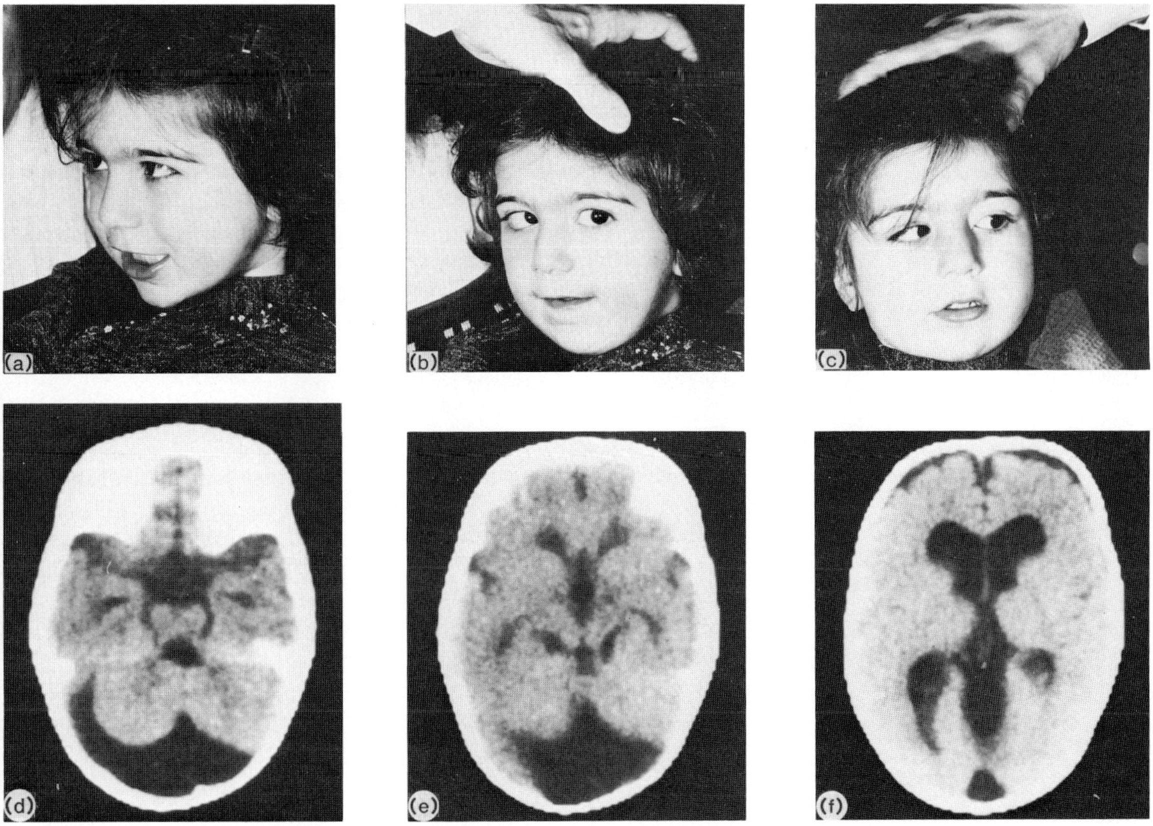

Fig. 6.7 Oculomotor apraxia. This child's eyes were noted almost from birth to be deviated to the left, but this improved as she grew up. When seen at 3 years of age, she was noted to have absent horizontal saccades and restricted vertical saccades, though pursuit was normal (a). When conjugate lateral movements were made head thrusts were first initiated, and when fixation was obtained the normal relationship between head and eyes was obtained by a slow head rotation with eyes fixed to the right (a). Attempted left gaze is initiated with a head thrust (b), until fixation on target is obtained and then the head straightens up (c). CT (d) demonstrated a hypoplastic cerebellum, overlaid by a very large cisterna magna, which separated the occipital lobes. The brain was generally atrophic or hypoplastic, particularly the upper midbrain and pretectal region. (CT courtesy of Dr K. Howlett, Consultant Radiologist, Charing Cross Hospital).

voluntary movements being first involved, then pursuit, and finally the oculovestibular. The vertical system organized at a pretectal level seems vulnerable in certain conditions (e.g. ophthalmoplegic lipidosis in children and progressive supranuclear palsy in adults) whereas in other conditions horizontal gaze is initially affected (e.g. Huntingdon's chorea, Wilson's disease, Gaucher's disease etc.). These conditions produce a characteristic supranulcear ophthalmoplegia with impaired saccadic and pursuit movements, but with relatively intact oculovestibular responses.

Horizontal supranuclear ophthalmoplegia

Bilateral involvement of the frontopontine system produces impaired saccadic movements in both directions with preservation of pursuit and oculocephalic movements (Fig. 6.6). Inability to generate voluntary saccades produces substitute oculocephalic responses. These include head thrusts, blinking and the substitution of vestibulo-ocular reflexes. Some patients with hereditary cerebellar syndromes particularly of the olivopontocerebellar type, which is sometimes evident on CT as cerebellar and brain stem atrophy (Fig. 6.20), may utilize head thrusts because volitional movements are affected more than pursuit and oculovestibular movements. Certain other conditions can produce saccadic abnormalities. In *Huntingdon's chorea*, CT demonstrates generalized cerebral atrophy, with a characteristic flattening of the caudate nuclei, manifest as focal, rounded enlargement of the frontal horns. *Wilson's disease*, hepatoleuticular degeneration, may produce no abnormality at CT, but low-attenuation cavities in the basal ganglia and high-attenuation zones, presumed to be due to copper deposition, have been reported (Kendall, Quiroga and Clavería, 1977). CT in *Gaucher's disease* is usually normal.

Oculomotor apraxia

Inability to generate adequate saccadic movements and the substitution of head movements and oculovestibular movements is termed oculomotor apraxia. Characteristic head thrusts are seen to move the eyes and when fixation is obtained the oculocephalic reflex allows the head to be straightened (Fig. 6.7). The defect may be congenital, in which case agenesis of the corpus callosum may be present: Orrison and Robertson (1979) described the CT findings of partial agenesis (Chapter 7) in one child with defective voluntary horizontal gaze and absent optokinetic responses in the horizontal plane.

6.5 BRAINSTEM CENTRES

Pathways from the frontal and occipital cortex descend in the internal capsule to the subthalamic region to terminate in the pretectal region for the control of vertical ocular movements, and in the paramedian pontine reticular formation (PPRF) for the control of horizontal eye movements.

The corticobulbar pathway from the frontal region decussates, whereas the occipital pathway is thought to project ipsilaterally. Horizontal ocular movements are generated in the pontine reticular formation on the same side and the ipsilateral VIth nerve nucleus is stimulated in the pons, whereas the contralateral medial rectus nucleus is stimulated via a pathway crossing the midline in the pons and passing to the midbrain via the median longitudinal fasciculus (MLF).

The cerebellum appears to function as a complex computer for the fine regulation and modulation of movements and appears to be concerned with saccadic, pursuit and oculovestibular movements.

Localization of lesions in the brainstem is facilitated by the anatomical separation of the 'centre' for vertical gaze in the pretectal region, from the 'centre' for horizontal gaze in the pons (Fig. 6.8).

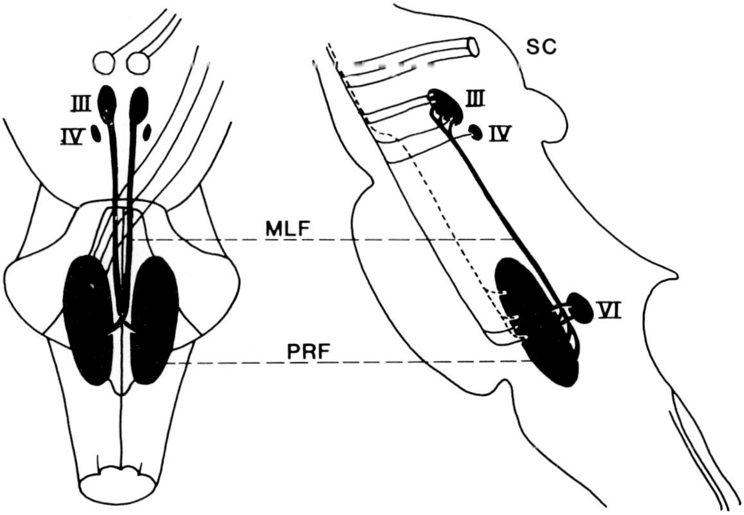

Fig. 6.8 Brainstem pathways for ocular motor control. Vertical gaze is organized at the level of the superior collicular (SC) and pretectum and descending fibres from the cortex pass to this region. Fibres concerned with horizontal gaze descend to the pontine reticular formation (PPRF). Cranian nerve nuclei: III, IV, V; MLF: median longitudinal fasciculus. (First published in *Scientific Foundations of Ophthalmology* (ed. Perkins and Hill), William Heinemann Medical Books Ltd., London, and reproduced with their kind permission).

6.6 HORIZONTAL GAZE DISORDERS

In a total pontine gaze palsy, the final common pathway for all inputs to the PPRF is destroyed so that the eyes do not move voluntarily, for pursuit, for optokinetic stimuli or on oculocephalic or caloric stimulation. Convergence should be retained if the integrity of the midbrain and IIIrd nerve are intact. Bilateral pontine disease may produce failure of gaze to either side, or the condition may occur unilaterally. In the absence of total destruction of the PPRF, gaze may be reduced in velocity or amplitude and the term pontine gaze paresis is used. Examination again demands assessment of the velocity of saccadic eye movements and the range of voluntary, pursuit and oculocephalic induced gaze.

Internuclear ophthalmoplegia

Total failure of adduction, or reduced velocity or range of adduction on attempted conjugate gaze, but with good adduction on convergence signifies an internuclear ophthalmoplegia. This is due to a lesion of the MLF, and is accompanied by varying patterns of nystagmus in the abducting eye and an overshoot of the eye on abduction (Fig. 6.9).

The integrity of convergence is essential for the diagnosis, and serves to differentiate an internuclear ophthalmoplegia from a fascicular IIIrd nerve palsy, or a lesion of the medial rectus muscle (e.g myasthenia, thyroid, granuloma). In the majority of patients, despite the finding of reduced convergence, clinical features or other brainstem signs usually suggest a lesion of the MLF. In addition the juxtaposition of the MLF and fascicular portion of medial rectus neurones means that both may be involved simultaneously.

A combination of a gaze palsy and an internuclear ophthalmoplegia (INO) has been termed the $1\frac{1}{2}$ syndrome (Fisher, 1967), due to the finding of gaze palsy or paresis to one side with half a gaze palsy (INO) to the other. In brainstem lesions the examiner must search diligently for components of gaze palsy, VIth nerve palsy and internuclear ophthalmoplegia. Intrinsic disease is usually responsible and includes vascular disease, demyelination and brainstem glioma.

Vascular lesions of the brainstem are usually of sudden onset; the constellation of physical signs accurately indicates the site of the lesion and the internuclear ophthalmoplegia is more likely to be unilateral. CT evaluation of the brainstem in intrinsic vascular disease is not rewarding, although the extremely rare *angioma* can be recognized as an irregular area of mixed attenuation, showing marked contrast enhancement.

Plaques of *multiple sclerosis* in the brainstem have not as yet been convincingly demonstrated by CT, but the presence of paraventricular low attenuation lesions in the cerebrum, which in the acute stage may show both mass effect and moderate to marked enhancement with intravenous contrast medium, may serve to confirm the diagnosis. *Central pontine myelinolysis* may, however, be recognized, as a central or bilateral paramedian area of low attenuation representing the corticospinal and corticobulbar tracts (Anderson *et al.*, 1979; Telfer and Miller, 1979).

Brainstem gliomas are usually manifest as expansion of the pons, with reduction in size of the pontine and cerebellopontine angle cisterns and flattening and posterior displacement of the

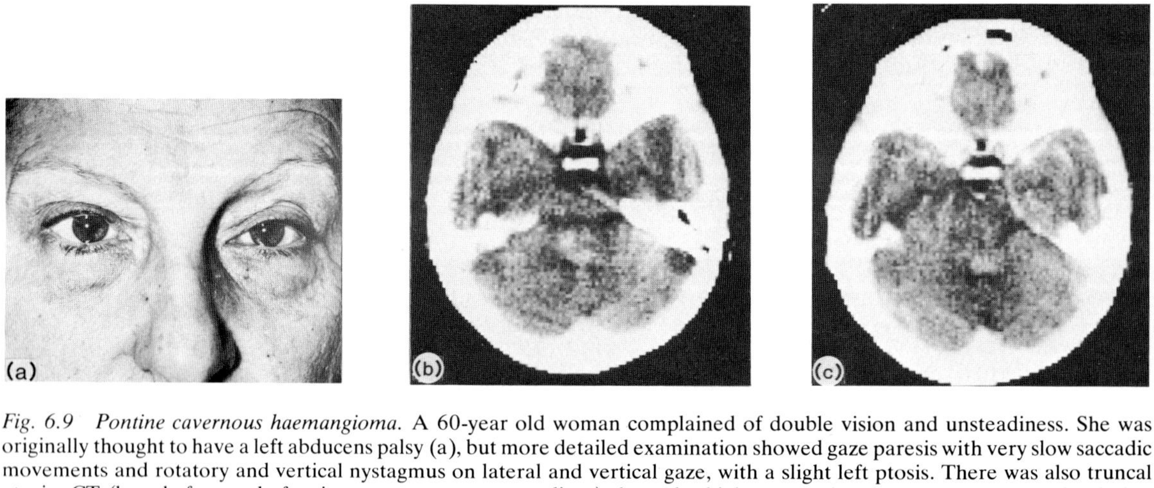

Fig. 6.9 Pontine cavernous haemangioma. A 60-year old woman complained of double vision and unsteadiness. She was originally thought to have a left abducens palsy (a), but more detailed examination showed gaze paresis with very slow saccadic movements and rotatory and vertical nystagmus on lateral and vertical gaze, with a slight left ptosis. There was also truncal ataxia. CT (b, c, before and after intravenous contrast medium) showed a high attenuation, poorly defined pontine lesion without pathological enhancement. Vertebral angiography was non-contributory. At surgery, the floor of the fourth ventricle was bulging, with prominent vessels and haemorrhagic staining. Histological examination showed a largely thrombosed cavernous haemangioma.

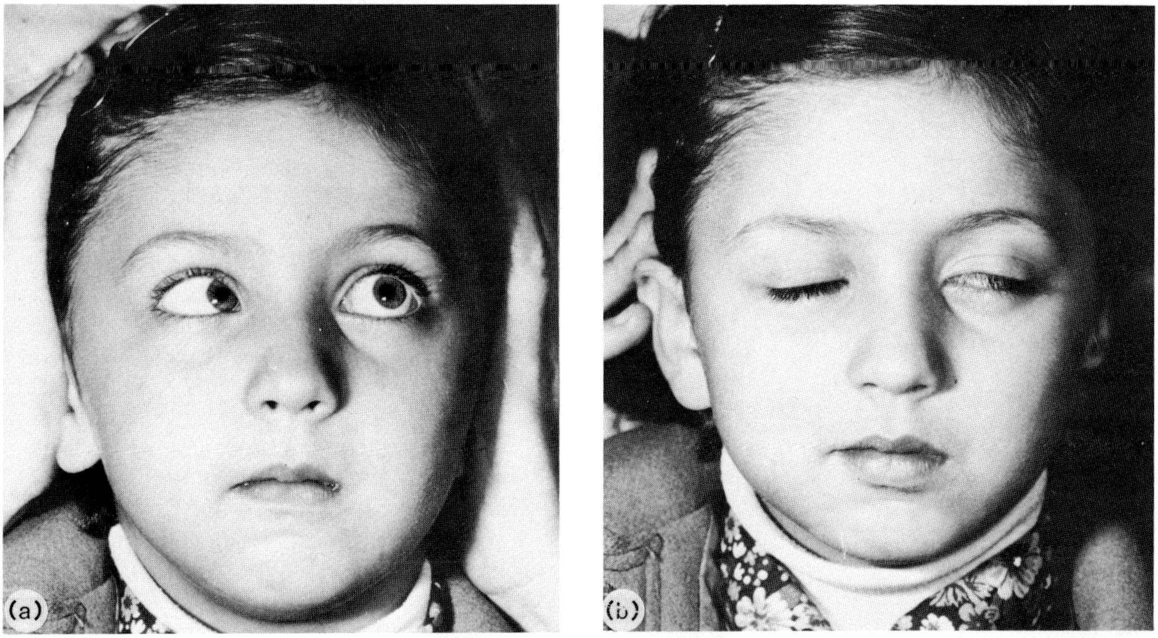

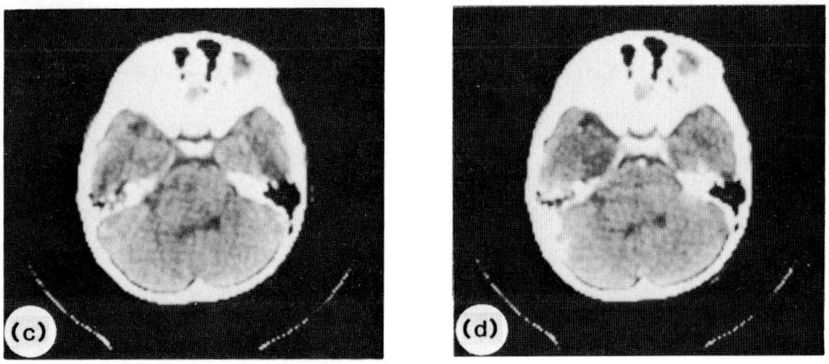

Fig. 6.10 Brainstem glioma. This child developed a convergent squint when she was 3 years old. Two squint correction operations were carried out, but after the second facial movements were noted to be impaired on the left side. Dysphagia, left hearing loss and left limb problems subsequently developed.

There was nystagmus on left and right gaze, and abduction of the left eye was limited (a). Bilateral facial weakness was more marked on the left (b). Palatal movements were poor and the voice was nasal. Cerebellar signs were present. CT (c) confirmed gross expansion of the pons, more marked on the left, with obliteration of the adjacent cisterns and compression of the fourth ventricle. There was no pathological contrast enhancement (d). Radiotherapy produced remarkable amelioration of signs.

fourth ventricle. They are characteristically of low attenuation, without marked increase after intravenous contrast medium. Rarely the pons may be calcified or show haemorrhages. Hydrocephalus is not generally a feature of pontine gliomas (Fig. 6.10).

Divergence paralysis

Horizontal diplopia in the distance, with clinical and oculographic features of bilateral symmetrical VIth nerve palsies suggests divergence paralysis. This is of significance because it is often due to raised intracranial pressure and we have seen it not only with benign intracranial hypertension, but also with subdural haematomas.

Vertical gaze disorders

Comprehension of the control of vertical eye movements is less elaborate than our understanding of the horizontal system. However, lesions in the pretectal region characteristically produce vertical gaze palsies. Elevated intraventricular pressure may produce impaired elevation of the eyes and a return to normal function may follow intraventricular drainage. This sign (the 'setting sun') is a feature of hydrocephalus.

Permanent failure of vertical gaze may be seen after vascular disturbances or trauma, but is characteristically seen with tumours of the pineal gland. In addition to failure of elevation, attempted up-gaze saccades may involve co-firing of other ocular muscles to produce the typical picture of convergence/retraction nystagmus. This sign is best elicited by using a downward rotating optokinetic drum. In addition, the clinician should search for pupillary signs (light-near dissociation), accommodative signs (reduced range of accommodation) and lid signs (Collier's sign).

This constellation of signs, classically the result of a pineal region tumour, rejoices under a variety of titles which include Sylvian aqueduct syndrome, Parinaud's syndrome, Koeber-Salus-Elshnig syndrome, dorsal midbrain syndrome.

The term 'pinealoma' has been used as a general term for tumours of the pineal gland, comprising 0.4 to 1% of all intracranial tumours, and these can be subdivided into two main subgroups:

1. *Teratomas*
   (a) Typical and teratoid
   (b) Atypical or germinoma

2. *Pinealomas*
   (a) Pineoblastoma
   (b) Pineocytoma

All these groups tend to present in children and young adults. Germinomas are the most common, and this group cannot be differentiated clinically from the other histological groups. The pineoblastoma is a more malignant tumour, and may show histological features resembling either medulloblastoma or retinoblastoma. Pineocytoma on the other hand is a more benign lesion which may present at a later age and is relatively resistant to radiotherapy. Recent evidence suggests a therapeutic shift from the current practice of ventricular shunting and radiotherapy towards biopsy and possible excision of the tumour (Herrick and Rubinstein, 1979).

Justification for this is demonstrated by the need for full radiotherapy, possibly involving the whole neuraxis in pineoblastoma, whereas the more benign pineocytoma is relatively insensitive.

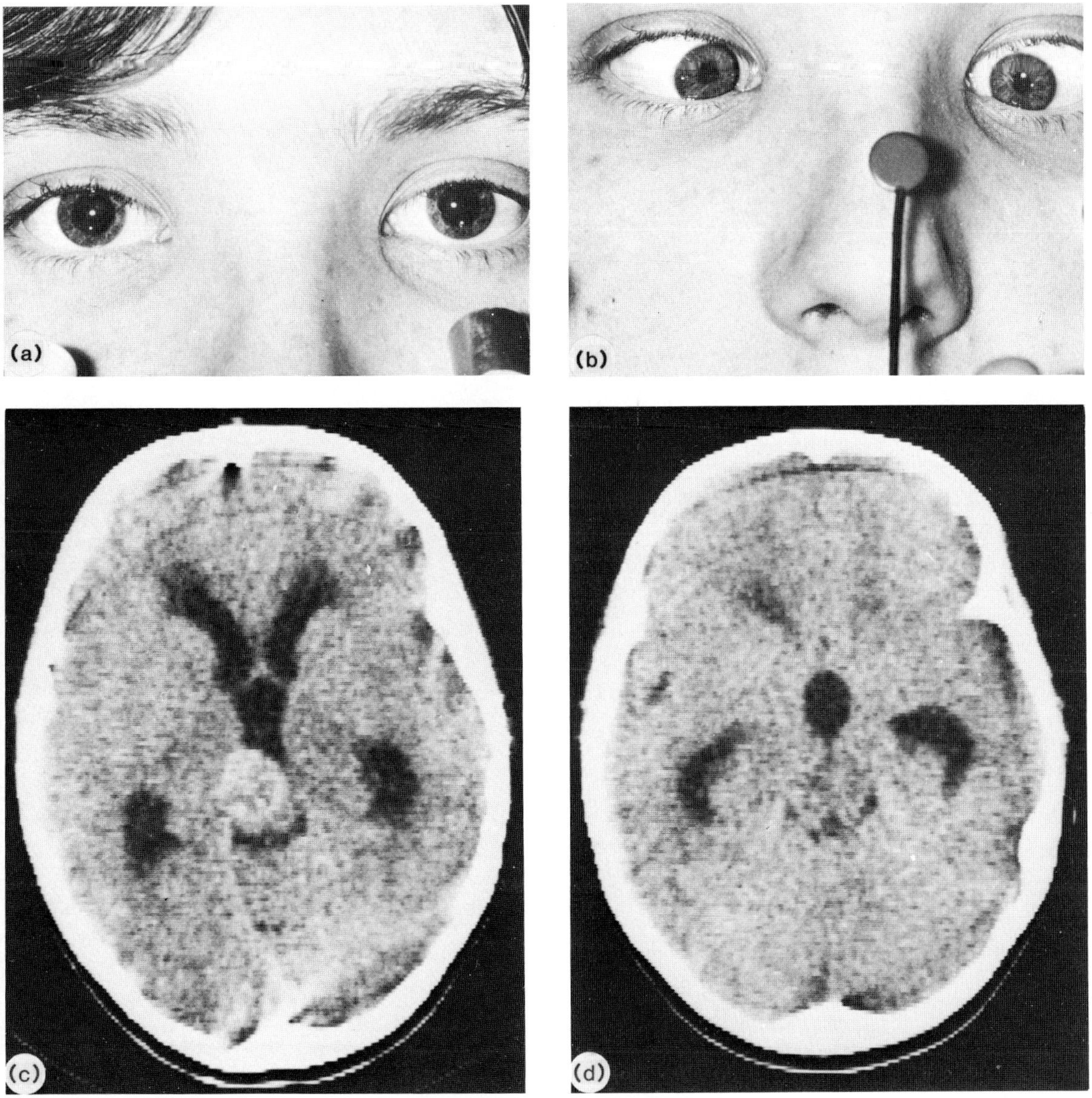

Fig. 6.11 Pineal tumour – pineoblastoma. An 11-year old boy presented with headaches. His pupils were unreactive to light (a), but reacted normally to accommodation (b). There was bilateral papilloedema. CT showed a rounded, high attenuation mass eccentrically placed in the upper midbrain (c,d), and obstructing the third ventricle to produce hydrocephalus (note the dilated temporal horns). Despite the considerable resemblance of this tumour to a radiosensitive germinoma, biopsy revealed a malignant tumour (pineoblastoma) with areas of pseudorosette formation similar to retinoblastoma. Resolution occurred with radiotherapy which included the whole neuraxis.

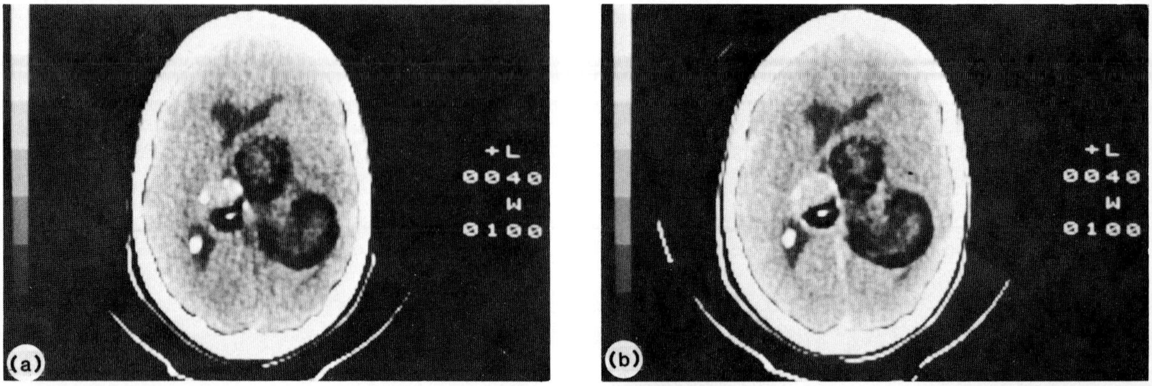

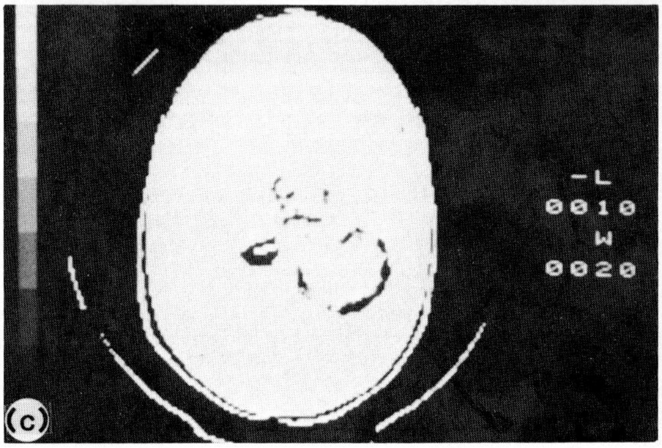

Fig. 6.12 Pineal tumour – teratoma. A boy of 14 presented with diplopia and symptoms of raised intracranial pressure. He showed light near dissociation, impaired upward gaze and bilateral papilloedema. There was no response to radiotherapy; he received surgical correction of his vertical deviation. CT (a) showed a massive, inhomogeneous, apparently cystic tumour, centred on the pineal region and extending to the right. There was minor contrast enhancement (b). Examination with a low level window (c) revealed that much of the contents were less dense than CSF, indicating that the lesion was teratomatous, containing fat. Complete removal was performed and the patient improved after the initial period.

Neuro-ophthalmic signs are frequent and diagnostically important. Ocular signs in a small group of patients showed:

Failure of elevation	100%
Light-near dissociation	100%
Retraction nystagmus	80%
VIth nerve palsy (pseudo)	50%
Skew deviation	30%

(Sanders and Bird, 1970).

We have seen one patient with rapid flutter-like movements of the eyes, and several patients presenting with features more typical of bilateral superior rectus or superior oblique palsies.

Bilateral papilloedema was noted in two thirds of a group of 33 patients with pinealomas whose CT scans were studied (Moseley *et al.*, 1979).

CT demonstrated increased attenuation in the region of the pineal gland in 23 patients and in ten the tumour was calcified. Four of the tumours were of reduced attenuation, while two were isodense with the surrounding brain. A clearly defined, rounded,

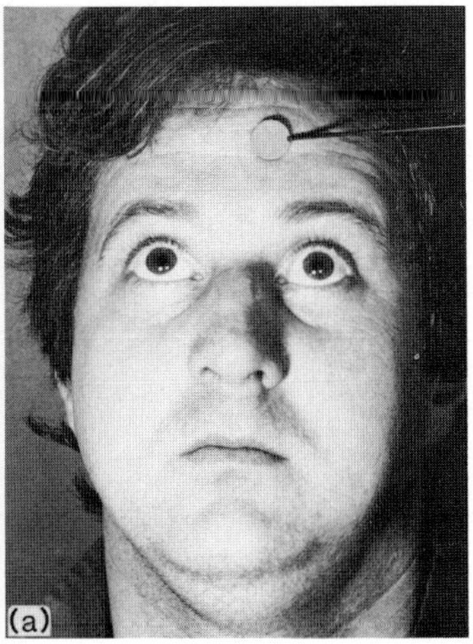

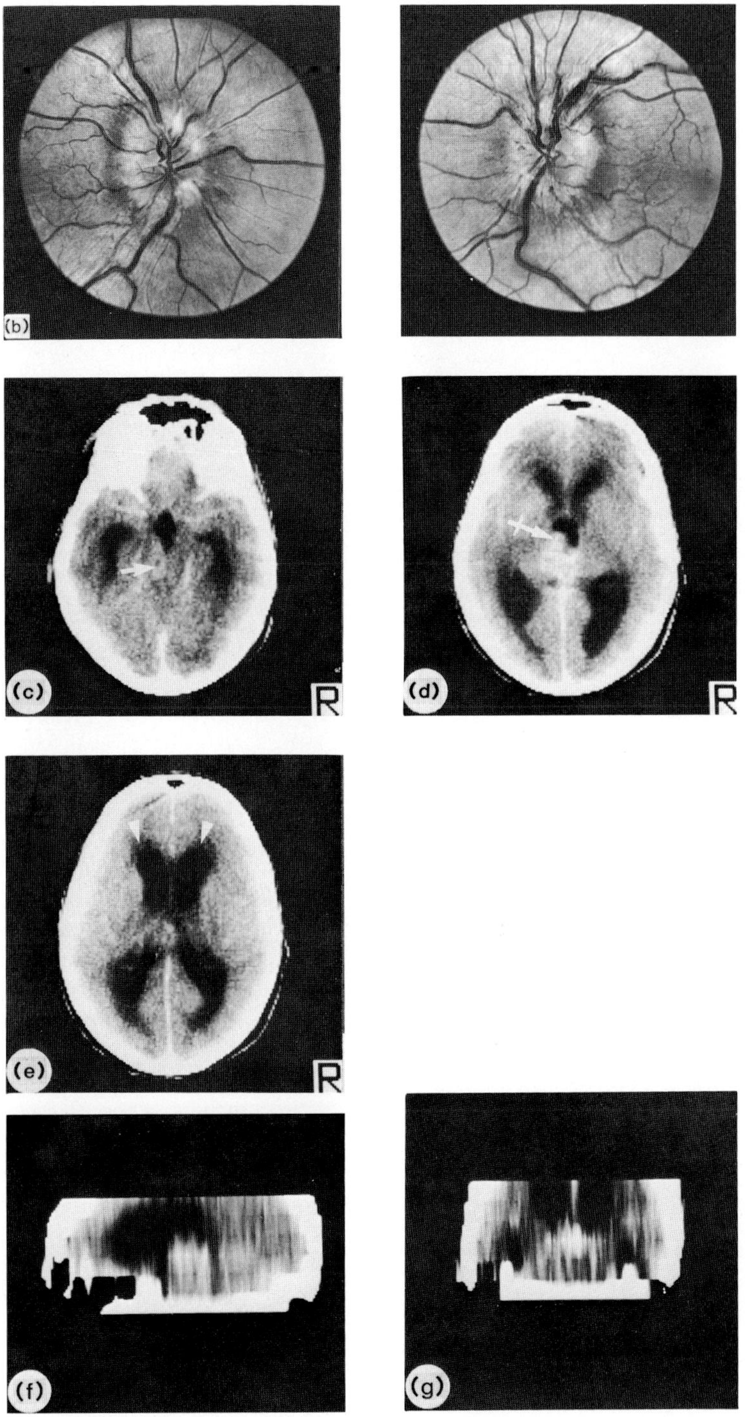

Fig. 6.13 Pineal tumour – presumed germinoma. Diplopia and headache were the presenting symptoms of a 33-year old man. He had restricted up-gaze (a) and convergence, retraction movements on performing upward saccades, light/near dissociation and bilateral papilloedema (b). CT (c–e, after intravenous contrast medium) showed a rather poorly-defined tumour extending downwards towards the left cerebral peduncle (arrow) and anterolaterally into the left thalamus (crossed arrow). There was moderate hydrocephalus, with periventricular lucencies (arrowheads). Sagittal (f) and coronal (g) reconstructions showed the extent of the tumour. Surgical excision of the tumour was deemed impossible and ventricular shunting and radiotherapy produced improvement.

usually smooth or slightly lobulated tumour mass bulging forwards into the dilated third ventricle and/or backwards into the quadrigeminal cistern was seen in 17, in two of which it seemed to be separate from the pineal gland itself (Fig. 6.11). Injection of intravenous contrast medium produced enhancement in the large majority of tumours, usually dense and homogeneous. Cystic tumours were rare, and lesions exhibiting marginal calcification without contrast enhancement were almost certainly teratomas (Fig. 6.12). In cases in which the mass was not clearly visualized, injection of contrast was of definite value in assessing spread into the adjacent thalamus (Fig. 6.13).

Hydrocephalus was present in 29 cases, and in eight patients it was unassociated with either papilloedema or optic atrophy. The hydrocephalus could be marked, and gross enlargement of the third ventricle in two patients produced bitemporal hemianopic field defects.

The differential diagnosis of the mass lesion demonstrated at CT must include a posteriorly orientated basilar tip aneurysm, an aneurysm of the vein of Galen, and a tentorial meningioma.

Treatment

These tumours were generally treated by ventricular shunting and radiotherapy without additional radiological investigation. Only 15 of the 33 patients described had angiography and pneumoencephalography in addition to CT, and six were treated solely on the CT findings. CT is particularly valuable in follow-up studies, and when shrinkage of the tumour and resolution of the hydrocephalus are demonstrated, it offers a non-invasive method of confirming the diagnosis of a radiosensitive lesion, probably a germinoma (Fig. 6.14). It is well recognized that seeding through the cerebrospinal fluid can occur, particularly to the region of the anterior end of the third ventricle (Fig. 6.15). In one patient with a histologically proven germinoma with apparent cure after radiotherapy, a parieto-occipital lesion developed which was thought to have arisen from spread along the track of a ventricular drain.

Onset of visual symptoms in cases of pineal region tumours is usually slow, but may be acute when hydrocephalus or vascular complications supervene. Chambers and McLennon (1978) described five surviving cases of an acute pericollicular syndrome, including what they termed ‘reflex blindness’, in which a haematoma was demonstrated at CT, within a 2 cm radius of the pineal in every case. The smallest was 0.8 cm in diameter, and confined to the tegmentum; the authors commented that narrow beam, overlapping cuts may be required to establish the diagnosis. All five patients showed grossly abnormal eye movements: one patient had a tonic deviation to one side, another had bilateral complete IIIrd nerve palsies and the remaining three had absent upgaze.

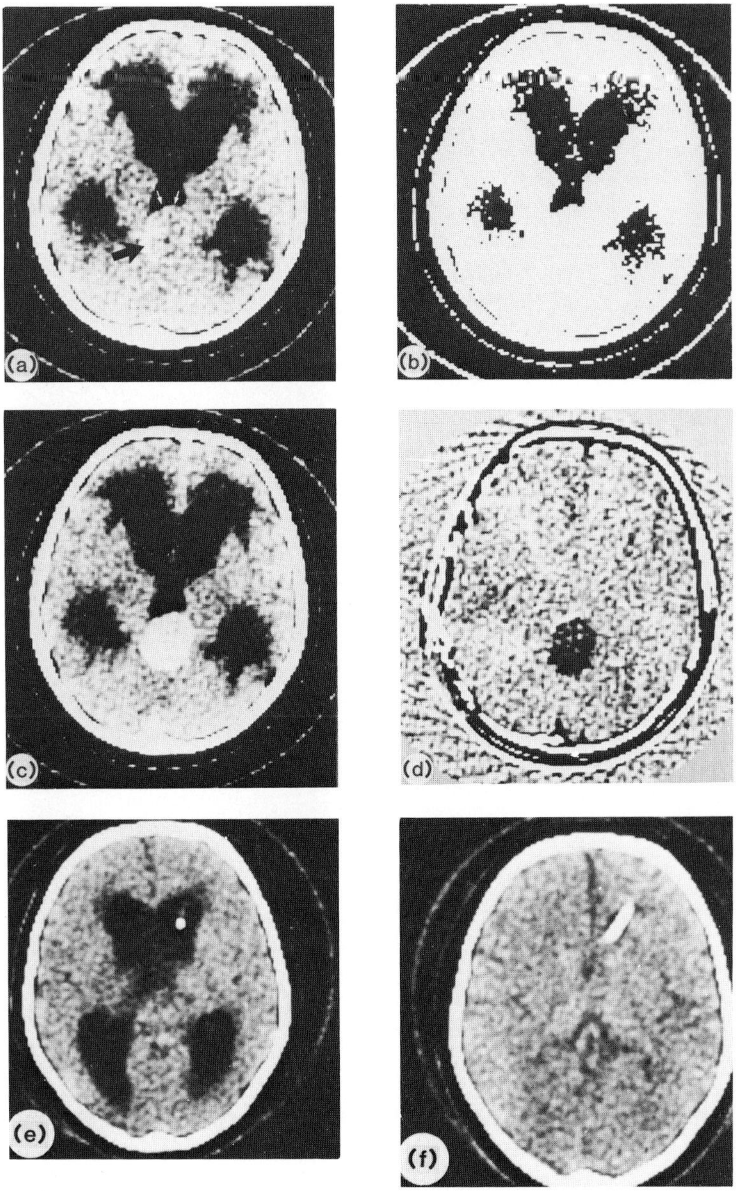

Fig. 6.14 Pineal tumour – presumed germinoma. A boy aged 8 years presented with a 10-week history of poor school performance, headaches, vomiting, unsteadiness and more recently of confusion. Examination showed gross bilateral papilloedema, with haemorrhages, light near dissociation, impairment of upward gaze and bilateral pseudo-abducens palsies. CT (a) showed a mass indenting the posterior end of the third ventricle (small arrows); there was a partial rim suggesting calcification (arrow). Marked periventricular lucencies (PVL) were present around the frontal and temporal horns, shown better by a narrow-window image (b). Marked contrast enhancement of the tumour occurred (c;d is a subtraction of (a) from (c)). The patient was treated by ventricular shunting (e; note disappearance of PVL before decrease in ventricular size) and external radiotherapy with excellent clinical and radiological results (f).

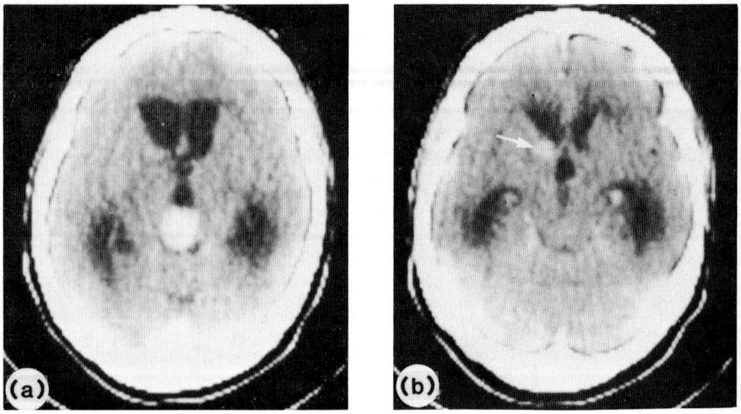

Fig. 6.15 Pinealoma with suprasellar seedling (presumed germinoma). A 62-year old man presented with headache and confusion. He was noted to have light near dissociation, defective up and down gaze and gait ataxia. The optic discs were normal, as were the visual fields. CT (a, b, after intravenous contrast medium) showed a rounded, enhancing mass in the position of the pineal, with a smaller, second lesion beneath the left caudate nucleus (arrow). The small areas of contrast enhancement within the temporal horns (in b) were thought to represent the choroid plexus.

6.7 MIDBRAIN LESIONS PRODUCING DISORDERS OF OCULAR MOVEMENTS

Lesions in the region of the midbrain can produce a complicated constellation of signs due to involvement of the descending fibres controlling horizontal gaze, the descending fibres and nuclei concerned with vertical gaze, and in addition pathways concerned with the lids, pupils, IIIrd and IVth cranial nerves and the 'collicular afferents and efferents'. Clinical differentiation between subthalamic, pretectal and midbrain lesions may be extremely difficult. The ocular motor abnormalities occurring with lesions in this situation, giving rise to the 'top of the basilar syndrome' were discussed by Caplan (1980) and include the following:

Disorders of vertical gaze

Upward or downward gaze may be involved either together or separately and in addition a skew deviation may be superimposed. Bilateral lesions are usually responsible, and isolated paralysis of down-gaze seems associated with posterior commisural lesions (Christoff, 1974), though bilateral lesions in the prerubral zone have also been suggested (Kompf *et al.*, 1979). Paralysis of up gaze may be associated with lesions medial and dorsal to the red nucleus (Halmagyi and Gresty, 1979). Experimental studies have attributed down-gaze palsy to a lesion of the rostral interstitial nucleus of the MLF, with more caudal lesions producing an up-gaze palsy, and the lesions need only be 1–2 mm to produce these signs (Bender, 1980).

Convergence abnormalities

The eyes may be in a convergent position due to increased tone in the medial recti producing the appearance of a pseudo-abducens palsy. Attempted rapid elevation may produce convergence and lier's sign (*vide infra*), oculomotor palsy, sometimes with somnolence, and midbrain corectopia of the pupils. The value of CT in accurate localization of these lesions has been documented.

A patient who was totally unable to look up or down on command or to refixate in the vertical plane after a stroke was subsequently shown by CT to have a widened third ventricle and low attenuation lesions in the dorsomedial part of the thalamus on both sides (Mills and Swanson, 1978), while another with similar eye movement disorders and bilateral ptosis showed enhancement after intravenous contrast medium in the same distribution (Halmagyi *et al.*, 1978). It was suggested in the latter case that the territory of the posterior thalamorubrothalamic or rubral artery was involved. The multiplicity of ocular motor signs makes anatomical localization extremely difficult, as in the patient shown in Fig. 6.16, in whom clinical diagnoses of myasthenia and myopathy were entertained prior to the CT studies.

Lesions producing midbrain and periaqueductal signs are often vascular and may present acutely or in a more chronic form. The anatomy of this region with perfusion from multiple small penetrating and circumferential branches of the terminal basilar artery may explain the variable clinical picture.

6.8 NYSTAGMUS

Oscillations of the eyes may be pendular when the speed is the same in each direction or 'jerk' when one direction has a fast component, which serves to define the nystagmus.

Congenital oscillation of the eyes may occur with absent or poor vision, when pendular features are present, or with adequate vision, when the nystagmus has a jerk pattern. Acquired nystagmus is a feature of subcortical derangement of neural function and is seen characteristically with brainstem, cerebellar and vestibular lesions. Particular types of nystagmus may provide important information of clinical localization.

This section will discuss types of nystagmus in which CT is indicated.

See-saw nystagmus

The combination of rotary and vertical nystagmus presents a characteristic appearance, particularly because the elevating eye intorts and the depressing extorts. Hence the designation and recognition is important because this represents a sign of a large mass in or near the optic chiasm (Fig. 6.17); such lesions are discussed further in Chapter 4. Developmental abnormalities (e.g. septo-optic dysplasia, Chapter 7) and trauma may also be responsible.

Russell's diencephalic syndrome

Severe marasmus, with vertical or rotatory nystagmus, in a baby should alert the clinician to the presence of a large hypothalamic lesion, usually a glioma (Chapter 4).

Gaze-evoked and gaze-paretic nystagmus

Gaze-evoked nystagmus is rapid, jerk type, enhanced by eccentric gaze, and increased by eccentricity (Alexander's Law). Gaze-paretic nystagmus is slower than jerk nystagmus and thought to reflect difficulty in maintaining eccentric gaze. A combination of both types in the same patient is suggestive of unilateral brainstem compression: the gaze-paretic nystagmus being due to pressure on the ipsilateral pons, and the contralateral gaze-evoked nystagmus to pressure on the ipsilateral vestibular system. This combination is usually due to a cerebellopontine angle tumour, of which the acoustic neuroma accounts for about 70% of cases, with meningiomas or metastases making up most of the remainder. Neuromas frequently have attenuation coefficients which are similar to those of the adjacent brain, be it normal or oedematous, and for this reason may be manifest at CT either by indirect signs, such as contralateral displacement of the fourth ventricle, or merely as a poorly-defined area of mixed or low attenuation anterolaterally in the posterior cranial fossa. Intravenous contrast medium almost invariably produces moderate to marked homogeneous increase in attenuation of the tumour, indicating its true extent, which may otherwise be difficult to assess (Fig. 5.6). Hydrocephalus is a not uncommon accompaniment, especially in older patients. Cerebellopontine angle meningiomas may be almost indistinguishable from neuromas at CT, but tend to be of higher attenuation before intravenous contrast medium. Improved demonstration of cerebellopontine angle lesions may be obtained by the use of intrathecal metrizamide (Fig. 6.18).

Asymmetric vertical oscillatory movements

Rapid small amplitude oscillatory movements, usually vertical or rotatory may be seen with visual loss. The movements may be asymmetrical and more marked in the eye with the greater reduction of vision. CT is useful to exclude a chiasmal glioma (Fig. 6.17) though other neurological causes of visual loss may be responsible.

Up-beat nystagmus

There are few satisfactory reports on this subject, but large amplitude up-beat movements increasing with elevation of the eyes have been attributed to anterior vermian lesions, whereas small amplitude up-gaze movements diminishing on elevation may be seen with intrinsic medullary disease, e.g. medulloblastoma (Fig. 6.19). Up-beat nystagmus may be seen in any condition that produces extensive brainstem dysfunction, when it is usually associated with other clinical signs.

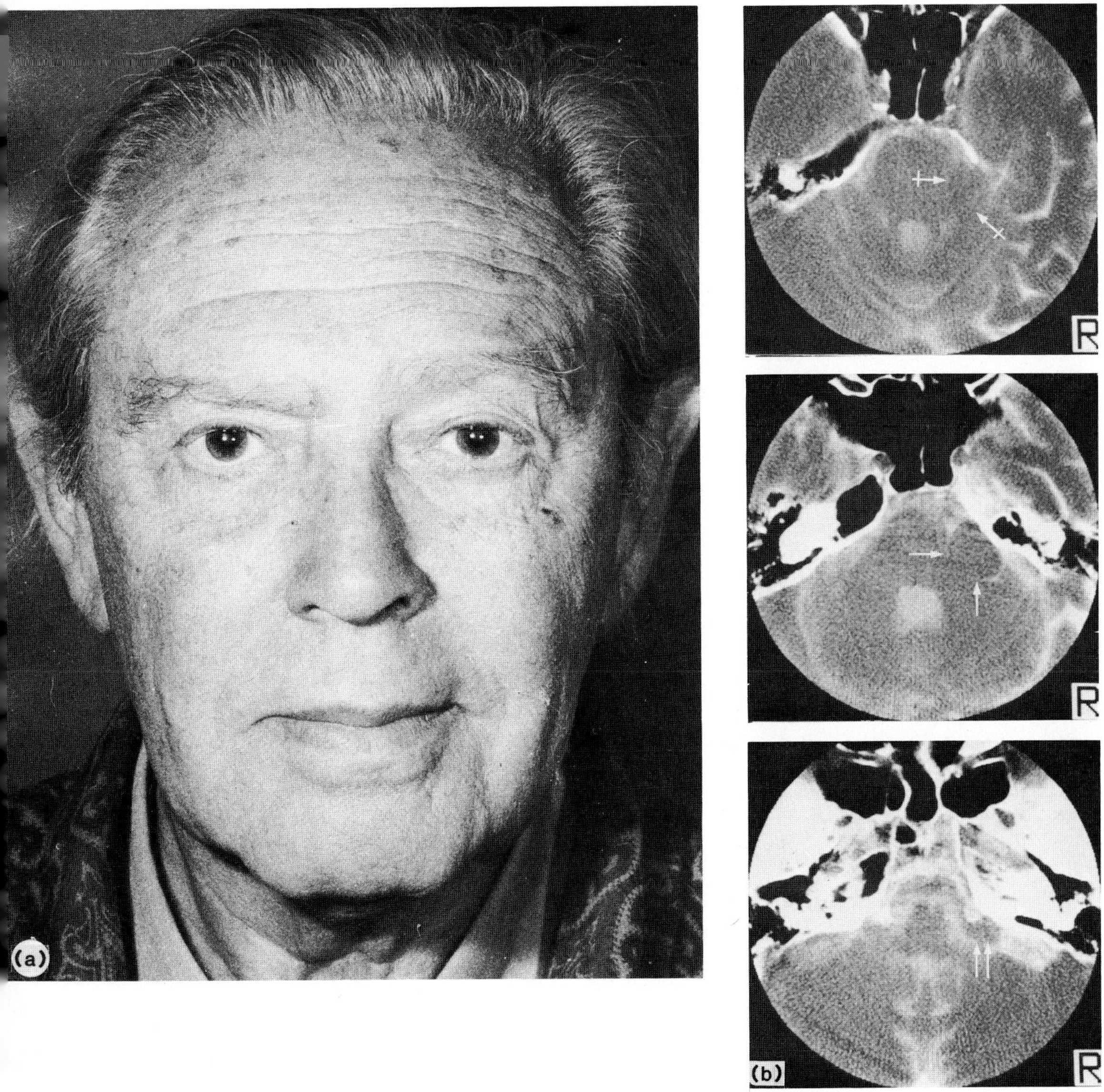

Fig. 6.18 Horizontal nystagmus – acoustic neuroma. A 76-year old man was seen with deafness in the right ear, giddiness and more recently loss of sensation and movement in the right side of the face (a). Ocular examination was normal apart from nystagmus on looking to the left, and looking upwards. Eye movement recordings showed nystagmus to the left with impaired pursuit to the left, and impaired pursuit upwards. Inhibition of the vestibulo-ocular reflex failed to occur when the head was rotated to the right. CT was carried out before and after intravenous contrast medium, and was thought to be normal. Because of the clear clinical picture, it was repeated with intrathecal metrizamide (b), revealing a rounded mass in the cerebellopontine angle (arrows) extending down to the pontomedullary junction (double arrow) and up to the tentorial hiatus (crossed arrows). At surgery a Schwannoma of the acoustic nerve was removed.

Down-beat nystagmus

This is defined as nystagmus in the primary position with the fast phase beating downwards, but similar aetiological factors may produce down-beat nystagmus only on looking eccentrically downwards. The finding of *isolated* down-beat nystagmus merits investigation to exclude:

Arnold-Chiari Type II malformation
(i.e. cerebellar tonsilar ectopia)
CT may reveal no definite abnormality. The fourth ventricle, and indeed all the posterior fossa structures, may appear low in position, but this is difficult to assess without coronal sections or sagittal reconstructions. With high resolution scans it may be possible to detect the presence of the cerebellar tonsils lying behind the medulla at the level of the foramen magnum; the normal cisterna magna cannot be seen. Myelography is, however, more reliable in this respect; where water-soluble contrast medium is used, it can be combined with CT (Fig. 6.20). Associated lesions may be shown by CT: hydrocephalus, craniocervical skeletal anomalies, meningocoele or syringomyelia.

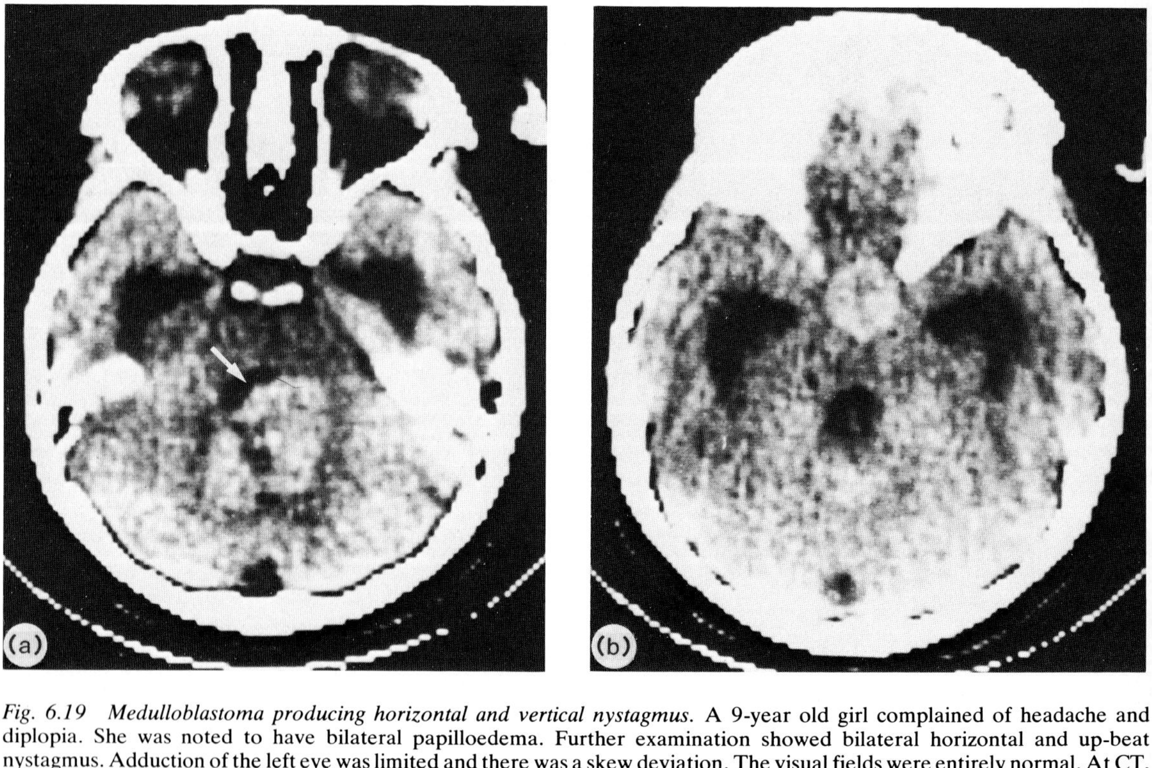

Fig. 6.19 Medulloblastoma producing horizontal and vertical nystagmus. A 9-year old girl complained of headache and diplopia. She was noted to have bilateral papilloedema. Further examination showed bilateral horizontal and up-beat nystagmus. Adduction of the left eye was limited and there was a skew deviation. The visual fields were entirely normal. At CT, an irregular tumour of increased attenuation was seen lying centrally in the cerebellum, compressing the fourth ventricle (arrow) and causing marked hydrocephalus. High sections showed further tumour lying directly above the sella turcica. A medulloblastoma was removed at operation.

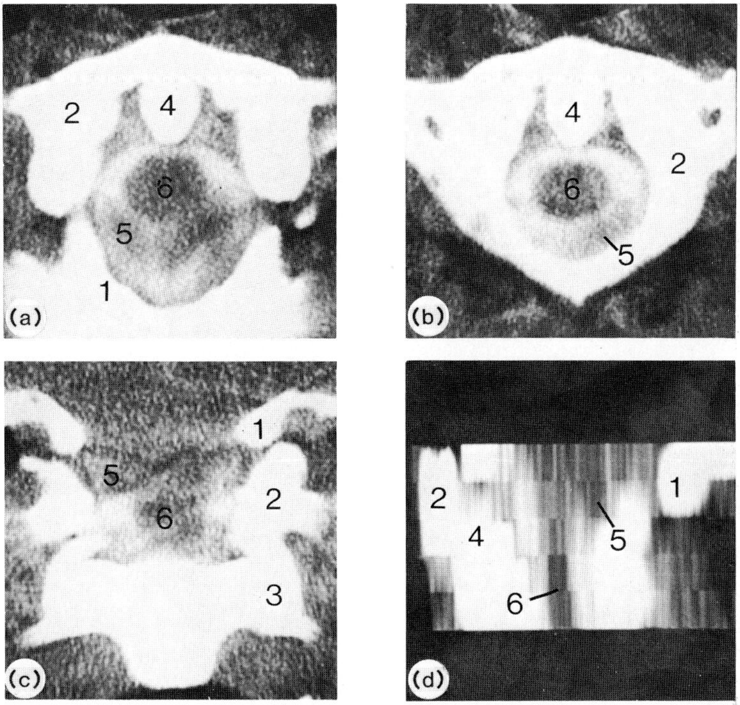

Fig. 6.20 Down-beat nystagmus – Arnold-Chiari malformation. Paroxysmal headache, engendered by emotional and physical excitement, was the presenting symptom in a 23-year old woman. The only abnormality on physical examination was down-beat nystagmus. CT (after metrizamide myelography) showed cerebellar tonsillar herniation (Arnold-Chiari malformation). (a,b) Axial sections at and below level of foramen magnum. (c) Coronal section, (d) midline sagittal reconstruction through foramen. (1) Margins of foramen magnum (basiocciput); (2) first cervical vertebra; (3) second cervical vertebra; (4) odontoid peg; (5) cerebellar tonsil; (6) cervical spinal cord.

Hereditary spinocerebellar degeneration
Atrophy of the cerebellum and upper spinal cord may be apparent (Fig. 6.21).

Other lesions
Other lesions within or near the brainstem (e.g. ependymoma, cherry red spot myoclonus syndrome) (Fig. 6.22).

It is important to realise that down-beat nystagmus may be seen with any diffuse brainstem process such as a glioma or demyelination, but in these conditions there are other ocular motor or neurological signs.

Ocular bobbing

Rapid, conjugate, downward jerking of the eyes is seen in severe bilateral brainstem disease, often associated with marked depression of conscious level. Massive intrinsic brainstem lesions such as haemorrhage, infarction or tumour, are commonly present, but compression by cerebellar or extra-axial haematomas has been reported.

Opsoclonus

This is a bizarre multidirectional, chaotic disturbance of eye movements, which may be due to a remote, non-metastatic manifestation of neuroblastoma (sometimes otherwise occult) in children or carcinoma in adults.

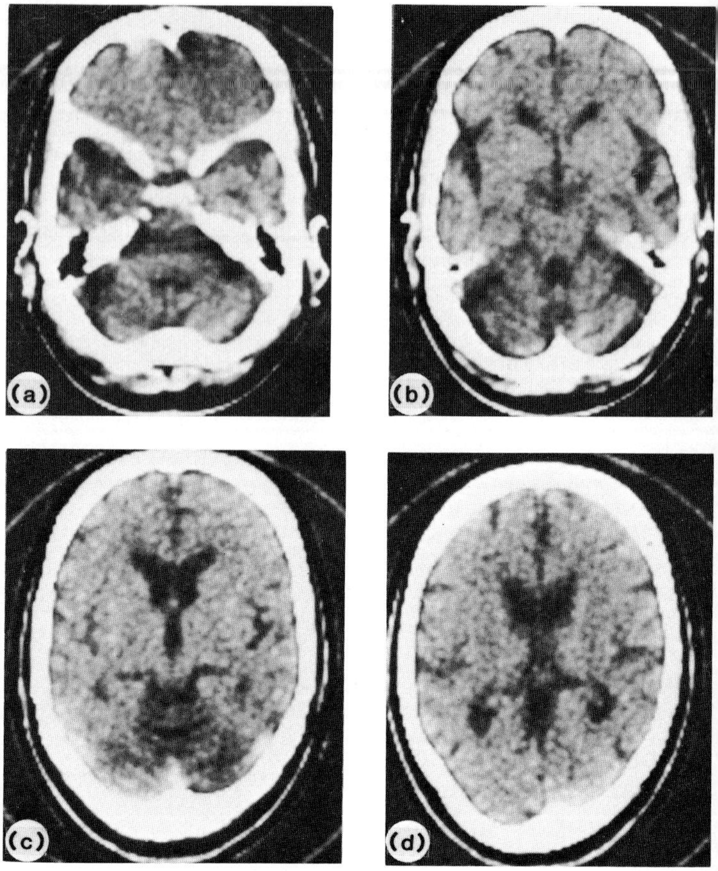

Fig. 6.21 Down-beat nystagmus – cerebellar atrophy. A 47-year old man showed a progressive cerebellar syndrome, with marked down-beat nystagmus, and dementia. CT (a–d) showed mild generalized cerebral atrophy, with gross cerebellar atrophy, affecting both hemispheres and the vermis. Note the inferior surface of the tentorium outlined by CSF in c.

6.9 CEREBELLAR LESIONS

Common conditions involving the cerebellum are:

1. Vascular disease.
2. Demyelination.
3. Spinocerebellar degenerations.
4. Tumours (e.g. astrocytoma).

The involvement of the cerebellum in saccadic, pursuit and vestibular ocular movements leads to a wide range of disordered eye movements in cerebellar disease. However, the close anatomical proximity and the abundant neural connections between the cerebellum and the brainstem make the differentiation between pure cerebellar and pure brainstem disease extremely difficult. Rare disorders such as flutter-like movements can be recognized with experience, but the clinician should observe nystagmus carefully for at least five minutes, to detect features of rebound nystagmus or periodic alternating nystagmus.

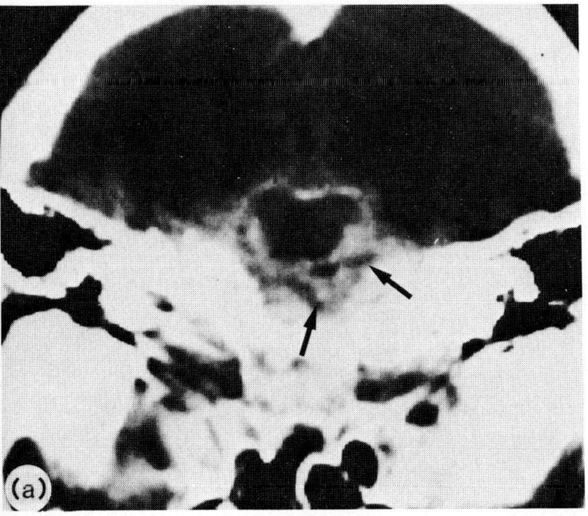

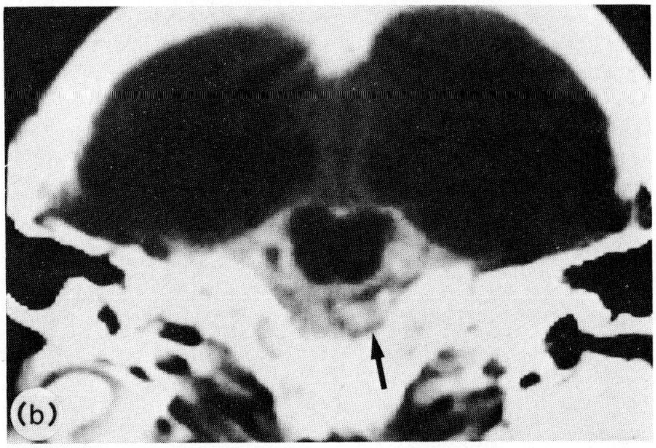

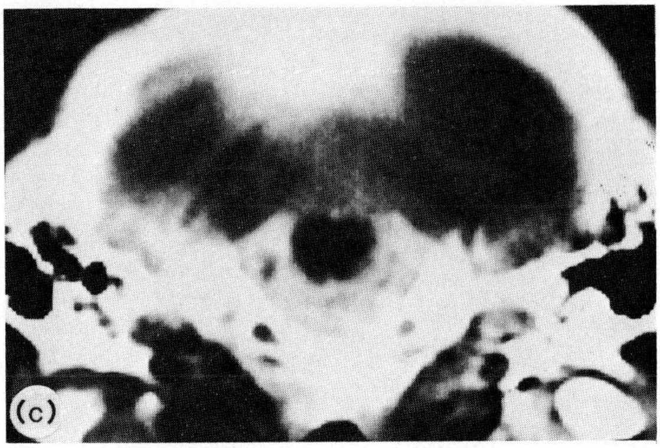

Fig. 6.22 Down-beat nystagmus – epidermoid tumour. A 30-year old woman presented with oscillopsia and subsequently developed gait ataxia and diplopia. She was found to have nystagmus, down-beating on laevo depression, she also had a left VIth nerve palsy. Repeated CT scans were negative; a further study was then carried out with intrathecal metrizamide (a–c). With the patient prone, an irregular filling defect was seen in the lower pontine cistern (arrows). An epidermoid was largely removed at surgery, after which the oscillopsia improved.

CT of cerebellar lesions generally provides accurate localization and the diagnosis of infarction or acute haemorrhage can be made with reasonable certainty, the CT features being identical to those of supratentorial lesions. Of the commonly seen tumours, astrocytomas, haemangioblastomas and metastases tend to arise in the cerebellar hemispheres; all may be cystic and show ring or nodular contrast enhancement. Medulloblastomas (Fig. 6.19) and ependymomas are characteristically solid tumours of increased attenuation, lying centrally in the position of the vermis or fourth ventricle and showing more or less homogeneous enhancement (Wilson and Moseley, 1977).

6.10 OCULARMOTOR NUCLEI AND NERVES (Fig. 6.7)

The ocularmotor nerve (IIIrd nerve). The ocularmotor nucleus lies ventral to the periaqueductal grey matter at the level of the superior colliculus. The rostrally placed superior rectus nucleus innervates the contralateral superior rectus muscle, while all other nuclei innervate the ipsilateral medial and inferior recti,

Fig. 6.23 IIIrd nerve palsy – posterior communicating artery aneurysm. A 63-year old woman suffered a subarachnoid haemorrhage, leaving her with a complete IIIrd nerve palsy (a). CT showed the aneurysm, five days after the ictus, slightly denser than the surrounding brain, anterolateral to the brainstem (b). There was questionable subarachnoid blood (open arrows). The aneurysm showed marked contrast enhancement (c) and was confirmed by angiography.

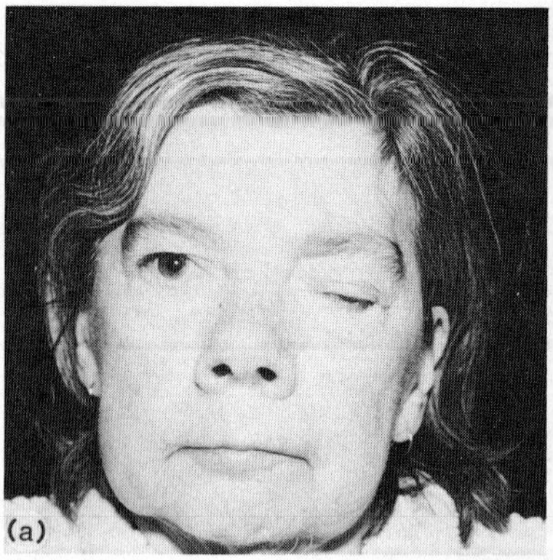

(a)

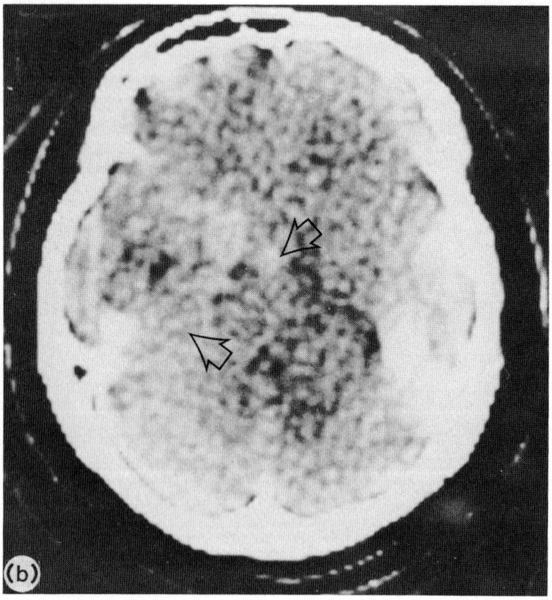

(b)

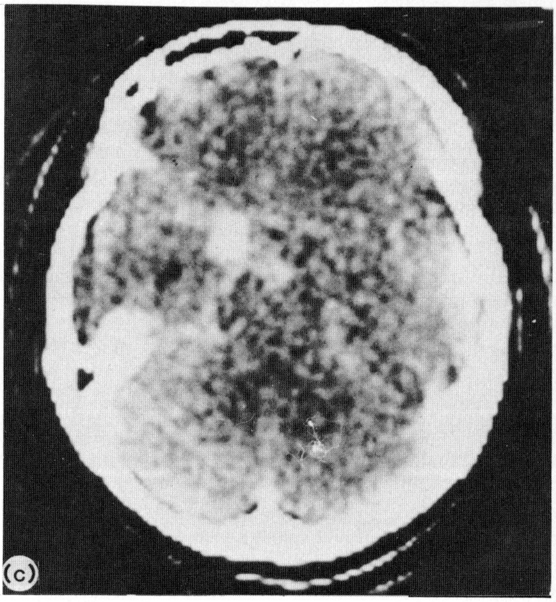

(c)

and the inferior oblique. The nerve fibres emerge through the midbrain, sweeping in an arc through the red nucleus to emerge in the interpeduncular fossa. The nerve then traverses the upper part of the cavernous sinus to enter the orbit via the superior orbital fissure.

Trochlear nerve (IVth nerve). The nucleus lies in periaqueductal grey matter caudal to the oculomotor nerve. Fibres cross after leaving the nucleus though there is some evidence of ipsilateral representation as well; decussation occurs in the superior medullary velum. This is the only nerve to decussate and emerge dorsally, which necessitates encircling the midbrain, crossing the superior cerebellar artery and entering the cavernous sinus. It enters the superior orbital fissure to innervate the superior oblique muscle.

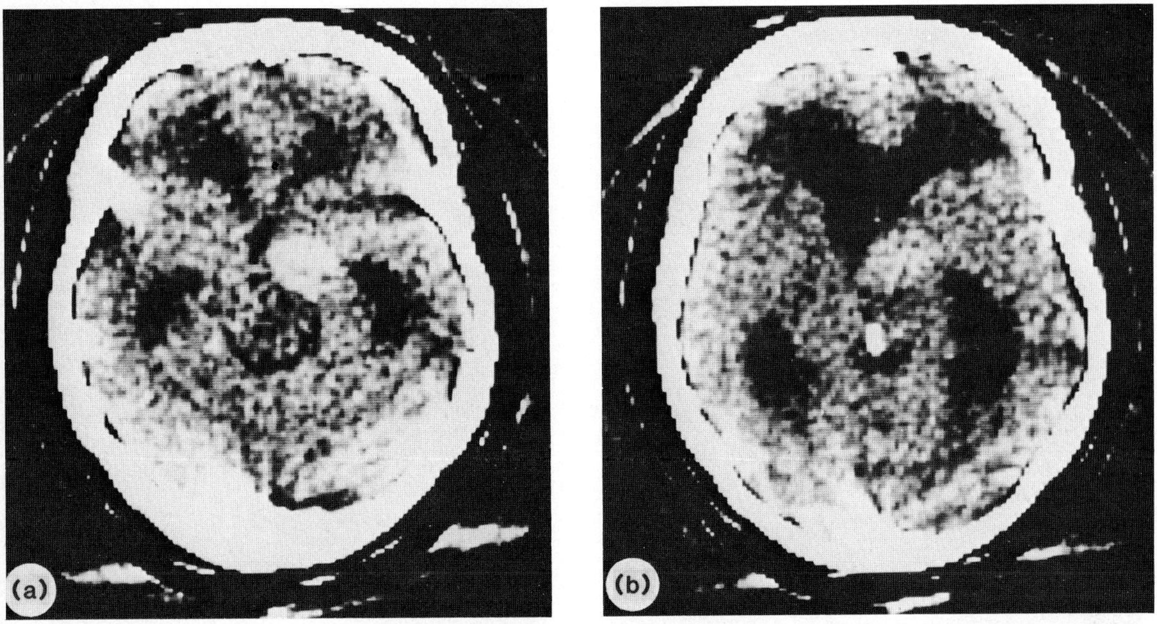

Fig. 6.24 IIIrd nerve palsy – terminal carotid artery aneurysm. A 56-year old woman suddenly lost consciousness and on recovering was found to have a right IIIrd nerve palsy. CT showed a rounded mass slightly denser than normal brain, lying to the right of the third ventricle, which was distorted (a) and causing obstructive hydrocephalus (b), with periventricular lucencies. Contrast medium was not given. This lesion was confirmed by angiography to be a large aneurysm arising from the internal carotid artery just distal to the ophthalmic artery.

Abducens nerve (VIth nerve). The nucleus is situated in the floor of the fourth ventricle lying in the eminence called the facil colliculus, due to looping of the facial nerve fibres around the VIth nerve nucleus. Emerging at the pontomedullary junction, the nerve climbs the clivus and crosses the inferior cerebellar artery. It traverses the petrosal sinus to enter the cavernous sinus under the petroclinoid ligament, and is in close apposition to the intracavernous carotid artery. Entering the orbit through the superior orbital fissue, it supplies the lateral rectus.

The ocularmotor nerves can be involved by pathological processes within the brain, intracranially, in the cavernous sinus, in the orbital fissure or within the orbit.

IIIrd nerve palsy

Nuclear lesions of the IIIrd nerve are rare and verification is difficult without pathological confirmation. Combined nuclear and fascicular lesions may result from intrinsic disease, either vascular or due to tumours such as gliomas or metastases. Fascicular IIIrd nerve palsies with contralateral hemiplegia (Weber's syndrome) or with contralateral tremor (Benedict's syndrome) emphasize the proximity of the IIIrd nerve to the corticospinal tracts and red nucleus respectively.

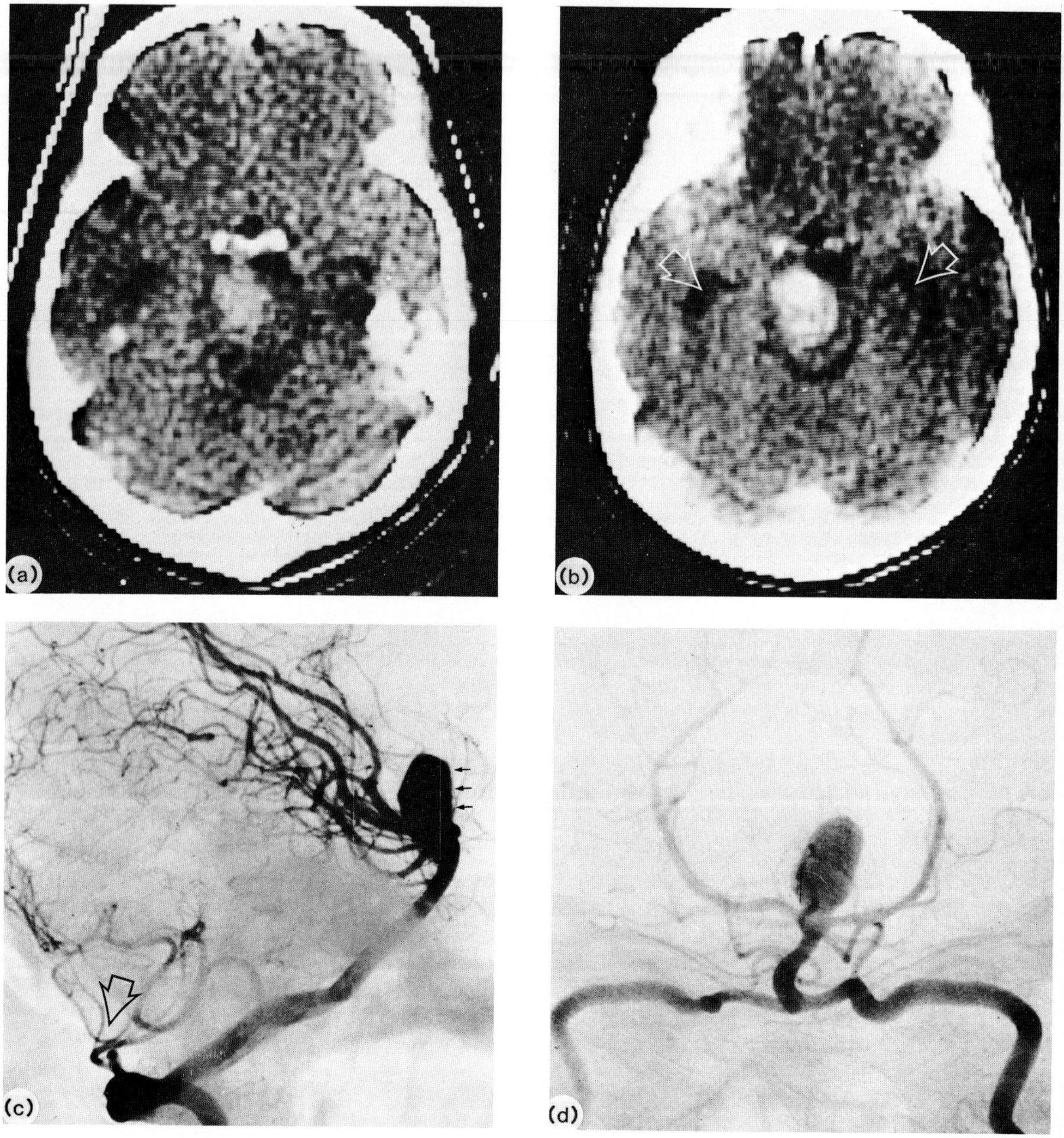

Fig. 6.25 Vertical gaze palsy – basilar aneurysm. A 51-year old man was admitted following the recent onset of diplopia; he had previously had four transient attacks over a 20-year period. The right pupil reacted slowly and he had bilateral ptosis, with complete failure of up and down gaze; neither eye could be adducted beyond the midline. He was drowsy, dysarthric and had a left cerebellar ataxia; the plantar responses were extensor. The CSF was xanthochromic. CT (a, before; b, after intravenous contrast) demonstrated a mass of higher attenuation than brain lying between the cerebral peduncles, markedly compressing the midbrain. It showed considerable eccentric contrast enhancement. Hydrocephalus was present (note the dilated temporal horns – open arrows). Vertebral angiography (c, lateral; d, half axial projections) confirmed the presence of a large saccular aneurysm at the tip of the basilar artery. Comparison of the apparent size of the aneurysm at CT and angiography indicates considerable mural thrombus. (Note the fluid level (small arrows) and evidence of tonsillar herniation (open arrow) in c). The patient subsequently developed a right rubral tremor.

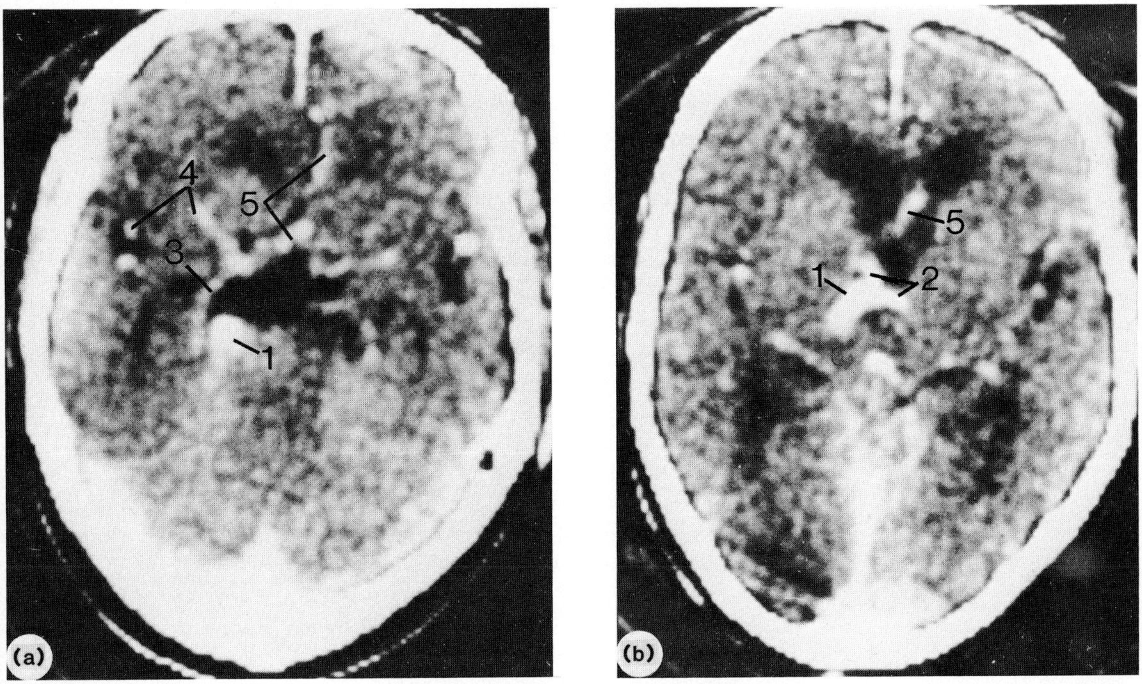

Fig. 6.26 IVth nerve palsy – basilar artery ectasia. A hypertensive man of 63 had been demented and ataxic; he complained of dysphagia and diplopia on down gaze. Examination showed a left IVth nerve palsy, dementia, ataxia, pyramidal and bulbar signs. Calcification was present on CT, and after intravenous contrast medium there was marked enhancement of ectatic basal arteries, especially the basilar. (1) Basilar; (2) posterior cerebral; (3) posterior communicating; (4) middle cerebral and (5) anterior cerebral arteries. There was mild hydrocephalus and hypertensive white matter low attenuation was present. Angiography confirmed the arterial ectasia.

The paired IIIrd nerves emerge in the interpeduncular fossa where they are in relationship to several vessels of consequence. The relationship to the posterior communicating artery accounts for the high incidence of sudden painful complete IIIrd nerve palsies due to aneurysms (Fig. 6.23). Though statistically the pupillary involvement is higher with aneurysms than microvascular infarction of the nerve, we have seen sufficient patients with pupil sparing IIIrd nerve palsies and aneurysms to make this rule less relevant to the individual case.

Since circulating blood has almost the same attenuation coefficients as normal brain, and as a relatively small aneurysm can produce a IIIrd nerve palsy, detection at CT may be difficult unless intravenous contrast medium is given. The aneurysm may appear as a circular area of increased attenuation posterolateral to the sella turcica but because of the proximity to the bones of the skull base, resolution is insufficient to detect small aneurysms. It may be argued that, since angiography will almost certainly be carried out in these cases, it is quite unnecessary to subject the patients to intravenous contrast medium injection;

we would subscribe to this view. If subarachnoid haemorrhage has occurred, the basal cisterns may be effaced or appear of high attenuation over a variable area; these changes are seen in almost 90% of cases examined within one week of the haemorrhage.

A case of primary aberrant regeneration of the IIIrd nerve, with abnormal innervation of the lids and pupils was described by Cox *et al.* (1979). CT showed a small parasellar lesion, denser with contrast enhancement, which was confirmed on angiography to be a posterior communicating artery aneurysm.

CT is more valuable in the larger terminal carotid or basilar tip aneurysms, which may involve the IIIrd nerves or in later stages produce other signs of rostral midbrain compression. (Figs. 6.24 and 6.25).

It was stated by Boeri and Passerini (1964) that ectasia of the basilar artery was almost invariably associated with at least a partial IIIrd nerve lesion, the side of affection of the nerve being determined by the tilt of the termination of the basilar artery. Moseley and Holland (1979), in their review of the clinical and radiological features of this condition, found that only two of 45 further cases were reported as showing IIIrd nerve palsies, while two patients had probable IVth nerve lesions (Fig. 6.26) and in nine the VIth nerve was involved. In the large majority of cases the cranial nerve palsies were unilateral; in saccular aneurysms of the basilar termination, both IIIrd nerves may be involved. The CT features of basilar artery ectasia are described in Chapter 4.

The IIIrd nerve may be involved in tumours of the basisphenoid, and a sphenoid sinus mucocoele may rarely produce optic nerve or IIIrd nerve compression, and when successfully recognized and treated produces gratifying results.

The IIIrd nerve is vulnerable to compression by basal cerebral tumours (Fig. 6.27) or when there is transtentorial uncal herniation. The latter can be recognized at CT by deformation of the brain stem, which is flattened on the affected side by the inferomedially herniated temporal lobe (Fig. 4.35) and by compression or absence of the ipsilateral ambient cistern, the chiasmatic cistern and the interpeduncular fossa. Asymmetry of the quadrigeminal cistern is also observed; in the early stages it may appear enlarged on the affected side, but it is subsequently obliterated (Osborn, 1977). Basal meningitis may also involve the IIIrd nerve (Fig. 6.28).

IVth nerve palsy

Isolated IVth nerve palsies are less common than IIIrd or VIth nerve palsies. Unilateral IVth nerve palsies may rarely be the presenting sign of tumours in the middle or posterior fossae in younger people, and in the older age groups are usually manifestations of a microvascular occlusion (Fig. 6.29). Bilateral palsies

Fig. 6.27 IIIrd nerve palsy – thalamic and midbrain glioma. A 45-yeard old man suddenly developed a typical left IIIrd nerve palsy with pupillary involvement (a). CT (b, before; c, after, intravenous contrast medium) demonstrated a glioma involving the left thalamus and third ventricular region. There was no evidence of haemorrhage.

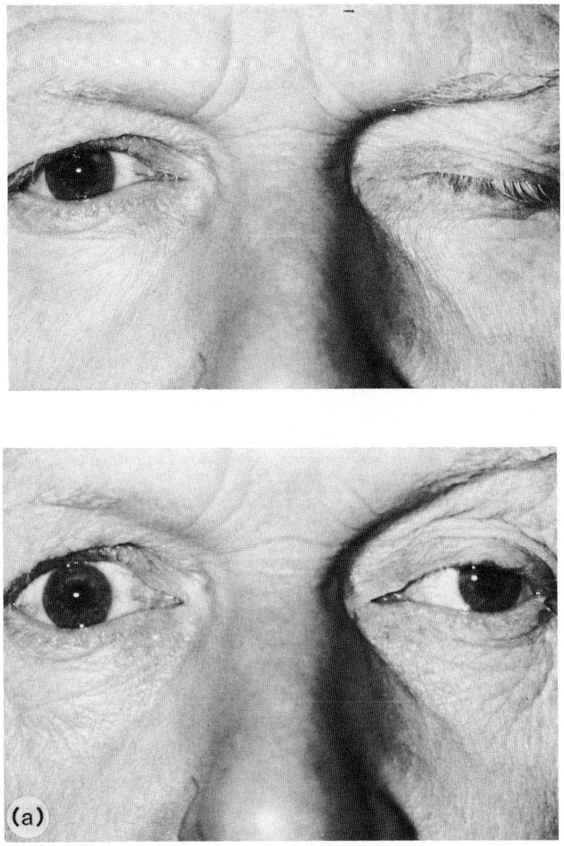

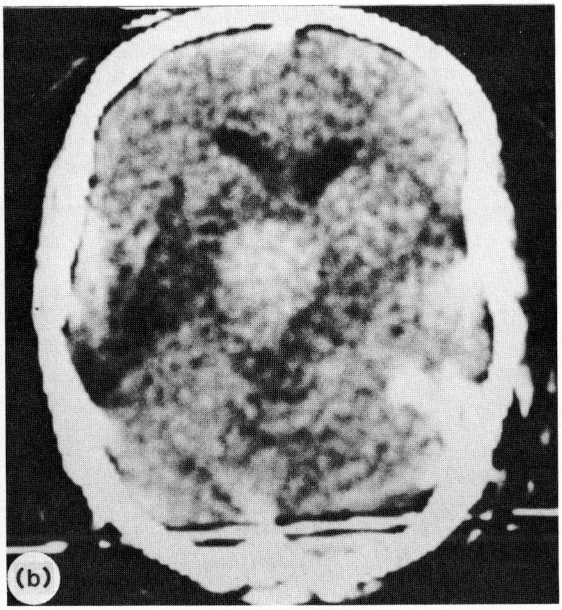

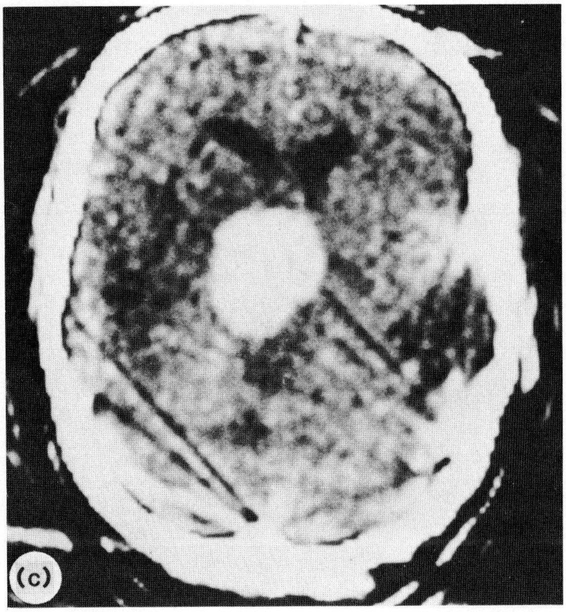

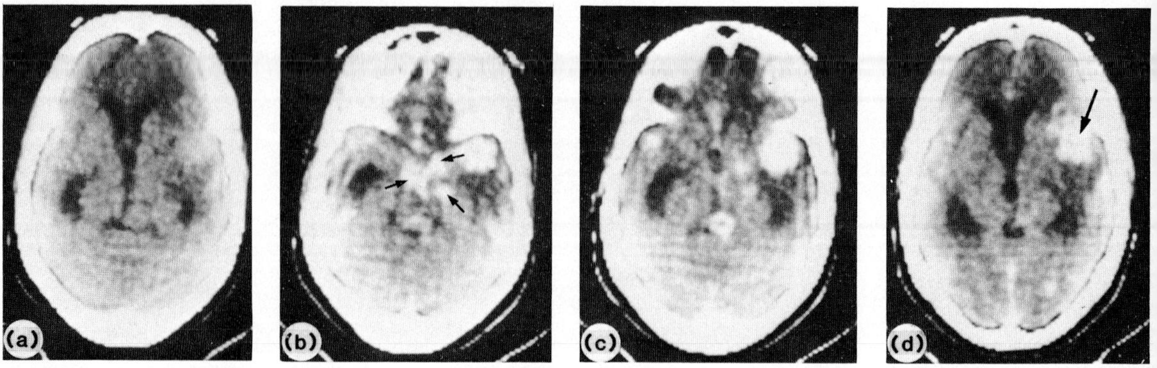

Fig. 6.28 IIIrd nerve palsy – tuberculous meningitis. Following pulmonary tuberculosis, a 32-year old Indian immigrant developed tuberculous meningitis which was extremely resistant to drug therapy. About one year after the onset, with generalized deterioration, she showed a right IIIrd nerve palsy. CT (a, before; b–d after intravenous contrast medium) showed white matter low-attenuation, and several tuberculomas, notably a multicystic lesion in the right Sylvian fissure (arrow). The lowest section (b) showed clear evidence of chronic granulomatous meningitis (small arrows).

are seen most frequently following trauma, particularly with direct falls on the vertex (e.g. after projection from a horse). In the occasional instance a tumour in the region of the superior medullary velum may produce bilateral IVth nerve damage. CT is therefore of value in excluding the rare space occupying lesion that may present with a IVth nerve palsy, and may be of value in traumatic cases. The majority of cases with microvascular and infiltrative lesions will show normal appearances.

VIth nerve palsy

Isolated sixth nerve palsies may be due to a wide variety of disorders in different sites, and rarely to a space occupying lesion, such as an intrinsic glioma (Fig. 6.10), a tumour arising from the basisphenoid (i.e. chordoma or carcinoma) or more rarely still, a tumour of the cavernous sinus. The VIth nerve is particularly vulnerable as it runs forward in relation to the petrous apex. Previously the major cause of VIth nerve lesions in this vicinity was ear infection, with mastoiditis or petrositis and lateral sinus thrombosis. Malignant destruction of the petrous apex is now the most common cause; affection of the sixth nerve as an isolated phenomenon is of course rare, but the basal CT cuts should be inspected carefully to detect bone lesions at the petrous apex in patients with appropriate symptoms and signs (Fig. 6.30). Tumours of the Gasserian ganglion (schwannoma) may also present with isolated ocular motor lesions, often involving the VIth nerve (Yamashita *et al.*, 1977) and occasionally the IIIrd or IVth nerves. Thus CT provides an essential part of the investigation, but generally with a low return. More common causes include microvascular disease, meningeal inflammatory disease and a number of cases may evade diagnosis despite

Fig. 6.29 Skew deviation. A 26-year old man awoke with diplopia, ataxia and dysarthria. The diplopia persisted and he noted that the left eyelid drooped, and that images appeared darker in the left eye. Visual examination was normal apart from the eye movements. There was a left hypertropia; present on elevation and depression, consistent with a skew deviation, but initially diagnosed as a IVth nerve palsy. CT was originally thought to be normal (b), but intravenous contrast medium showed a small enhancing lesion posteromedially in the left thalamus. Vertebral angiography was normal. CSF and VER studies were normal, suggesting that a small infarct was more likely than an episode of demyelination.

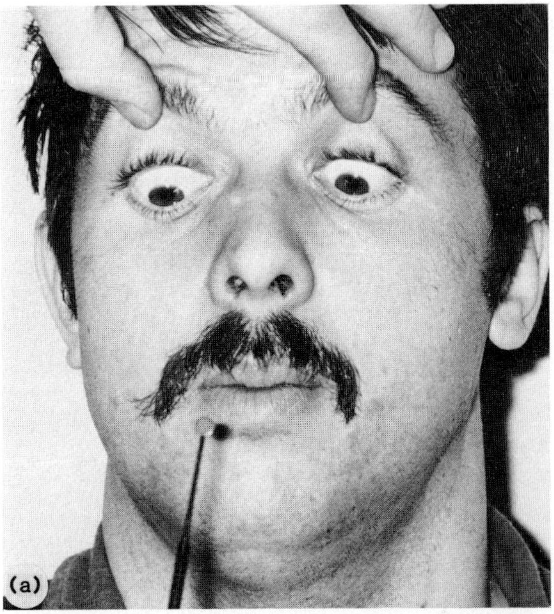

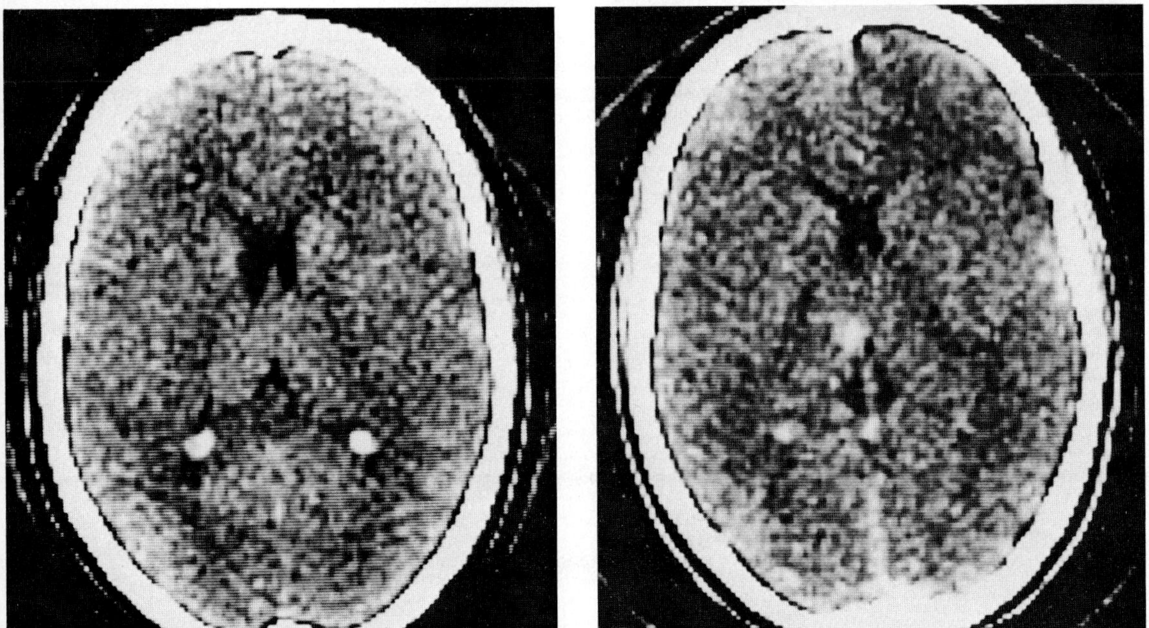

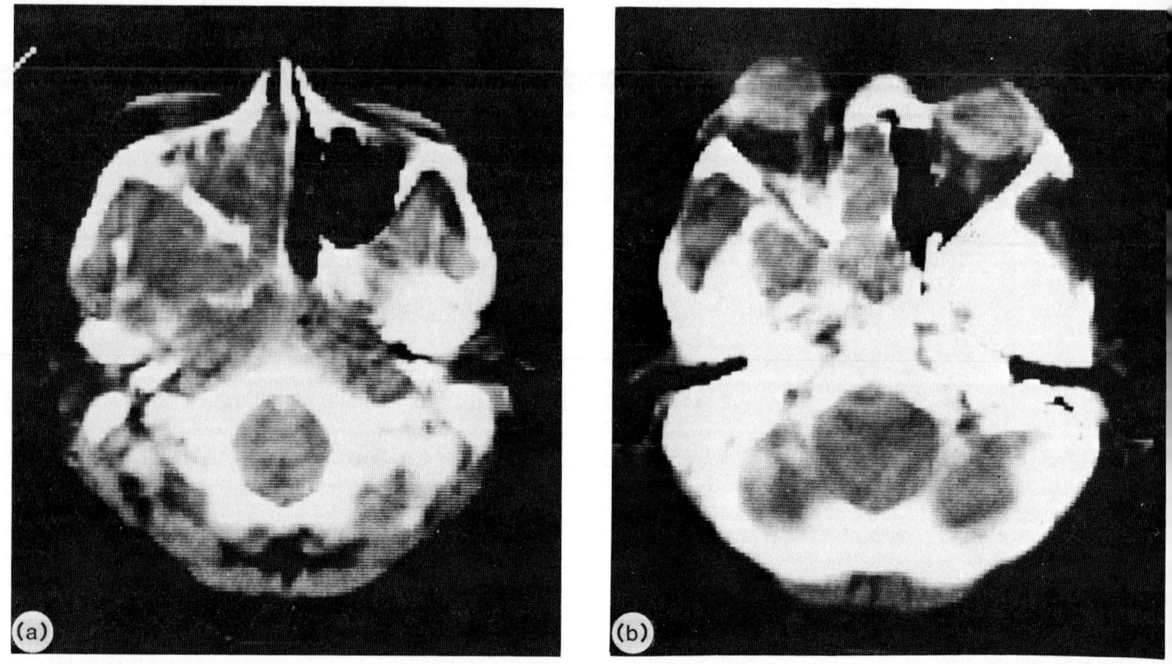

Fig. 6.30 *VIth nerve palsy – meningioma invading skull base.* A sphenoid wing meningioma had been treated surgically seven years previously, when the patient was aged 49. She returned complaining of proptosis, diplopia and hearing loss. Examination confirmed gross proptosis, a left VIth nerve palsy and a bulging left drum. CT showed massive destruction of the skull base, tumour filling the sphenoid and left ethmoid and maxillary sinuses and the nasal cavity.

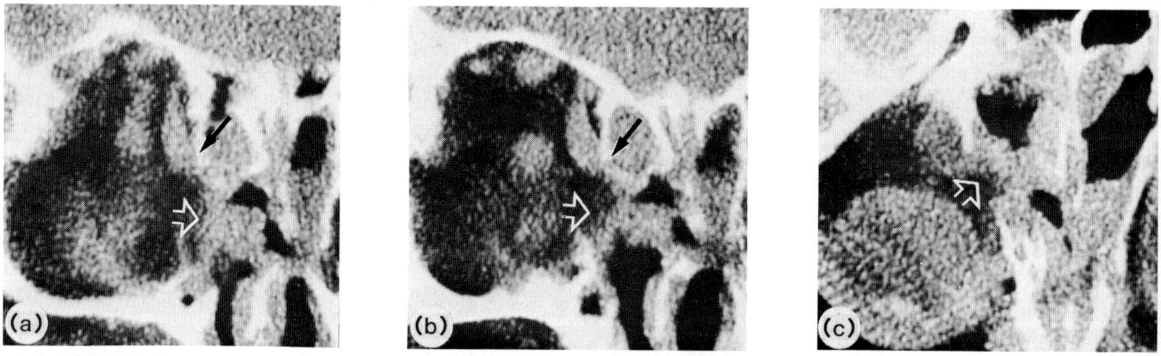

Fig. 6.31 *Pseudoabducens palsy – trapped medial rectus.* Abduction was grossly limited immediately following an operation for inflammatory disease of the ethmoid sinuses in a middle-aged man. Attempted abduction caused an increase in intraocular pressure, indicating tethering. CT (a,b, coronal; c, axial sections) showed a large defect in the lamina papyracea (open arrows) surrounded by inflammatory tissue to which the medial rectus muscle (arrows) appeared adherent (note lack of movement between a and b).

extensive investigation. The clinician should always exclude developmental anomalies and local infiltrative conditions of the orbit, or specific disease of the ocular muscles (e.g. myasthenia).

Pseudoabducens palsy should always be considered, but other midbrain or orbital signs are usually present. Infiltration or granulomatous change in the medial rectus simulating an adbucens palsy has been seen in two recent patients, and thyroid disease is well recognized. Adherence of the medial rectus to the orbital wall following ethmoidal surgery may also produce a pseudoabducens palsy (Fig. 6.31).

Cavernous sinus lesions

Lesions in the cavernous sinus region usually produce multiple cranial nerve signs but may present with isolated ocular motor nerve involvement. Causes include inflammatory disease, intracavernous aneurysm (Fig. 6.32) thrombosis, meningioma and metastasis (Fig. 6.33).

Inflammatory disease

Inflammatory disease may be due to either specific infection or non-specific granuloma. The spectrum of granulomatous disease extending from scleritis anteriorly to inflammation of the cavernous sinus and adjacent dura posteriorly has already been described (p.28).

The term Tolosa-Hunt syndrome, as noted, describes granulomatous infiltration of the cavernous sinus, and although such eponyms provide an arena for diagnostic showmanship it can be argued that they close the mind to other diagnostic possibilities. The clinician should localize a lesion into anterior, middle and posterior cavernous sinus syndromes. A trial of steroids may be indicated if investigations are negative, though a therapeutic response to steroids will still not confirm any particular diagnosis. Biopsy of the cavernous sinus may be resorted to, but is likely to exacerbate the cranial neuropathies (Unsold *et al.*, 1980). As has been mentioned previously, minor differences in the attentuation coefficients or enhancement characteristics of the cavernous sinus region are difficult to assess. Bone erosion is similarly difficult to diagnose unless extensive.

Tumours

Meningiomas within the cavernous sinus are also difficult to diagnose. The same difficulties in demonstrating the lesion are encountered as with granulomas in this region. In both conditions, orbital phlebography with attention to the cavernous sinus may be valuable in establishing accurate localization. However, differentiation of inflammatory disease of the cavernous sinus from meningioma or even the rare metastasis may be difficult (Fig. 6.34).

Fig. 6.32 Giant intracavernous aneurysm. This 60-year old lady illustrates the classical history of an intracavernous aneurysm. *1969*: left VIth nerve palsy, *1973*: partial left IIIrd nerve palsy, (left corneal sensation reduced); *1975*: left V_1 and V_2 reduced sensation; progressive left visual loss to no perception of light; *1980:* left ptosis, and almost complete ophthalmoplegia, with fixed semidilated pupil (a); loss of sensation V_1 and V_2; left eye blind but upper temporal loss in the *right* eye. CT (b–d) shows a large, rounded mass of slightly increased attenuation, with irregular plaques of calcification. With a wide window (e) the mass is seen to be enlarging the superior orbital fissure (arrow) and eroding the basisphenoid (crossed arrow) and petrous apex (double arrow). Intravenous contrast medium produces only peripheral enhancement (f; g is a subtraction of c from f), indicating that the large aneurysm is almost entirely filled with clot.

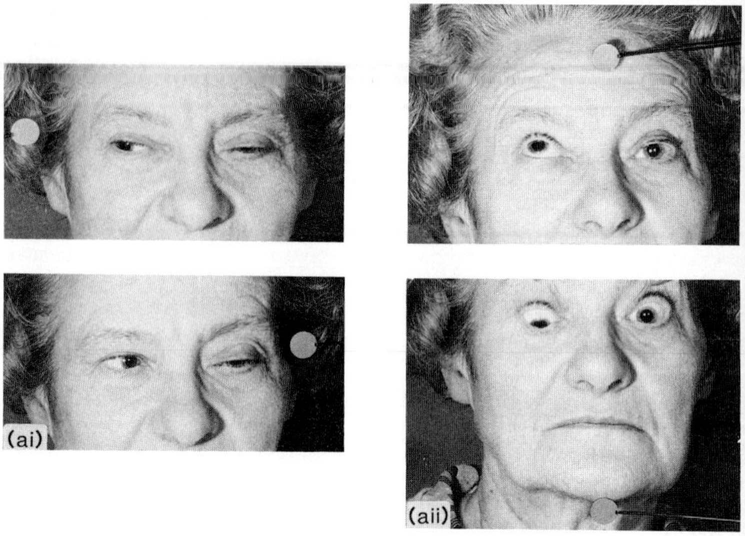

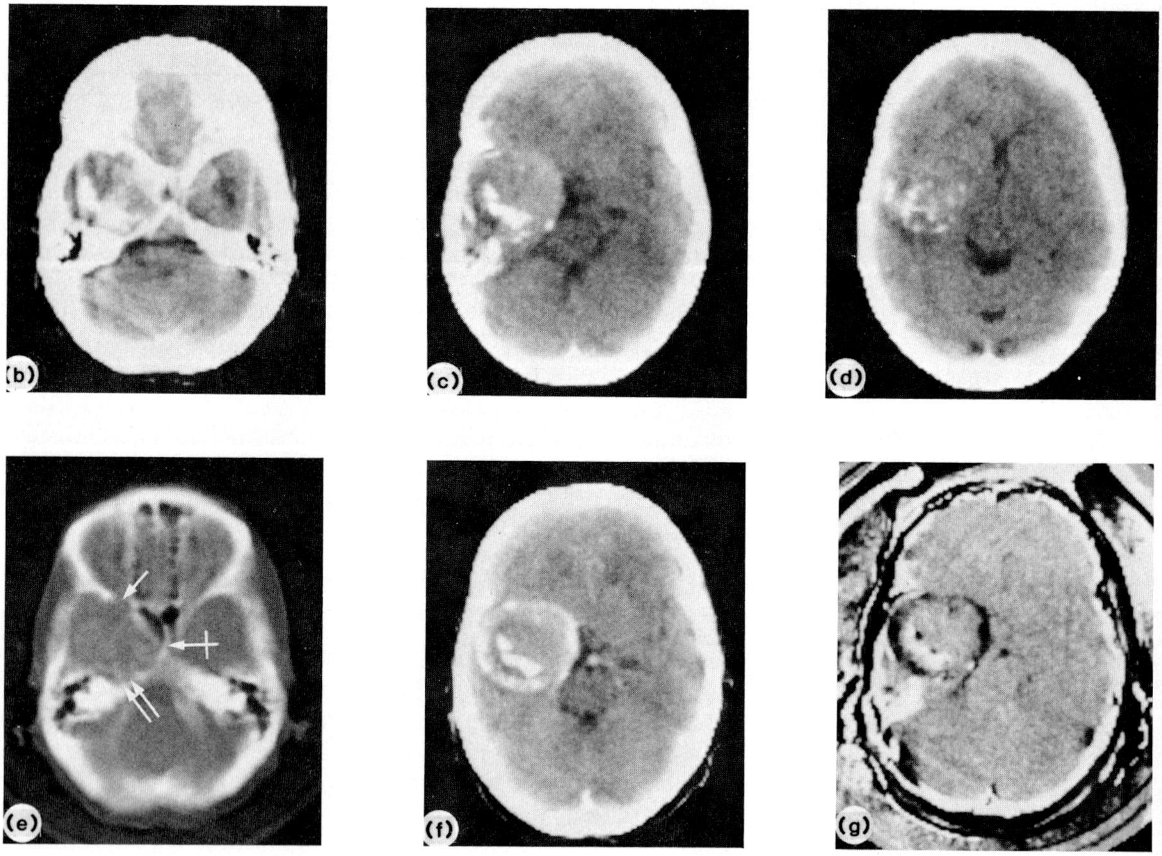

Fig. 6.33 Ophthalmoplegia – cavernous sinus syndrome. This 70-year old woman was operated on for bronchial carcinoma at aged 61 and received radiotherapy for a carinoma of the larynx at the age of 68. One year later she developed a right ptosis and frontal headaches. Visual acuity was normal, but she showed an almost total right ophthalmoplegia with a non-reacting pupil, but the Vth nerve was normal. Plain skull radiographs were normal, but CT showed abnormal uptake of contrast medium alongside the sella and extending towards the petrous apex on the right; the left superior ophthalmic vein was prominent. The patient died one month later despite further radiotherapy and post-mortem examination showed disseminated bronchial carcinoma, with a deposit to the right of the sella. (a) before, (b) after intravenous contrast medium.

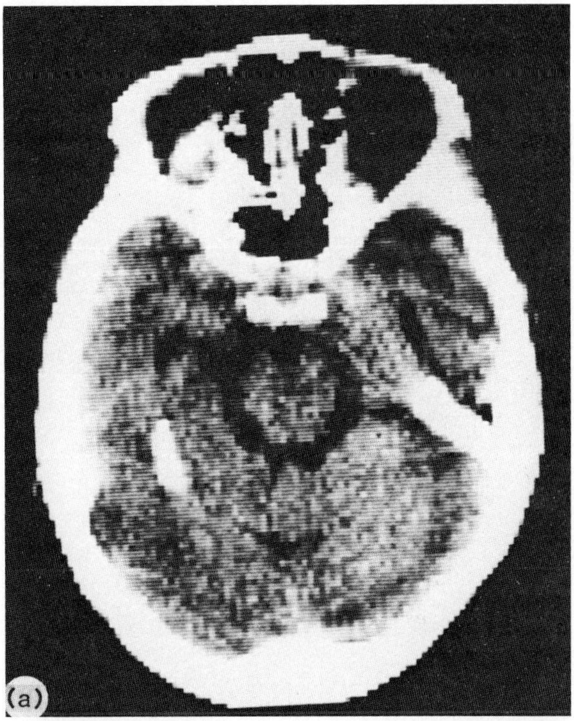

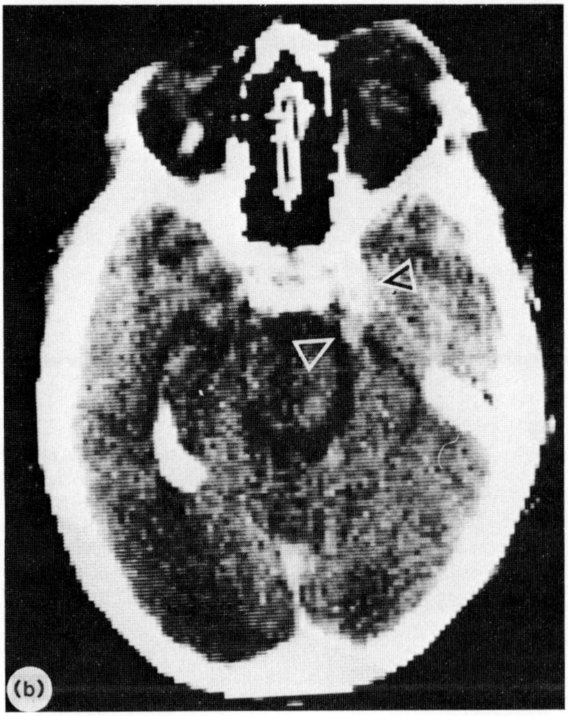

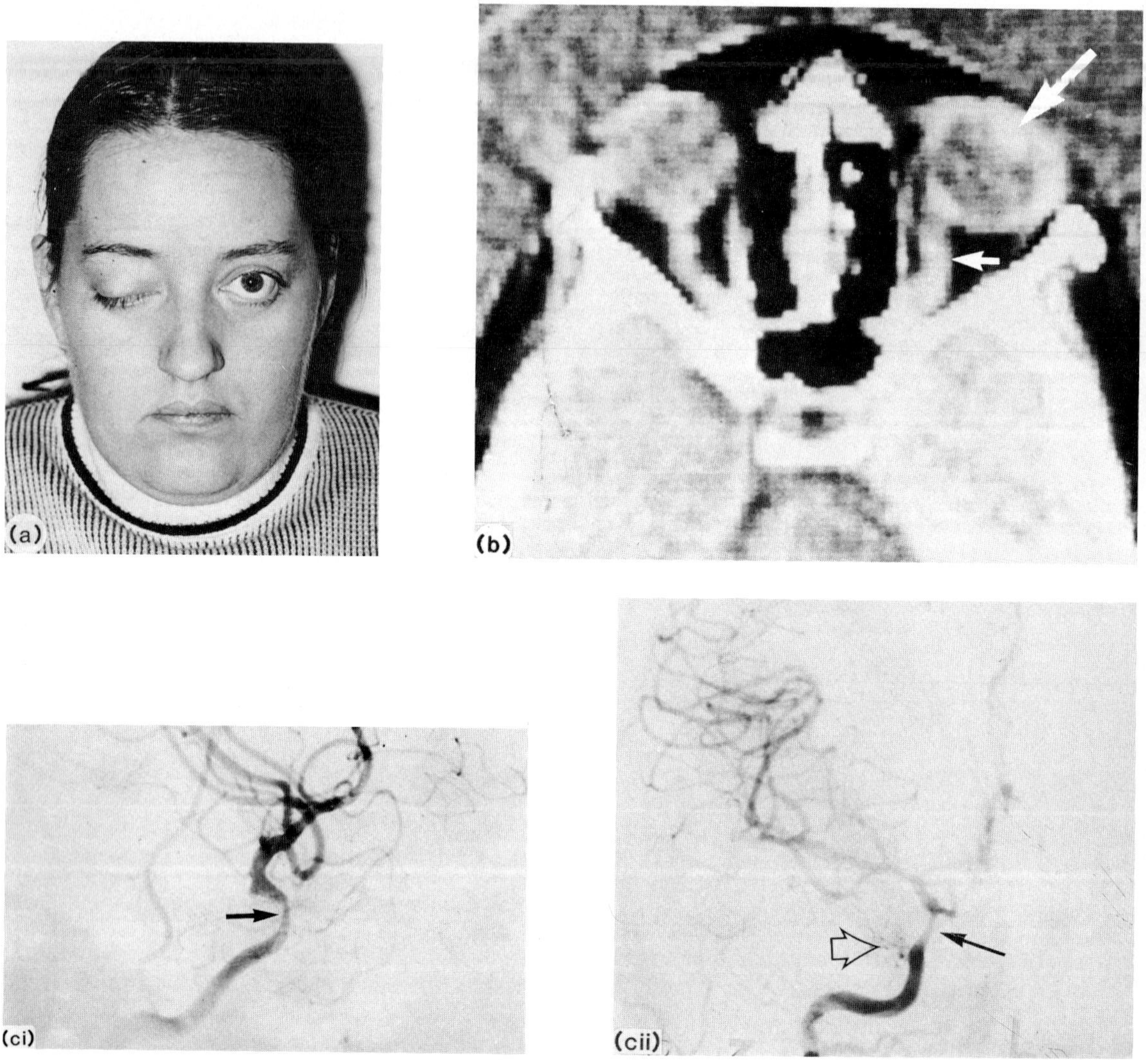

Fig. 6.34 Ophthalmoplegia with cavernous sinus/orbital granuloma. This 33-year old woman presented with complete right visual loss and an ipsilateral IIIrd nerve palsy (a). There was a vague history of prior left visual disturbance. Skull radiographs were thought to show sphenoid wing hyperostosis, while CT (b) showed an expanded, dense optic nerve (arrow). Note abduction, shown by lens position (larger arrow). Carotid angiography (c) demonstrated stenosis of the internal carotid artery (arrow) and abnormal vessels arising from it (open arrow). The ophthalmic artery filled only on external carotid injection (crossed arrows). Air encephalography was thought to show a flattened mass overlying the right anterior clinoid process. After three months, the patient had developed a VIth nerve palsy on the right, but the ptosis had resolved (d). CT now showed marked progression, with intense enhancement of the optic nerve, spreading onto the posterior surface of the globe (arrows) and extending along the right side of the tentorium (arrowheads) (e). These appearances were thought to represent a meningioma, but exploration revealed a non-specific granuloma. The diagnostic significance of the previous left-sided problems and of the variable clinical picture had not been fully appreciated. (Reproduced from paper in *Topics in Neuro-Ophthalmology* (ed. H.S. Thompson), Williams and Wilkins, Baltimore, 1979).

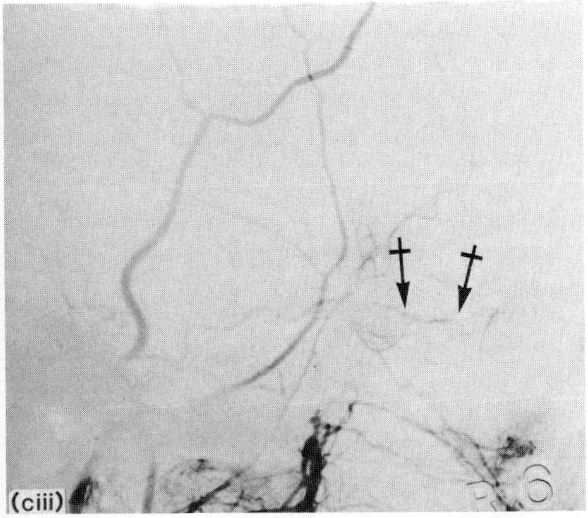
(ciii)

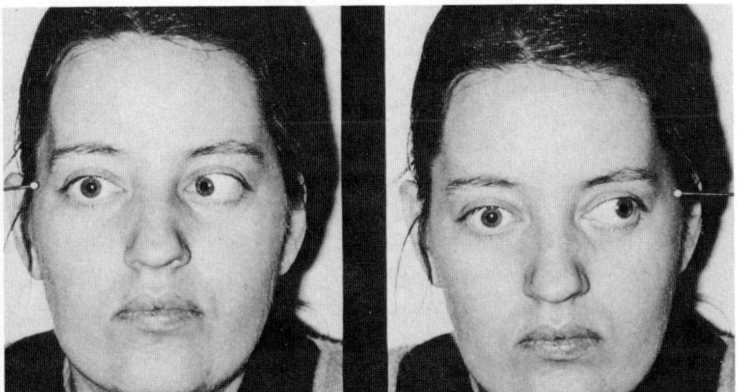
(d)

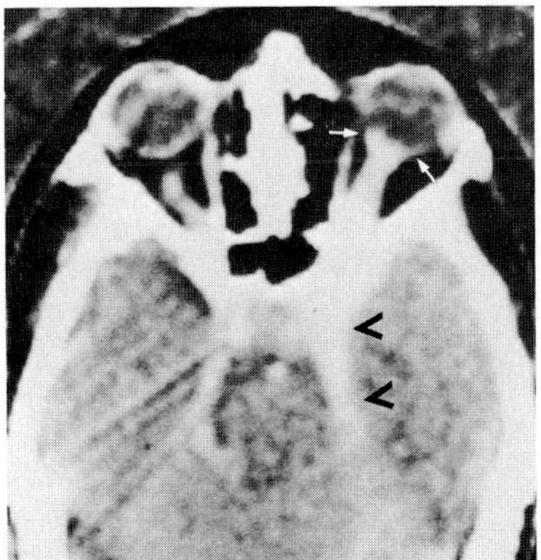
(e)

Carcinoma of the nasopharynx with invasion of the base of the skull, orbital fissure and cavernous sinus is an important cause of ocular motor nerve lesions. There is a high incidence in the Chinese (Fig. 6.35) of squamous carcinoma, whereas woodworkers have a predilection for adenocarcinoma (Acheson *et al*., 1968). Despite this recognized association, we have recently seen a patient who worked for 40 years with hard woods (beech, etc.), who developed a nasopharyngeal reticulum cell sarcoma.

About one third of patients with carcinoma present with diplopia, and about 5% with visual loss, usually monocular. Narasimha and Chandran (1979) found cranial nerve involvement in about 40% of a large series of cases. The VIth nerve is the most commonly involved, probably because of its inferomedial position, but any combination of ocular motor nerve palsies, including total ophthalmoplegia, may be observed. Horner's syndrome and proptosis complete the picture. CT shows more or less extensive irregular bony destruction affecting principally the basisphenoid, but in advanced cases the ethmoid and basiocciput are also involved. The adjacent paranasal sinuses, especially the sphenoid sinus, are obliterated and replaced by material of soft-tissue attenuation. Low sections, or coronal sections, will be required to demonstrate the tumour mass projecting into the nasopharynx (Fig. 6.36). Intravenous contrast medium injection is of little use in delineating the extracranial extent of the tumour, but can be extremely useful when there is an intracranical mass.

Cavernous sinus aneurysms

Intracavernous aneurysms provide a unique example of the evolution of an aneurysm within a venous sinus. Rupture may occur in the early stages to produce a spontaneous carotid–cavernous fistula, but if this does not occur progressive enlargement follows. The initial presentation is often with a VIth nerve palsy and this may be followed many years later by signs of a IIIrd or IVth nerve palsy. Finally the Vth nerve is involved, and upward extension may produce visual loss. The evolution of these changes has been fully documented (Barr *et al*., 1971), and the case illustrated here shows the classical features terminating in a totally blind eye from upward extension, epilepsy and a temporal lobe field defect from lateral extension, and involvement of all the contents of the cavernous sinus (Fig. 6.32).

Pituitary adenoma should also be considered in this context. In one series (Moseley *et al*., 1979), about one quarter of patients with pituitary adenomas or craniopharyngiomas showed cranial nerve involvement. There was solitary affection of the IIIrd, Vth or VIth nerves in half of these cases, the remainder having multiple lesions. The IIIrd nerve was most commonly involved, the IVth least often and never alone, while the Vth and VIth

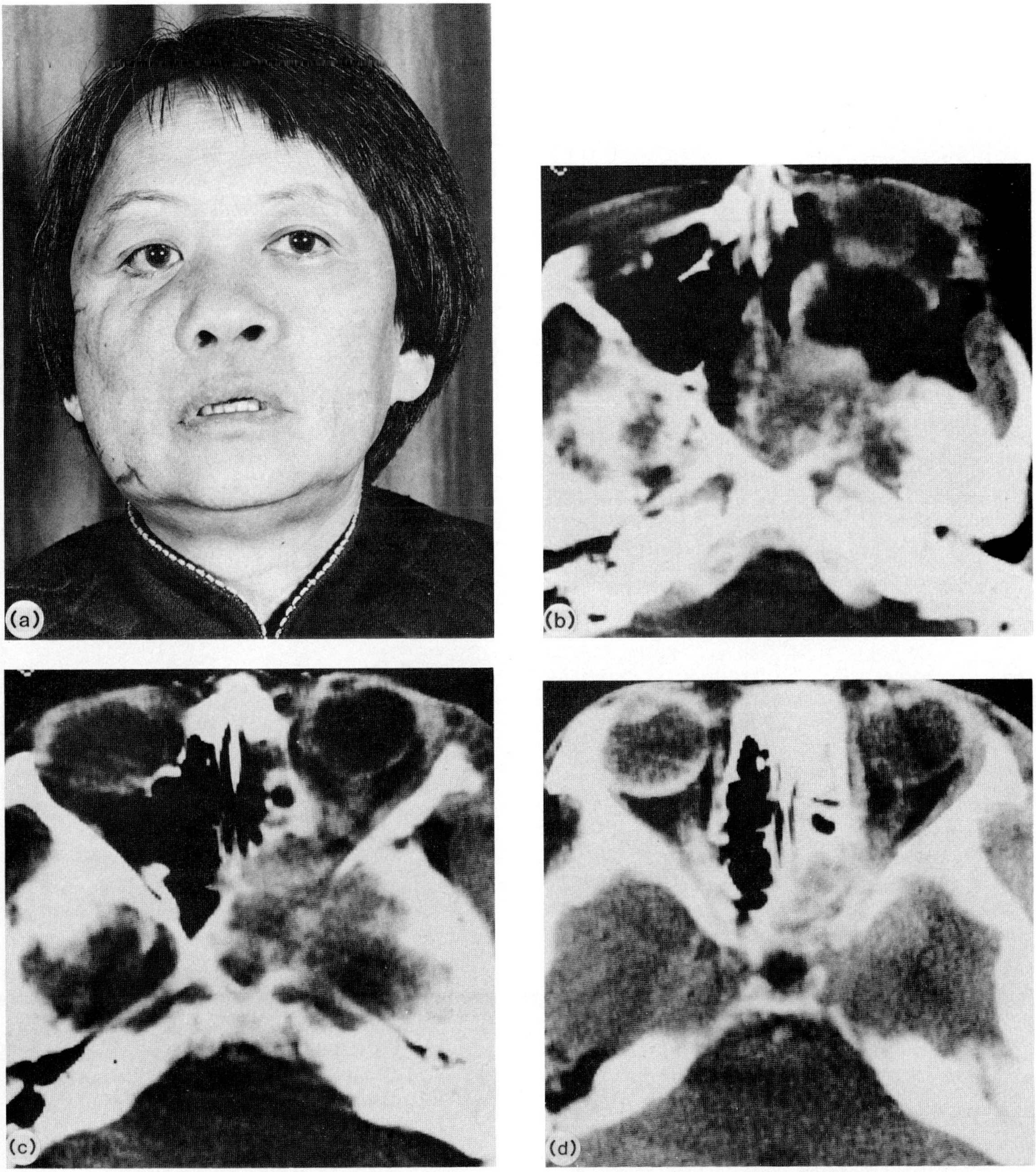

Fig. 6.35 Ophthalmoplegia – orbital apex (nasopharyngeal carcinoma). A 69-year old Chinese woman developed a swelling on the cheek, shown by biopsy to be due to a squamous carcinoma. This progressed relentlessly, producing total blindness and external ophthalmoplegia on the right side (a). CT at the level of nasopharynx (b) through sphenoid sinus (c) and at the level of the anterior clinoid processes (d). There is extensive destruction of bone (compare right and left side in c), which is replaced by a soft-tissue mass. (Destruction of the right maxillary antrum is partly iatrogenic.)

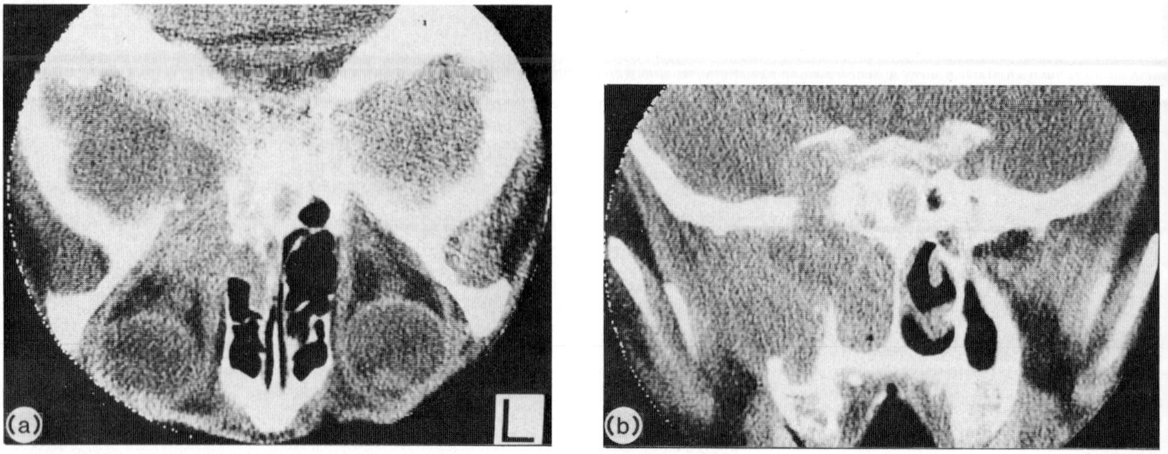

Fig. 6.36 Cavernous sinus and orbital apex syndrome (squamous carcinoma). A 60-year old man who had worked for 30 years in the asbestos industry was found to have squamous carcinoma in cervical nodes three years before the CT study. He presented with a short history of numbness of the face and mild proptosis. Visual acuity was reduced to 6/60 on the right with generalized loss of all isopters in the visual field, and all movements were limited. Pupillary responses were reduced to both light (indirect) and accomodation. There was right disc oedema. Sensation was diminished in the first two trigeminal divisions. CT (a, axial; b, coronal sections) showed destruction of the right orbital apex and basisphenoid extending into the posterior ethmoid cells and maxillary antrum. A soft tissue filled the latter, the right nasal cavity, sphenoid sinus and infratemporal fossa.

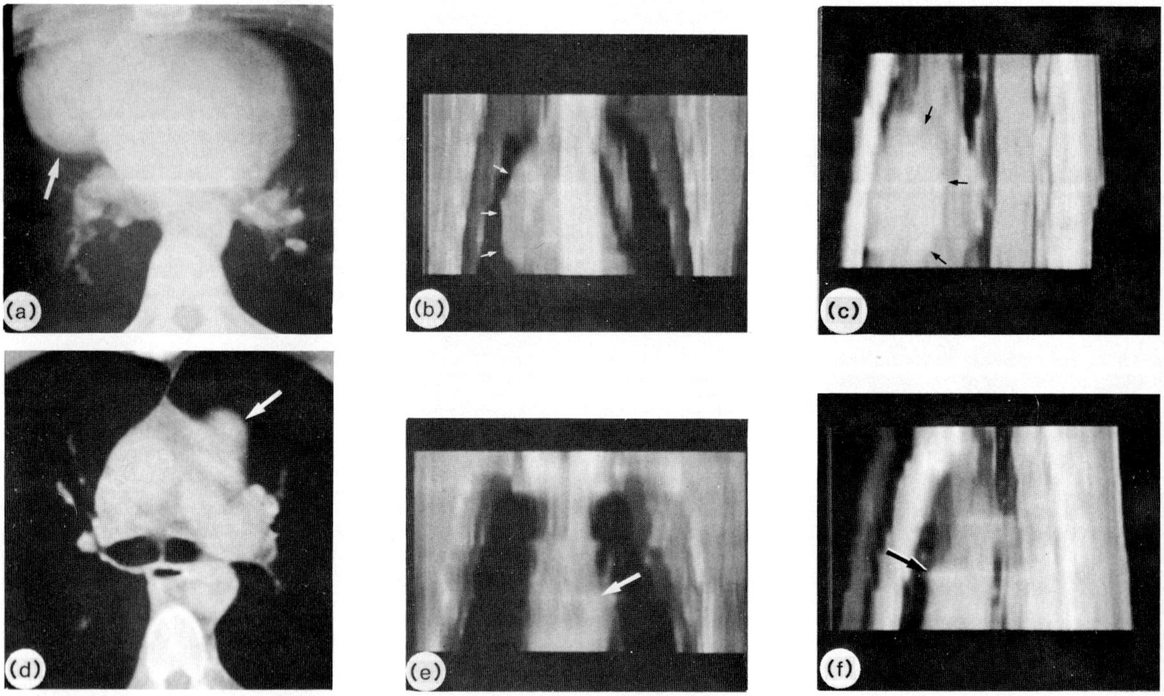

Fig. 6.37 Thoracic CT in two cases of myasthenia gravis. (a–c) Very large thymoma (arrows) in right lower zone (in body scans the patient's right is on the reader's left). (a) Composite of six axial sections, showing rounded mass alongside the heart, against the anterior chest wall. (b, c,) Composite coronal and sagittal reconstructions, equivalent to PA and lateral chest films. (d–f) Smaller tumour (arrows) in classical position anterior to left pulmonary artery. This lesion was not clearly shown on chest radiographs.

nerves were affected with equal frequency. Three of four patients with Vth nerve lesions had craniopharyngiomas.

6.11 DISORDERS OF THE OCULAR MUSCLES

Myasthenia gravis

This diagnosis should be suspected in any patient with ptosis or an unusual ocular motor problem. Diplopia is the commonest presenting symptom in this disease, and in patients with 'ocular myasthenia' the effects are confined to the ocular muscles. Involvement of the eyes can be unilateral, and may produce any combination of signs usually suggestive of brainstem disease including nystagmus. Once the diagnosis is suspected, CT plays no part in confirming it, but can be useful in showing enlargement of the thymus, which occurs in at least 20% of patients with myasthenia (Fig. 6.37); thymectomy even when a thymoma is not present is a valuable therapeutic measure.

Inflammatory disease

This may involve either one or several ocular muscles and may be due to thyroid disease, granulomatous disease or orbital myositis (see Chapter 3). In certain clinical situations where lesions are situated in relation to the orbital apex it may be important to show whether the ocular motor problems are due to orbital disease or involvement of the cranial nerves. Assessment of the intraocular pressure in eccentric gaze is useful; the forced duction test has not been helpful in our hands. Thus, in monocular elevator palsy CT may demonstrate a mass, or abnormal muscles (e.g. thyroid disease) or a blow-out fracture, which serves to localize the lesion and differentiate it from the rare monocular elevator palsy of neural origin (Figs. 6.38–6.41). Similarly we have suspected a IIIrd nerve lesion in a patient with anisocoria and adduction weakness, until a CT scan demonstrated a granuloma around the lateral rectus. We have also seen an elderly man, known to have amyloidosis, who apparently developed bilateral VIth nerve palsies, without other abnormalities of the nervous system. CT of the orbits showed thickened medial rectus muscles on both sides, probably due to infiltration by amyloid, and presumably limiting abduction of the eyes (Fig. 6.42).

6.12 PUPILLARY ABNORMALITIES

Evaluation of pupillary function is an integral part of the neuro-ophthalmic examination, providing objective information on the afferent visual system. Pupil tone changes constantly due to changes in illumination, accommodation and other external or emotional influences. Afferent pupillary information is con-

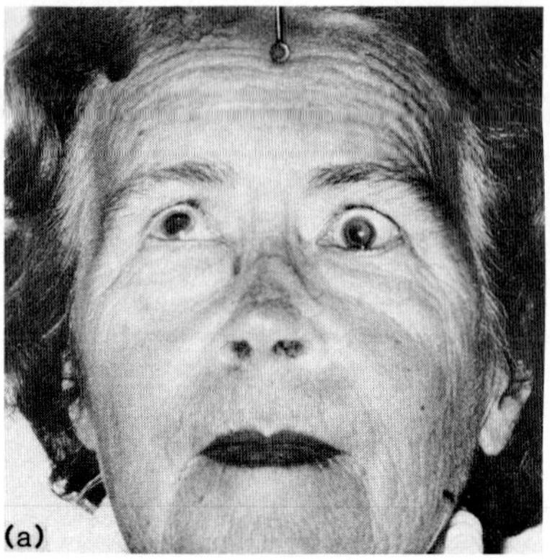

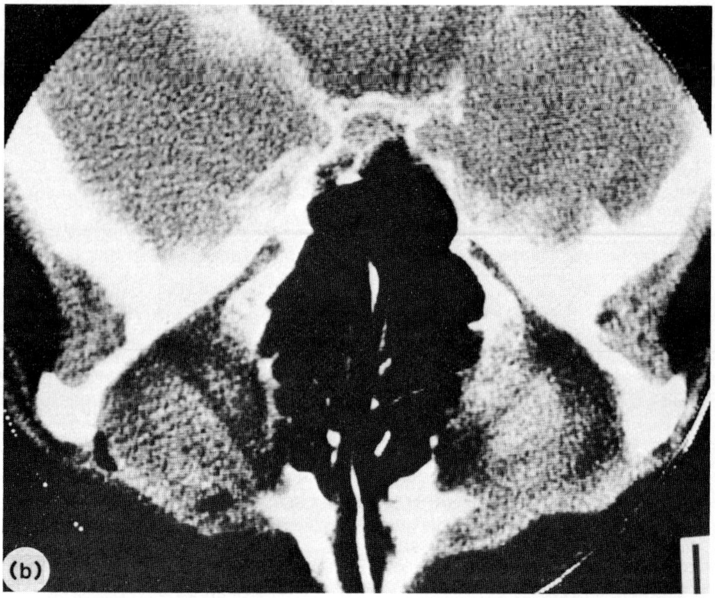

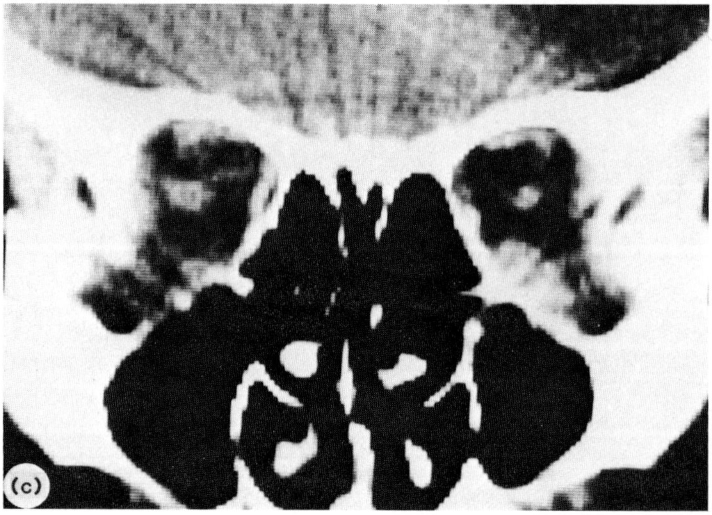

Fig. 6.38 Monocular elevator palsy – orbital metastasis. This 62-year old woman gave a history of double vision on up gaze for two months. There was no proptosis, but elevation of the left eye was limited (a), with increase in intraocular pressure, indicating tethering, on attempted up gaze. Thyroid function was normal, but she had had a radical mastectomy two years previously. CT showed a mass lying inferiorly in the left orbit, obscuring the inferior rectus muscle, particularly anteriorly. The mass was poorly shown by axial scans (b) and coronal sections (c) were necessary for detection. She was treated by local radiotherapy. (See also Figs. 6.39–6.41).

veyed in the optic nerve, traverses the chiasm, but leaves the tract before the lateral geniculate body to reach the rostral midbrain via the brachium of the superior colliculus. Complicated intercalated neurones connect each side with the centrally placed Edinger-Westphal nucleus (accommodation – anterior; convergence – posterior), and efferent neurones pass with the IIIrd nerve and lie superficially. They reach the ciliary ganglion via the inferior division of the IIIrd nerve, and after a synapse in the

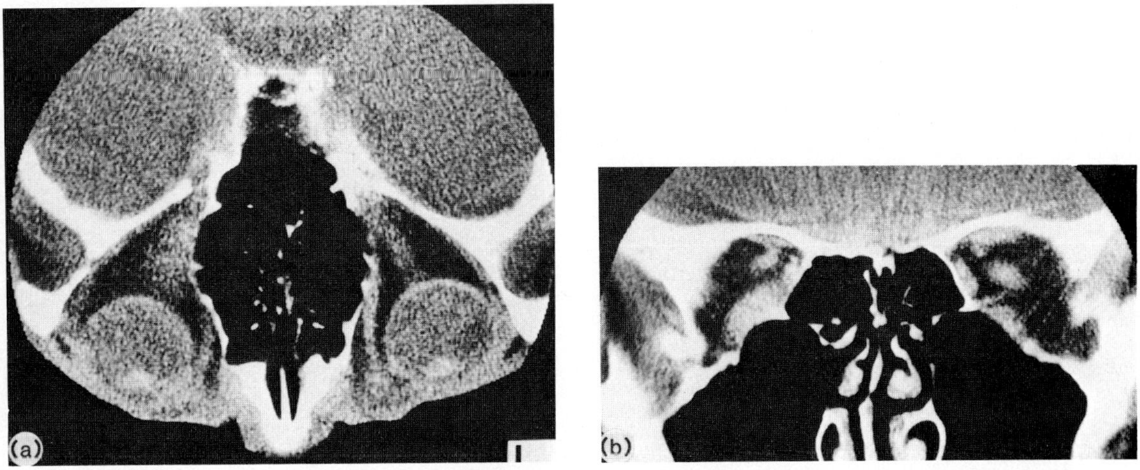

Fig. 6.39 Monocular elevator palsy – thyroid eye disease. A 49-year old man had shown impaired elevation of the right eye for one year; intraocular pressure increased on attempted elevation, suggesting tethering. Lid retraction was present and thyroid cytoplasmic antibodies were positive at 1:10. CT showed isolated enlargement of the right inferior rectus muscle (a). Coronal section (b) showed the superior rectus and levator palpebrae superioris muscles to be thinner on the affected side; the optic nerve was elevated indicating that gaze was directed downwards, while the left optic nerve was in the primary position.

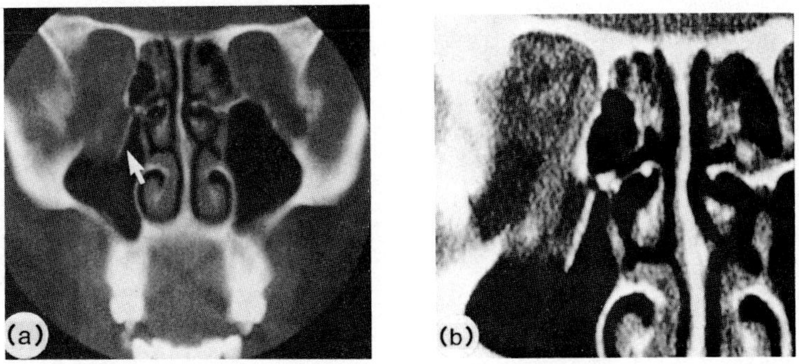

Fig. 6.40 Monocular elevator palsy – orbital blow-out fracture. A 28-year old man received a blow to the face, after which he suffered from numbness of the cheek and diplopia. On examination one month after the injury there was mild enophthalmos and limited elevation of the right eye; sensation was impaired in the V_2 distribution. Plain radiographs showed a mass in the antrum, but did not demonstrate a definite fracture. Axial CT sections were unhelpful, but coronal sections (a) clearly showed depression and medial displacement of a fragment of the floor of the right orbit (arrow). The same section imaged to show the soft tissues (b) strongly suggested downward herniation and probably entrapment of the inferior rectus muscle.

ganglion the terminal neurone reaches the iris and ciliary body via the short ciliary nerves.

Sympathetic (pupillodilator fibres) reach the iris after a complicated journey starting in the hypothalamus. Neurones synapse in the ciliospinal centre of Budge (C8-T2) and second order neurones emerge with T1 rootlet to join the sympathetic chain. After lying in close relationship with the apex of the lung the fibres ascend to the superior cervical ganglion. Third order neurones then ascend with the internal carotid artery and enter the orbit to reach the eye via the ophthalmic artery and with Vth nerve branches.

The clinician rarely has to resort to CT to assist him in the diagnosis of pupillary problems. Anisocoria is probably the

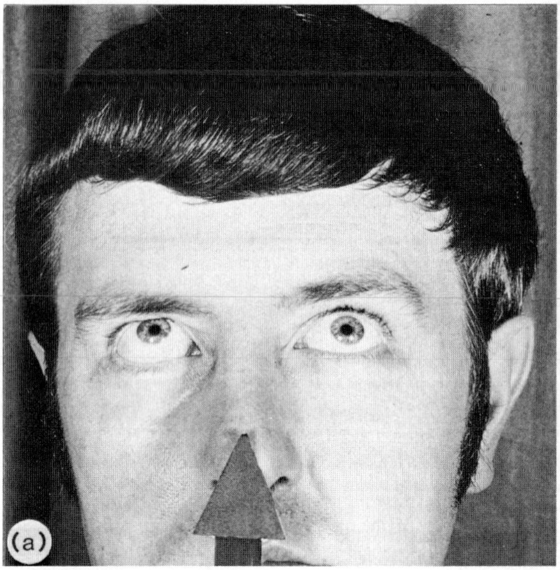

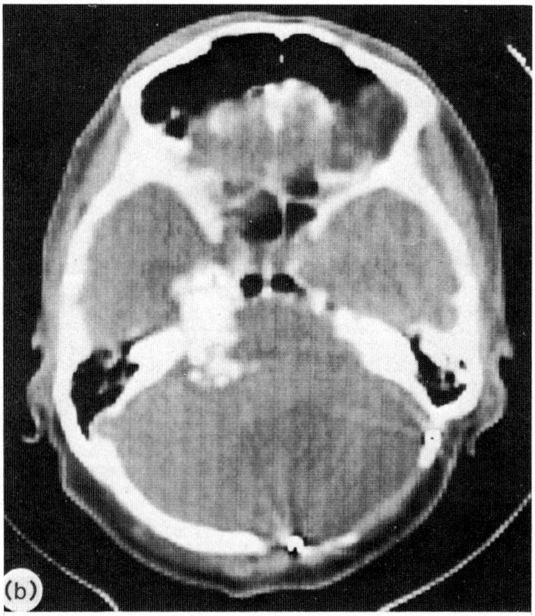

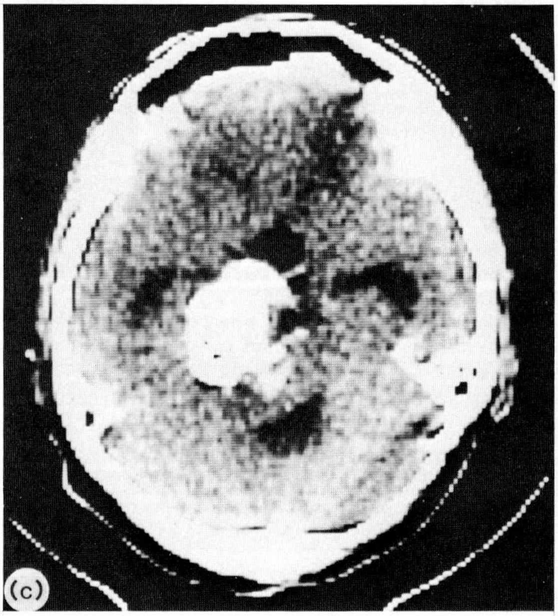

Fig. 6.41 Monocular elevator palsy (chordoma). A chordoma arising from the basisphenoid was partially removed when the patient was aged 31. Eight years later he returned with altered sensation down the right side. Examination showed evidence of a recurrence, including bilateral horizontal nystagmus, rotatory nystagmus on right gaze and limited elevation of the left eye (a) with diplopia. CT showed a massive, calcified tumour extending from the left cerebellopontine angle, forwards through the petrous apex into the middle cranial fossa (b) and upwards into the left suprasellar region (c). There was hydrocephalus, including the forth ventricle. In (b) note the texture of the tumour calcification, better shown with a wide window, and the right occipital craniectomy with surgical clips. This patient had persistent failure of elevation of the left eye and there were no signs to suggest an orbital cause.

commonest problem, and it is not surprising in view of the complicated neural pathways that almost a quarter of healthy people have some difference in the size of their pupils. Furthermore it is rare for disparities in pupillary size alone to present clinically without other signs of localizing value. Clinical data about pupillary problems will be followed by some contributions that CT can make.

Argyll-Robertson pupils

These are small, irregular pupils, usually bilateral, and a feature of neurosyphilis. They exhibit light-near dissociation, with a poor or absent response to light and a usually brisk near response. The site of the responsible lesion has defied localization, but is usually attributed to the pretectal region; serological tests are mandatory.

CT may provide other evidence of neurosyphilis, including cerebral atrophy, hydrocephalus or focal cerebral granulomas (gummas). Granulomata are seen as isodense lesions surrounded by reduced attenuation, which show increased attenuation after intravenous contrast. These appearances are, however, non-specific, being seen with other ganulomata such as tuberculosis and sarcoidosis (Godt *et al.*, 1979).

Midbrain pupillary signs

Bilateral failure of the pupillary light response, with preservation of accommodation and pupils in the dilated or mid-dilated position, merits a search for well defined neuro-ophthalmic signs, which are discussed on p.200 but briefly repeated here owing to the importance of early diagnosis of pinealomas:

1. Reduced range of accommodation.
2. Reduced elevation of the eyes.
3. On attempting elevation a convergence of retraction movement can be elicited.
4. Retraction nystagmus on following a downward rotating optokinetic drum.

Horner's syndrome

This consists of mild ptosis, lower lid ptosis and miosis. There is occasionally autonomic disturbance of the same side of the face if the sympathetic chain is damaged prior to the origin of the external carotid artery.

The syndrome may be central (first neurone), preganglionic (second neurone) or postganglionic (third neurone). A recent review of 120 cases (Grimson and Thompson, 1979) showed the following incidence:

Preganglionic	41%	(commonest cause is malignancy)
Postganglionic	34%	(vascular headache or trauma)
Undetermined	12%	
Congenital	10%	
Central	3%	

Pharmacological tests may confirm a diagnosis of Horner's syndrome, and instillation of cocaine 5% fails to produce dilatation on the affected side. Localization may be facilitated by hydroxyamphetamine 1% which fails to dilate the postganglionic

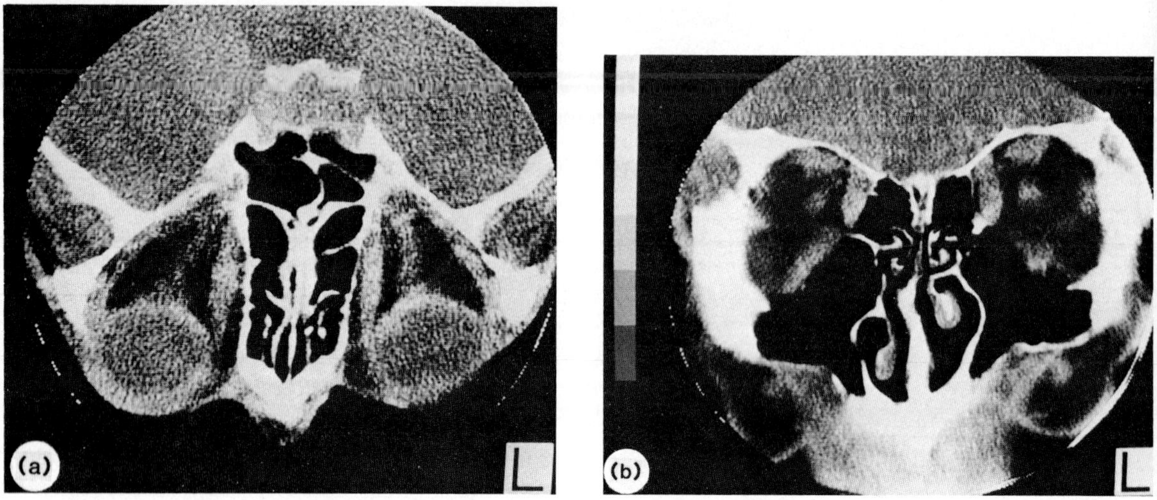

Fig. 6.42 Ocular muscles – infiltration by amyloid. A 58-year old man was seen with syncopal attacks and amaurosis fugax. Diplopia had commenced one week prior to admission. Examination suggested bilateral VIth nerve palsies, but CT showed this to be due to medial rectus thickening. Other ocular muscles also appeared slightly thickened, e.g. the right inferior rectus. Systemic investigations indicated a diagnosis of amyloid, and myocardial biopsy showed amyloid infiltration of the myocardium. His cerebral and ocular symptoms were attributed to emboli arising from the damaged myocardium.

Horner's pupil, but dilates central and preganglionic Horner's.

Preganglionic Horner's syndrome

Preganglionic Horner's syndrome is important to recognize because of the higher incidence of malignant disease, often from pulmonary or breast carcinoma.

Postganglionic Horner's syndrome

Postganglionic Horner's syndrome is usually caused by carotid disease, trauma to the cervical region, or lesions in the cavernous sinus region where concomitant involvement of other ocular motor nerves may also be involved (i.e. IIIrd nerve). In carotid occlusion CT shows cerebral infarction in the majority of cases Radü and Moseley, 1978). A postganglionic Horner's syndrome was not seen with orbital disease in any of the cases reported by Grimson and Thompson (1979).

Central Horner's syndrome

This is rare and almost invariably associated with other brainstem signs (e.g. Wallenberg's syndrome, syringomyelia). A syrinx may be demonstrated on CT as a central zone of reduced attenuation in a collapsed or expanded spinal cord. Metrizamide, injected into the subarachnoid space, concentrates in this central cavity from about six hours after injection. An Arnold-Chiari malformation (p.213) frequently coexists. CT is less satisfactory for examination of the lower brainstem, i.e. the pons and medulla oblongata, because of artefacts caused by interfaces between the dense petrous bone and the adjacent structures, but also because marked clinical deficit can result from small lesions in this region.

6.13 LID ABNORMALITIES

Lid retraction with upper midbrain lesions (Collier's sign).
Lid retraction is usually a sign of local orbital disease (e.g. thyroid, lymphomatous infiltration) but may also be seen with pretectal lesions. CT may therefore demonstrate a vascular or infiltrative lesion in the upper midbrain region (Fig. 6.43).

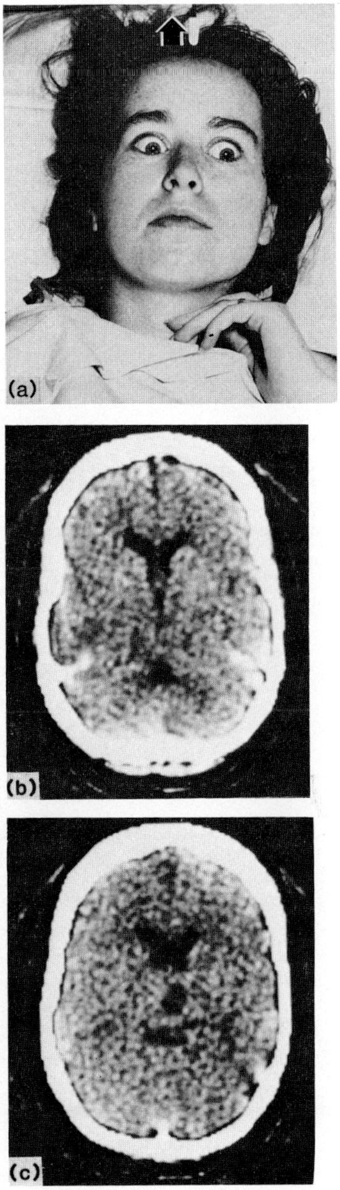

Fig. 6.43 Collier's sign (tonic lid retraction). A 27-year old woman collapsed suddenly, after which she showed marked lid retraction and failure of up gaze (a, attempted up gaze; note pointer beside arrow) which persisted for several months. CT at the onset showed a haemorrhage (from a basal arteriovenous malformation) and subsequent studies (b,c) demonstrated a low-attenuation post-haemorrhagic cavity in the right thalamus.

Lid nystagmus
Two main types of lid nystagmus have been described, one occurring with horizontal gaze movements, and the other with convergence (Pick's nystagmus). The pathophysiology is poorly understood, but we have recently seen a patient with a large tentorial meningioma and gross papilloedema who exhibited this abnormality (Fig. 6.44) (see over).

REFERENCES

Acheson, E.D. Cowdell, R.H., Hadfield, E. and Macbeth, R.G. (1968), Nasal cancer in woodworkers in the furniture industry. *Br. Med. J.* (June 8th), 577–96.

Anderson, T.L., Moore, R.A., Grinnell, V.S., Itabashi, H.H. (1979), Computerized tomography in central pontine myelinolysis. *Neurology*, **29**, 1527–30.

Baloh, R.W., Yee, R.A.D. and Honrobia, V. (1980), Optokinetic nystagmus and parietal lobe lesions. *Ann. Neurol.*, **7**, 269–76.

Barr, H.W.K., Blackwood, W. and Meadows, S.P. (1971), Intracavernous carotid aneurysms. *Brain,* **94**, 607–22.

Bender, M.B. (1980), Brain control of conjugate eye movements. *Brain,* **103**, 23–70.

Boeri, R. and Passerini, A. (1964), The megadolichobasilar anomaly. *J. Neurol. Sci.*, **1**, 475–84.

Caplan, L.T. (1980), Top of the basilar syndrome. *Neurology,* **30**, 72–9.

Chambers, A.A. and McLennon, J.E. (1978), Pericollicular syndromes. *Neuroradiology*, **16**, 547–8.

Christoff, N. (1974), A clinicopathological study of vertical eye movements. *Archs Neurol.*, **31**, 1–8.

Cox, T.A. Wurster, J.B. and Godfrey, W.A. (1979), Primary aberrant oculomotor regeneration due to intracranial aneurysm. *Archs Neurol.* **36**, 570–1.

Daroff, R.B. and Proost, B.T. (1978), In *Neuro-Ophthalmology* (Glaser, J.S. ed.), Harper and Row, Maryland.

Fisher, C.M. (1967), Some neuro-ophthalmological observations. *J. Neurol. Neurosurg. Psychiat.*, **30**, 383–92.

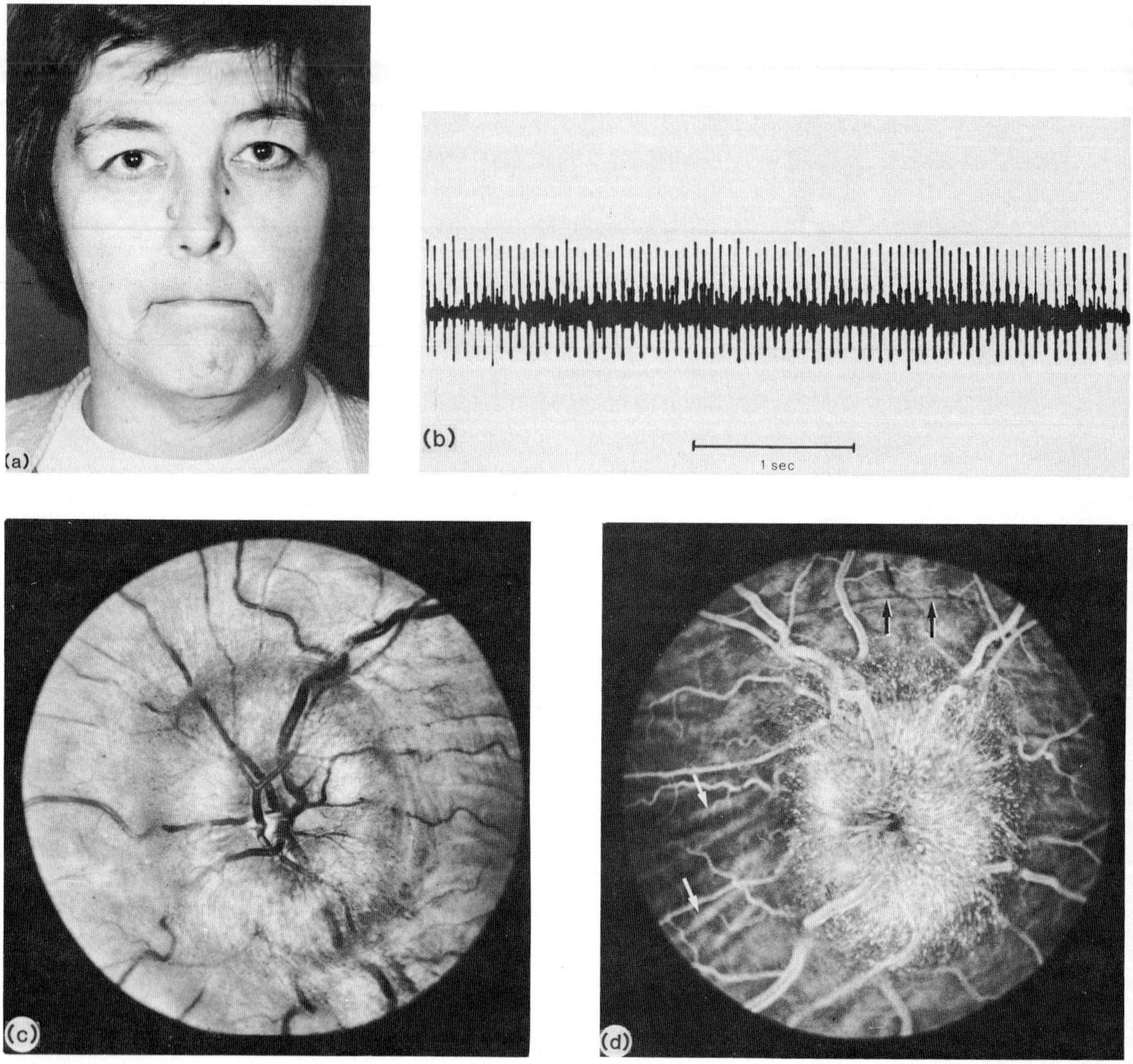

Fig. 6.44 Lid nystagmus. This 51-year old woman, complaining of headaches and mild confusion, showed normal ocular movements (a), but had lid nystagmus, aggravated by any eye movement, with constant firing of the orbicularis oculi (b). Chronic bilateral papilloedema was present (c, left eye), and flourescein angiography (d, right eye) showed choroidal striae, both folds (white arrows) and wrinkles (dark arrows). CT confirmed the grossly expanded optic nerve sheaths (e) and showed a tenorial meningioma on the right side (f) before (g) after contrast medium. A direct coronal postinjection section (h) shows a minor extension into the tentorial hiatus (arrows). (1) Free border of tentorum; (2) falx cerebro; (3) petrous ridge; (4) left lateral ventrical containing choroid plexus; (5) midbrain.

Gilner, L.I. and Avin, B. (1977), A reversible ocular manifestation of thalamic haemorrhage. *Archs Neurol.*, **34**, 715–16.

Godt, P., Stoeppler, L., Wischer, U. and Schroeper, M.M. (1979), The value of computer tomography in cerebral syphilis. *Neuroradiology*, **18**, 197–200.

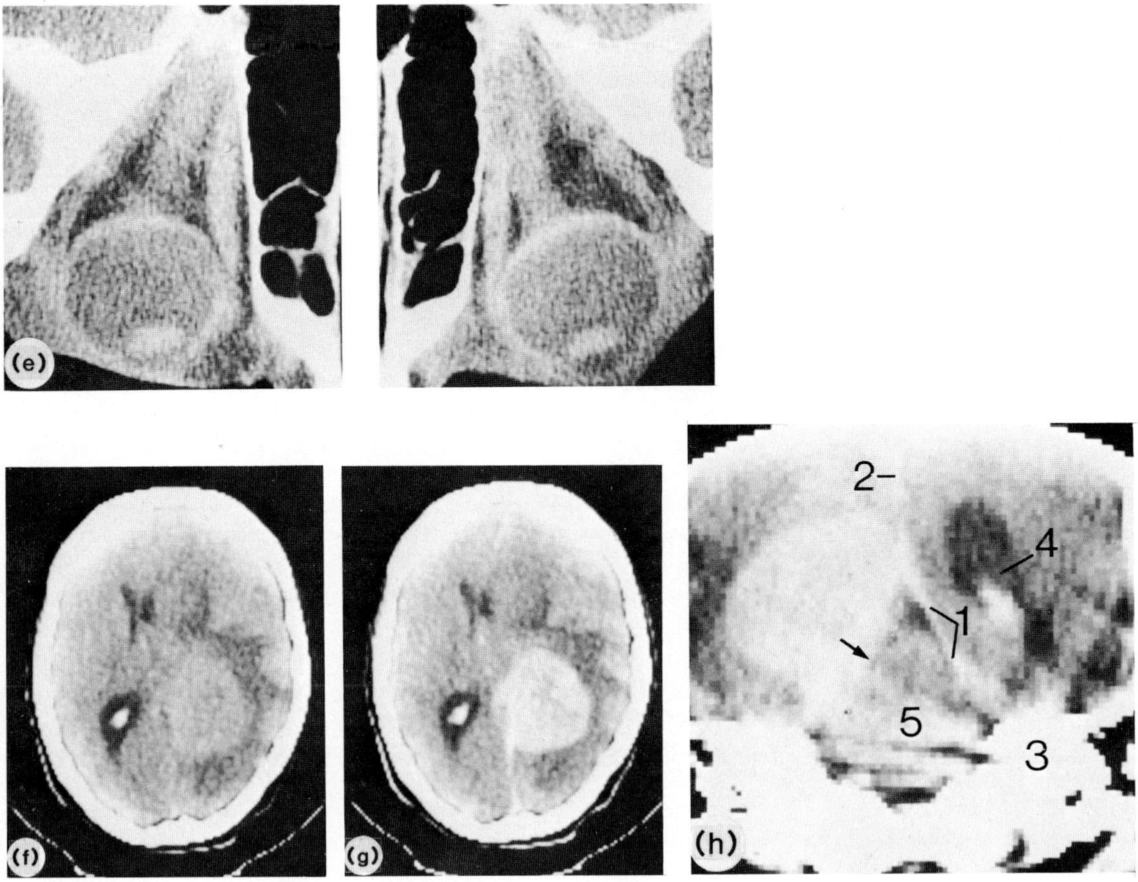

Grimson, B.S. and Thompson, H.S. (1979), Horner's syndrome: overall view of 120 cases. In: *Topics in Neuro-Ophthalmology*, (ed. H.S. Thompson), Williams and Wilkins, Baltimore, pp.151–6.

Halmagyi, G.M., Evans, W.A. and Hallinan, J.M. (1978), Failure of downward gaze. *Archs Neurol*, **35**, 22–26.

Halmagyi, G.M. and Gresty, M.A. (1979), Clinical signs of visual vestibular interaction. *J. Neurol. Neurosurg. Psychiat.*, **42**, 934–9.

Herrick, M.K. and Rubinstein, L.J. (1979), The cytological differentiating potential of pineal parenchymal neoplasms (true pinealomas), *Brain*, **102**, 289–320.

Kendall, B.E., Clavería, L.E. and Quiroga, W. (1977), CAT in Leukodystrophy and neuronal degeneration In: *First European Seminar on Computerised Axial Tomograhy in Clinical Practice* (eds. G.H. du Boulay and I.F. Moseley. Springer-Verlag, Berlin.

Kompf, D., Pasik, T., Pasik, P. and Bender, M.B. (1979), Downward gaze in monkeys. *Brain*, **102**, 527–58.

Mills, R.P. and Swanson, P.D. (1978), Vertical oculomotor apraxia and memory loss. *Ann. Neurol.*, **4**, 149–53.

Moseley, I.F. and Holland, I.M. (1979), Ectasia of the basilar artery. *Neuroradiology*, **18**, 83–91.

Moseley, I.F., Sanders, M.D., Karoutas, G. and Radue, E.W. (1979), CT scan in neuro-ophthalmology. In: *Topics in Neuro-Ophthalmology*, (ed. H.S. Thompson), Williams and Wilkins, Baltimore, pp.302–17.

Narasimha, G. and Chandran, C. (1979), Ocular and trigeminal involvement in nasopharyngeal carcinoma. *Aust. J. Ophthal.*, **7**, 147–50.

Neville, B.G.R., Lake, B.D., Stephens, R. and Sanders, M.D. (1973), A neurovisceral storage disease with vertical supranuclear ophthalmoplegia and its relationship to Niemann-Pick disease. A report on 9 patients. *Brain*, **96**, 97–120.

Orrison, W.W. and Robertson, N.S. (1979), Congenital oculomotor apraxia. *Archs Neurol.*, **36**, 29–31.

Osborn, A.G. (1977), Diagnosis of descending transtentorial herniation by cranial computed tomography. *Radiology*, **123**, 93–96.

Radü, E.W. and Moseley, I.F. (1978), Carotid artery occlusion and computerised tomography. *Neuroradiology*, **17**, 65–69.

Sanders, M.D. and Bird, A.C. (1970), Supranuclear abnormalities of the vertical ocular motor system. *Trans. Ophthal. Soc. U.K.,* **90**, 433–50.

Sanders, M.D. and Wybar, K.C. (1969), Vertical supranuclear ophthalmoplegia with compensatory head movements. In: *Transactions of the Consilium Europaeum Strabismi Studio Deditum Congress*, London.

Telfer, R.B., Miller, E.M. (1979). Central pontine myelinolysis following hyponatremia. *Ann. Neurol.*, **6**, 455–6.

Unsold, R., Safran, A.B., Safran, E. and Hoyt, W.R. (1980), Metastatic infiltration of nerves in the cavernous sinus. *Neurology*, **37**, 59.

Weiskrantz, L., Warrington, E.K., Sanders, M.D. and Marshall, J. (1974), Visual capacity in the hemianopic field following a restricted occipital ablation. *Brain*, **97**, Part IV, 709–28.

Wilson, J.L. and Moseley, I.F. (1977), A diagnostic approach to cerebellar lesions, In: *First European Seminar on Computerized Axial Tomography in Clinical Practice* (eds. G.H. Du Boulay and I.F. Moseley), Springer, Berlin, pp.123–33.

Yamashita, J., Asato, R., Handa, M., Nakao, S. and Ogata, M. (1977), Abducens nerve palsy as initial symptom of trigeminal schwannoma. *J. Neurol. Neurosurg. Psychiat.*, **40**, 1190.

7 · Heredofamilial developmental and metabolic disorders

The orbits and optic pathways may be involved by a variety of craniocerebral malformations and developmental anomalies (Lindenberg, 1967). Since the affection of these structures is often a minor part of the whole, only those conditions will be considered in which CT is useful or shows characteristic abnormalities.

7.1 MIDLINE DEVELOPMENTAL ANOMALIES

Defects of the development of midline structures of the brain and meninges produce a wide range of abnormalities of interest to the ophthalmologist.

Meningocoeles and encephalocoeles

Failure of closure along the dorsal midline results in exposure of the neuraxis and spinal column, with lesions being more common in the occipital region, although they also occur in the frontal region. The term meningocoele is used when meninges are present without neural tissue and meningomyelocoele and encephalocoele when neural tissue is also ectopic. CT is of limited value in assessing the content of meningocoeles unless intrathecal contrast medium is used, but may be of value in demonstrating associated cerebral malformations, or hydrocephalus, often the result of aqueduct stenosis. We have seen one case in which an occipital encephalocoele and meningomyelocoele were associated with hypoplasia of the optic nerves.

Nasal encephalocoeles occur in association with marked *hypertelorism*, and when a mass is present at the medial margin of the orbit in a child, the diagnosis of frontoethmoidal encephalocoele should be entertained prior to exploratory surgery.

Colobomata

Colobomata may also be associated with encephalocoeles, though the association is extremely rare. CT provides no diagnostic information about the globe, which resembles that of high myopia (Fig. 7.1), though coronal cuts of the sphenoid region are important to exclude basal encephalocoele. Lesions in the skull base may be small (Fig. 7.2).

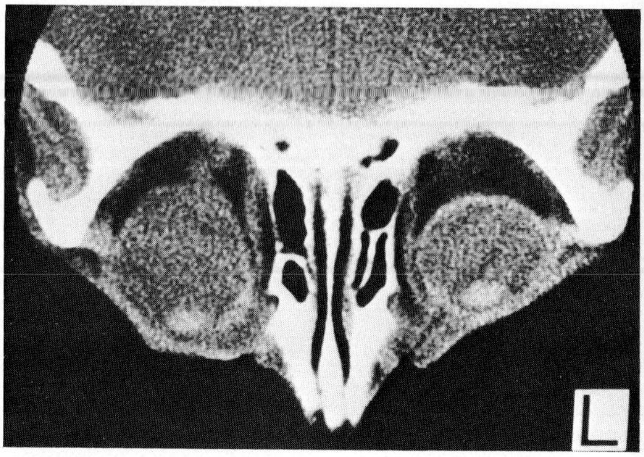

Fig. 7.1 High myopia. A 51-year old woman presented with chiasmal compression due to a suprasellar meningioma. The right eye showed 20 dioptres of myopia; the left was normal. CT shows a normally-shaped left globe (transverse diameter 25.3 mm, longitudinal diameter 23 mm), but the right is elongated (transverse diameter 26.5 mm, longitudinal 32.2 mm) and obviously not spherical. The right retrobulbar space is therefore reduced, and the optic nerve on that side appears more tortuous.

Patients with hypertelorism (abnormally wide spacing of the orbits) may show abnormalities such as exophthalmos, eyelid defects, cleft palate etc., without there being any associated intracranial abnormality. Binocular fusion can be impossible in extreme cases. Bilateral VIth nerve palsies are sometimes present and field defects or optic atrophy may result from stretching of the nerves or narrowing of the optic canal. If cosmetic surgery (Tessier's operation) is undertaken, it is important to be aware of the possibility of the facial deformity being associated with an anterior midline basal encephalocoele (Fig. 7.3). CT can be of great value in this respect, by showing the integrity of the basal structures. It should be noted that where hypertelorism is present, the frontal lobes normally lie low down between the orbital roofs and may simulate an encephalocoele; they are usually identifiable as bilaterally symmetrical linear structures. However, coronal sections are helpful if doubts remain.

Sphenopharyngeal encephalomeningocoele
This may also show hypertelorism, but in addition there is a midline defect in the pharynx or palate. Distortion of the nerves and chiasm may produce visual loss and optic disc colobomata have been described.

Anencephaly
This results from failure of development of the cerebral hemispheres and though compatible with life the visual system may be intact at a subcortical level.

Hydrancephaly
This is associated with incomplete development of the cerebral hemispheres which may be due to vascular obliteration, but the skull and meninges appear normal. The absent hemispheres are

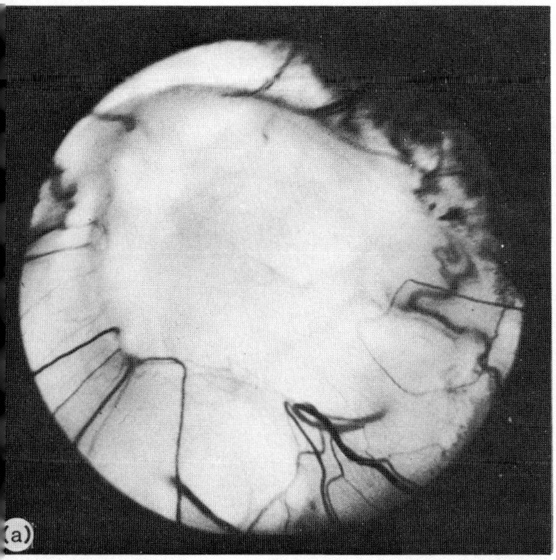

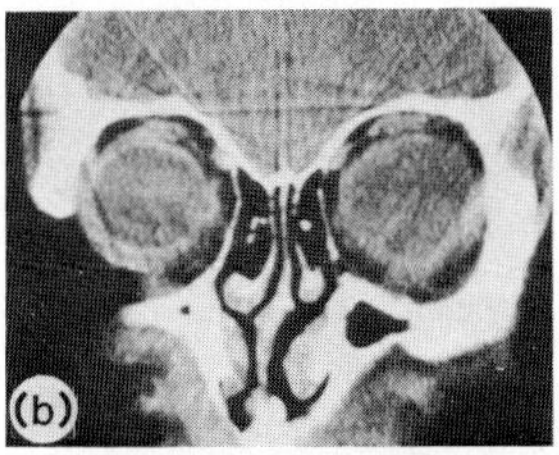

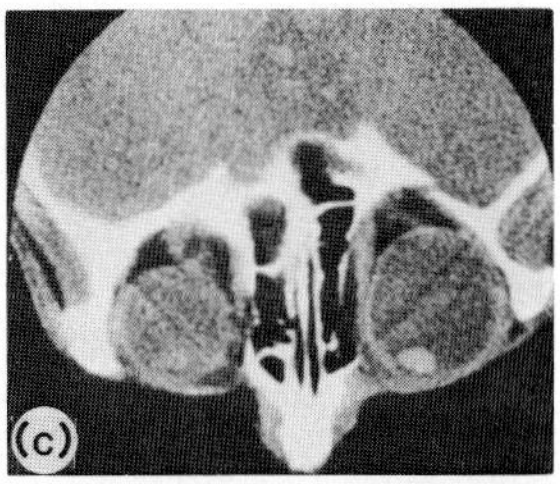

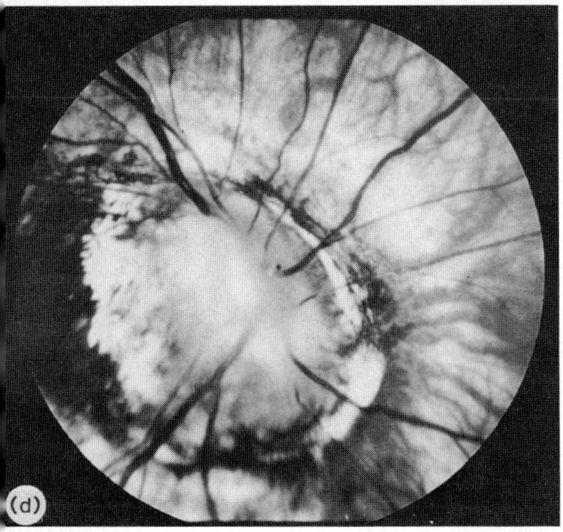

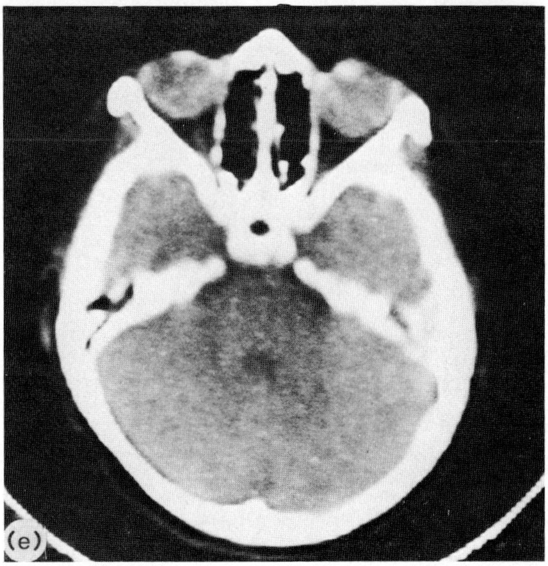

Fig. 7.2 Coloboma of the disc and peripapillary region. Case 1. A large unilateral coloboma and posterior staphyloma was seen in a young man (a). CT showed marked enlargement of the globe in both axial and coronal scans (b). No bone defect could be detected in the base of the skull. *Case 2*. A similar lesion was seen in a 14-year old girl with bilateral colobomata and anomalous tissue of the discs (d). She had an isolated deficiency of growth hormone and was below the 2nd precentile in height. CT showed a small defect in the floor of the sella due to a central meningocoele (e). (Case 2 courtesy of Mr D.S.I. Taylor).

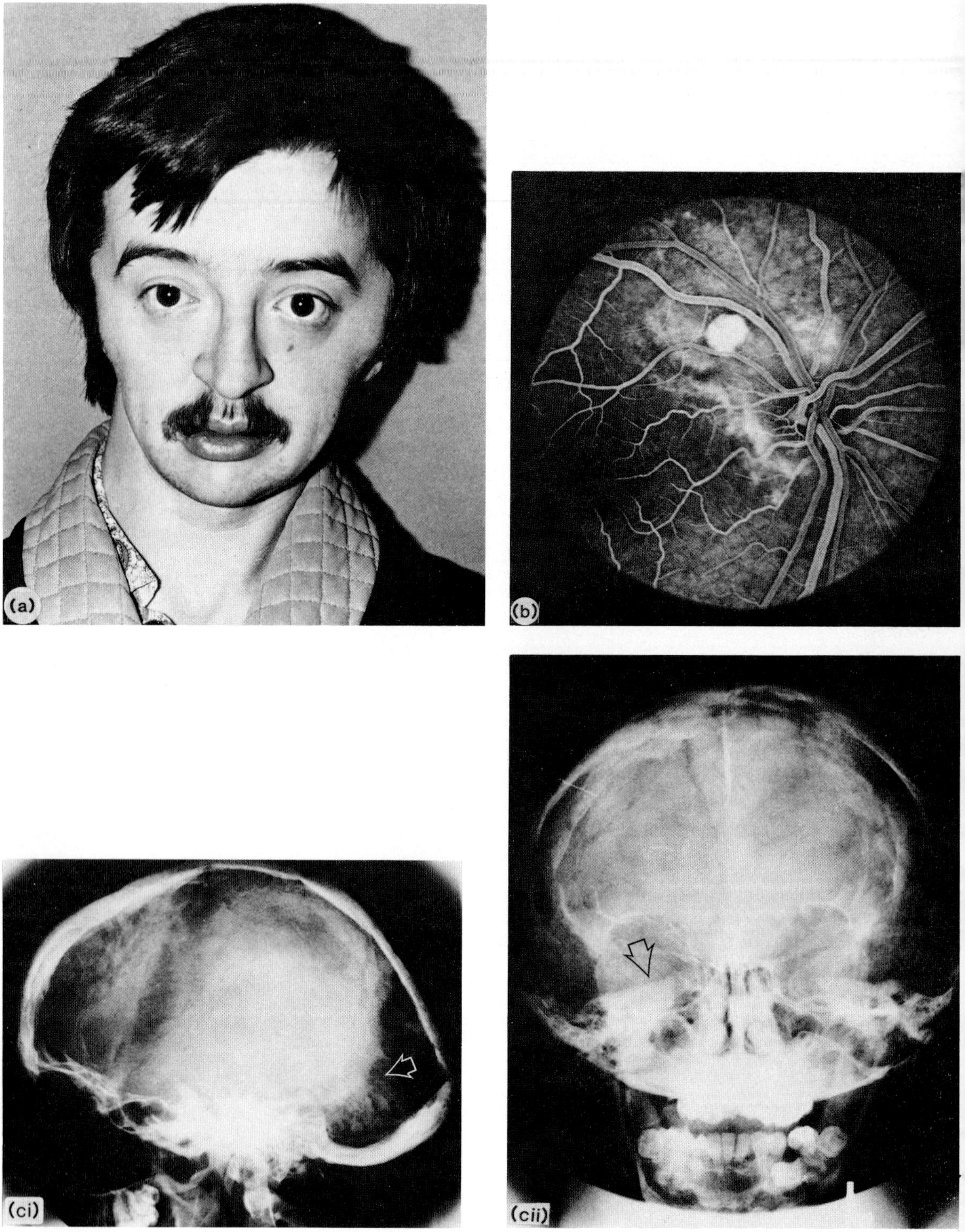
(a)
(b)
(ci)
(cii)

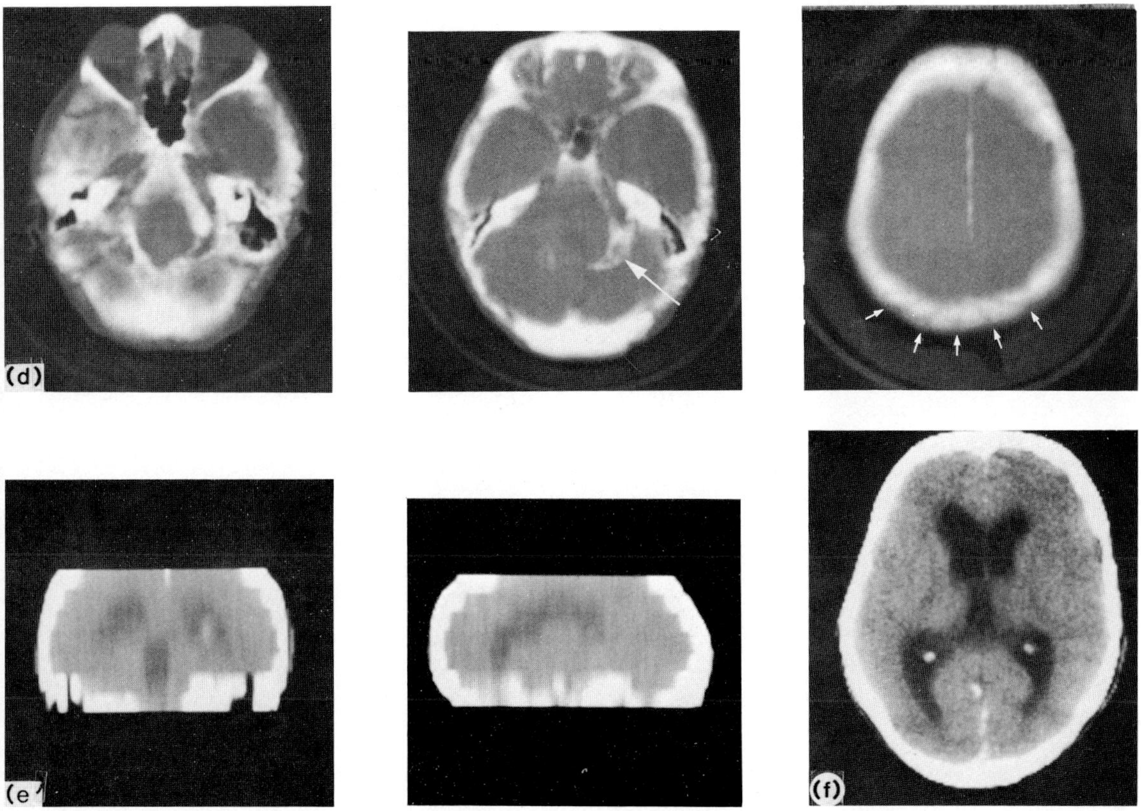

Fig. 7.3 *Hypertelorism: Cleidocranial dysostosis.* This young man was admitted for investigation of pressure headaches. His skull was abnormal in shape (a) with marked hypertelorism and mild exophthalmos. At 5 years of age, he had had an operation for a divergent squint, and was now noted to have impaired upgaze and bilateral nystagmus on lateral gaze. In addition, he had peripapillary disciform lesions (b, right eye fluorescein angiogram). Skull radiographs (c) showed the typical features of cleidocranial dysostosis, with prominent Wormian bones (white open arrow) and basilar invagination: note upward slope of petrous ridge (black open arrow). CT (d) confirmed these bony changes, showing the projection into the posterior fossa of the basiocciput (arrow) (small arrows, Wormian bones). It also demonstrated the abnormal form of the skull (compare e with c). Furthermore, it showed moderate hydrocephalus (f) for which ventricular shunting was carried out after a trial of conservative therapy.

replaced by cerebrospinal fluid. CT in a typical case is shown in Fig. 7.4.

Arrhinencephaly or holoprosencephaly

This group of midline facial and cerebral abnormalities comprises abnormalities of the olfactory bulbs, anterior visual system, nose and lips, and the cerebral abnormality is related to abnormal development of the prosencephalon. The severe form should be suspected when hypotelorism is present and there may be cyclopia, though milder forms are more common manifesting as septo-optic dysplasia. In addition there are combinations of arrhincephaly, encephalocoele, facial clefts and ocular abnormalities with the 13–15 Trisomy syndrome.

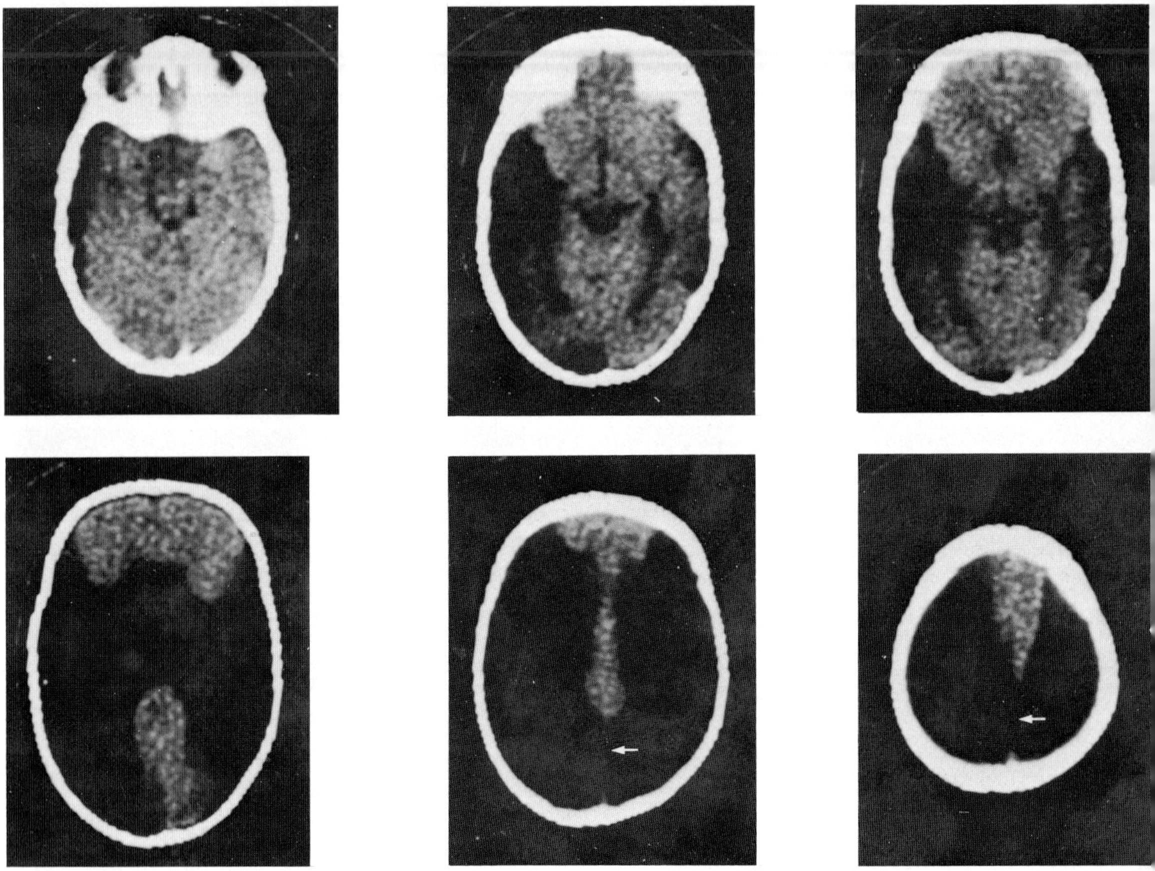

Fig. 7.4 *Hydranencephaly.* A young child with global retardation and a large head. The lower part of the brain, up to the inferior frontal lobes is relatively normal, but the remainder of the cerebrum is replaced by CSF, apart from a small rim of tissue anteromedially. The falx cerebri (arrows) is present.

Congenital cataract is a feature of this syndrome and of other genetic diseases, e.g. the 17–18 Trisomy syndrome and Down's syndrome. It also occurs sporadically. We examined a boy with unilateral congenital cataract whose sister had an optic nerve glioma. CT showed microphthalmia on the affected side, increased thickness of the sclera and raised attenuation coefficients in the sclera and lens. The optic nerve on the affected side appeared thinner than its fellow (Fig. 7.5).

Septo-optic dysplasia

The ophthalmologist has a vital diagnostic role in the diagnosis of the blind child. Recognition of hypoplasia of the optic discs should obviate other investigations apart from CT and continued endocrine follow-up. This condition can be readily separated from the congenital amaurosis of Leber on clinical grounds.

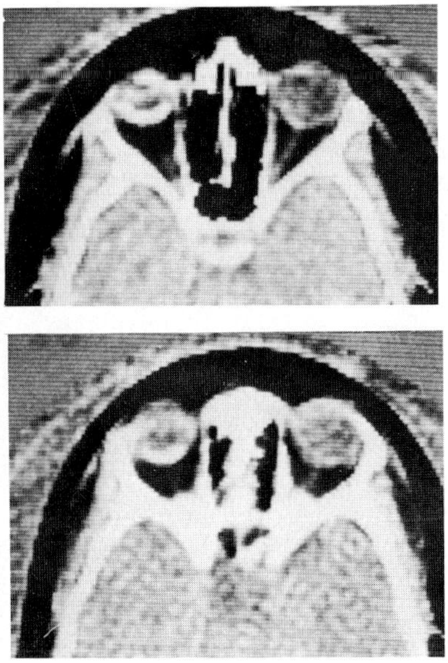

Fig. 7.5 Congenital cataract on left (see text).

Although De Morsier (1956) introduced the term and described the developmental nature of the condition, the pathological features of the first case were from an 83-year old brain. The syndrome includes absence of the septum pellucidum in combination with abnormal development of the optic nerves, chiasm or tract. Abnormal development of the olfactory bulb producing anosmia, with hypopituitarism and hypoplastic discs has also been described.

Embryology

Total aplasia of the nerve results from failure to incorporate mesoderm into the optic stalk at the 4–10 mm stage. Hypoplasia results from an abnormal development of retinal ganglion cells at a slightly later stage. The anterior diencephalon develops into the olfactory bulbs, septum pellucidum, corpus callosum and anterior visual system.

Ocular features

The ophthalmologist usually sees this condition in blind babies or children and those with less severe involvement may be referred later by endocrinologists for mild visual disturbances. Optic disc hypoplasia may be unilateral or bilateral and the discs are small, usually with a double rim. Nerve fibres are reduced in the retina, and the retinal vessels are sparse, with a paucity of the smaller branches. Hypoplasia of the nerve may occur as an isolated phenomenon, representing part of a spectrum (Frisen and Holmegaard, 1978) or be associated with a variety of other anomalies ranging from porencephalic cysts to Duane's syndrome.

Abnormal ocular movements may be present with pendular nystagmus, but see-saw nystagmus has been described.

General features

Early development may be normal, but endocrine disturbance may become manifest over the early years, as an isolated hormone deficiency or panhypopituitarism. Recent interest has been directed towards aetiological factors and maternal ingestion of anticonvulsants or quinine has been suggested, and also the presence of maternal diabetes or prediabetes.

CT

CT examination in the fully-developed syndrome of septo-optic dysplasia reveals optic nerves of abnormally small diameter (confirmed on coronal sections), a large chiasmatic cistern, and absence of the septum pellucidum. The latter can be differentiated from acquired absence by the form of the anterior horns; in the congenital variety, their anterior border is flat, rather than tapering down to the normal point of insertion of the septum. We have seen a case with an absent septum pellucidum and partially

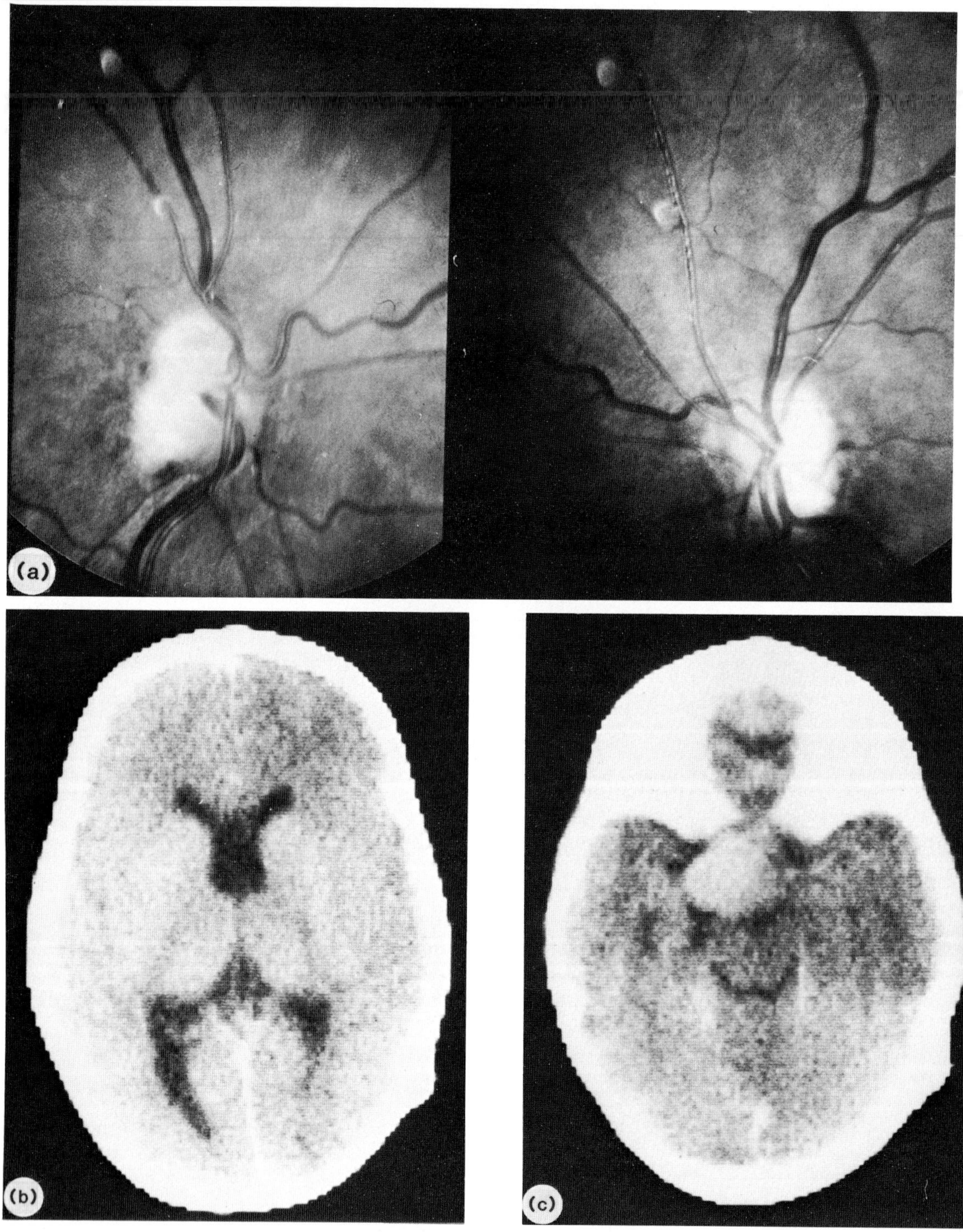

Fig. 7.6 Optic nerve hypoplasia with optic chiasm glioma. A girl aged 7 years had always had poor vision, and more recently had complained of headaches. Visual acuity was grossly reduced in both eyes, and the fields were constricted. The optic discs were small with an unusual shape and paucity of retinal neurones (a). CT (b) confirmed the absence of a septum pellucidum (note the rounded form of the frontal horns anteromedially) but also revealed a large suprasellar mass, isodense with brain and showing homogeneous contrast enhancement (c).

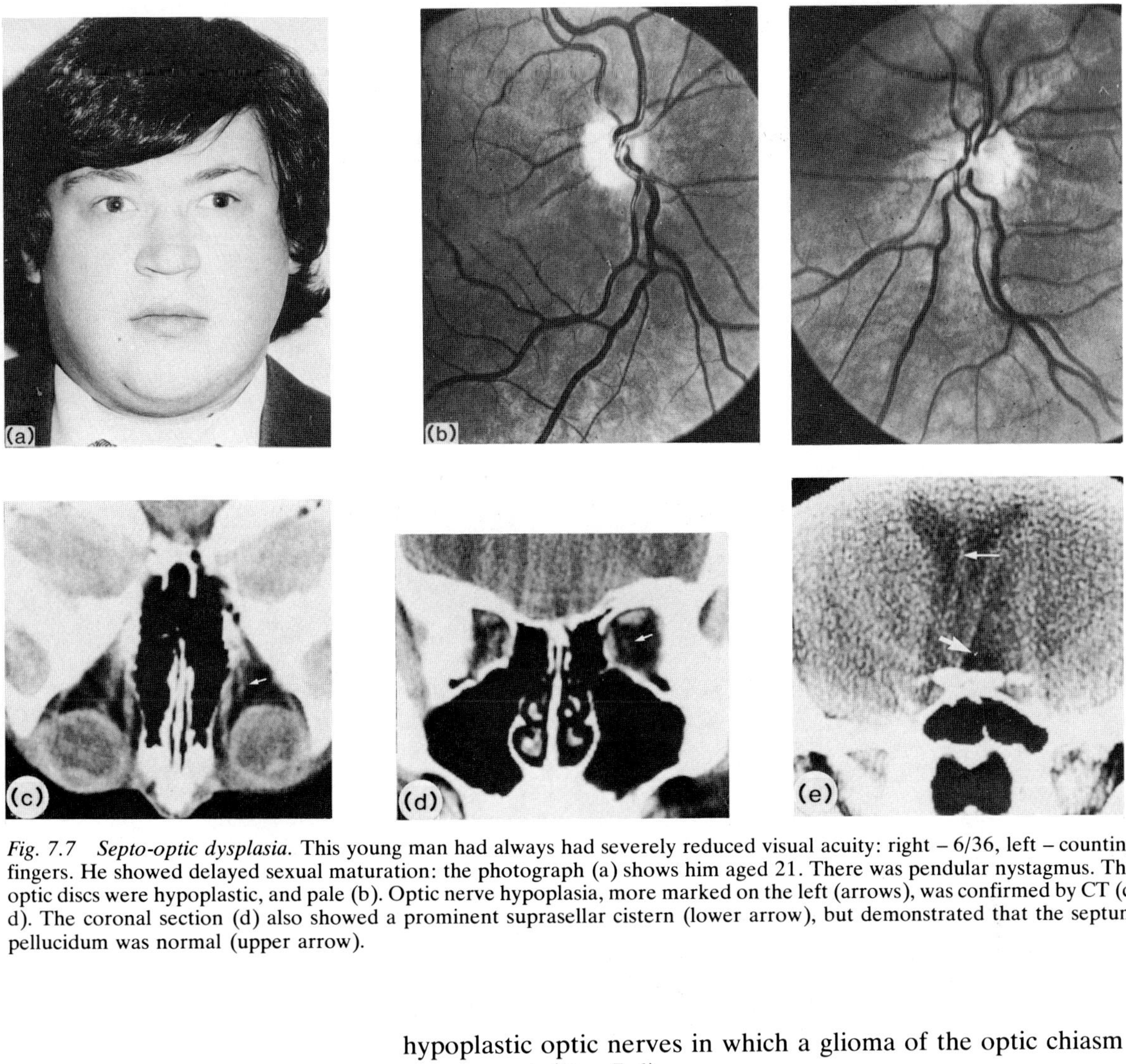

Fig. 7.7 Septo-optic dysplasia. This young man had always had severely reduced visual acuity: right – 6/36, left – counting fingers. He showed delayed sexual maturation: the photograph (a) shows him aged 21. There was pendular nystagmus. The optic discs were hypoplastic, and pale (b). Optic nerve hypoplasia, more marked on the left (arrows), was confirmed by CT (c, d). The coronal section (d) also showed a prominent suprasellar cistern (lower arrow), but demonstrated that the septum pellucidum was normal (upper arrow).

hypoplastic optic nerves in which a glioma of the optic chiasm was present (Fig. 7.6).

There have been several reports of hypoplastic discs with a normal septum pellucidum, so that this is not an essential ingredient of the syndrome (Sanders and Brook, 1974; Fig. 7.7). Lebuisson *et al*. (1979) described the findings in eight patients with optic disc hypoplasia, all with poor vision. Six were thought to be normal at CT while two patients with unilateral hypoplasia showed optic nerves which appeared of smaller diameter on the affected side. In one of the latter, the asymmetry was incontrovertible, but in the other, apparent asymmetry on the axial scans was not confirmed by coronal sections.

Aicardi's syndrome

This occurs in girls with a single dominant gene on the X chromo-

Fig. 7.8 Agenesis of the corpus callosum. This 2-year old child had hypertelorism and disordered eye movements and right ptosis (a). The head was abnormally rounded. Agenesis of the corpus callosum was shown at CT (b), with gross separation of the lateral ventricles, and a large posterior fossa cyst, separating the occipital horns and extending into the quadrigeminal cistern. There were atrophic cortical changes. (c) A coronal section in another case demonstrates the upward extension of the third ventricle (arrow) between the lateral ventricles, whose medial borders are abnormally concave.

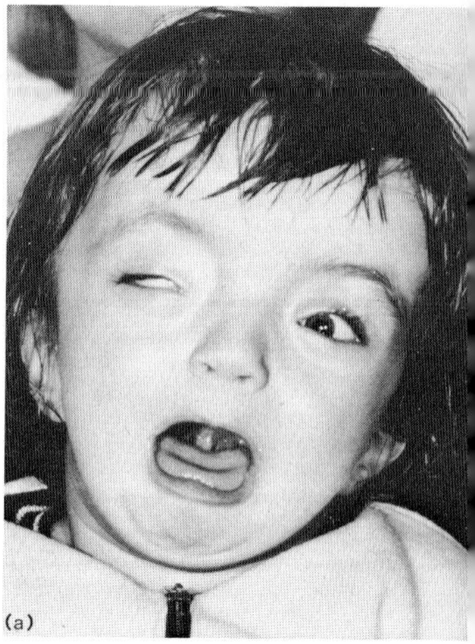

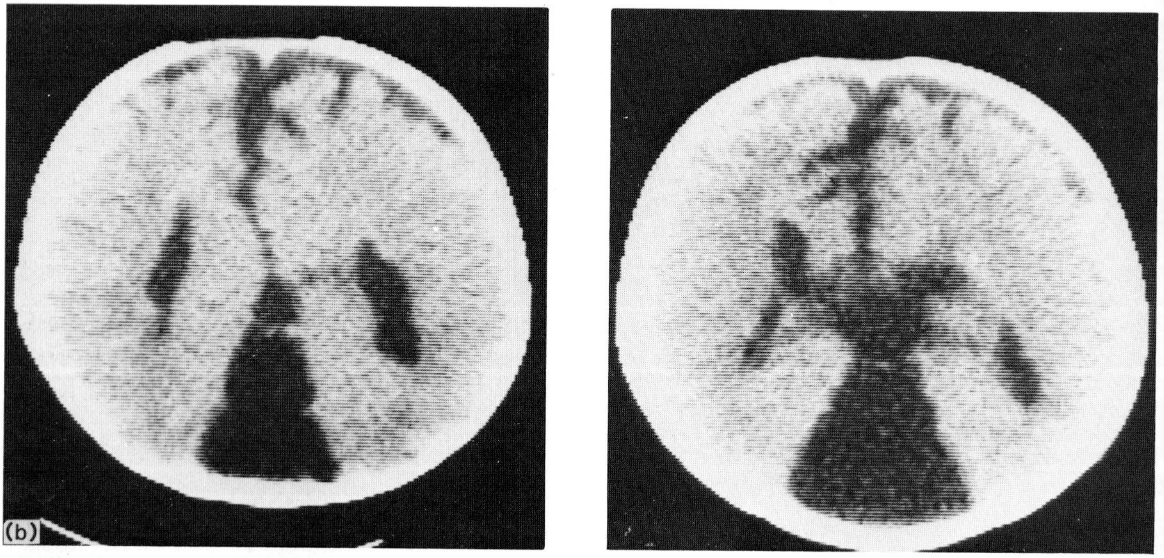

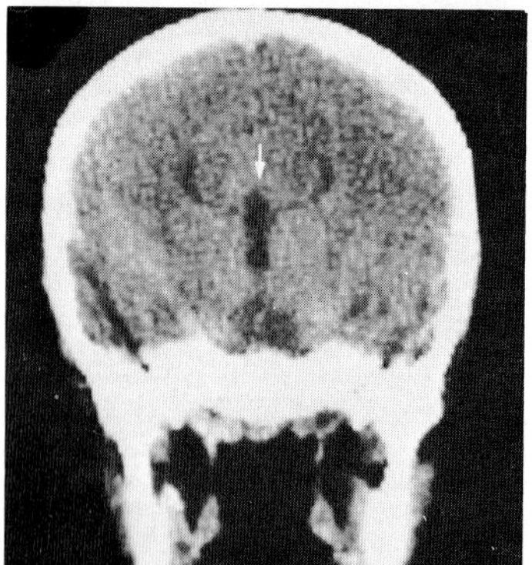

some and carries a poor prognosis in boys. Clinical features classically include infantile spasms, and chorioretinal lacunae. Additional ocular features include optic disc colobomata and hypoplasia of the disc. Microphthalmos and persistent pupillary membrane may be present, as may dysplastic retinal tissues.

The orbital CT examination reveals hypoplastic optic nerves; in one patient thought to have this syndrome, a retrobulbar mass was present. Intracranial abnormalities include agenesis of the corpus callosum and ectopia of grey matter (Limnaios *et al.*, 1979).

Agenesis of the corpus callosum is relatively common, frequently seen without other congenital anomalies (Bull, 1967), but forming part of more complex malformations such as Aicardi's syndrome (Fig. 7.8). The cardinal feature is marked separation of the lateral ventricles, whose medial borders are not in contact; an enlarged third ventricle extends up between them in the midline. The lateral ventricles are often abnormally shaped, with dilatation of their caudal portions. The septum pellucidum is absent, as is the falx cerebri.

7.2 LESIONS PRINCIPALLY AFFECTING THE SKULL

Craniostenosis

This developmental abnormality results in early fusion of cranial bones to produce asymmetrical skull appearances, in addition to facial anomalies such as hypoplastic maxillae, cleft palate etc. The failure of normal skull growth may result in raised CSF pressure, producing papilloedema and visual loss. The orbits may be shallow so that the eyes are prominent and often divergent.

Various terms describing the shape of the skull are used from oxycephaly (tower skull), to brachycephaly (broad skull), but in addition other abnormalities such as syndactyly are described (Apert's syndrome; Fig. 7.9).

Crouzon's craniofacial dystosis

This well-defined abnormality consists of craniostenosis, hypertelorism, and facial abnormalities with hypoplastic maxillae, hooked nose and prognathism. The ocular abnormalities include exophthalmos due to small orbits and visual loss due to papilloedema or optic nerve compression.

Facial dysplasias

Disorders of the first visceral arch produce abnormalities of the face, which comprise a number of components occurring individually or in combination. The full syndrome is seen as mandibulofacial dysostosis comprising obliquity of the palpebral fis-

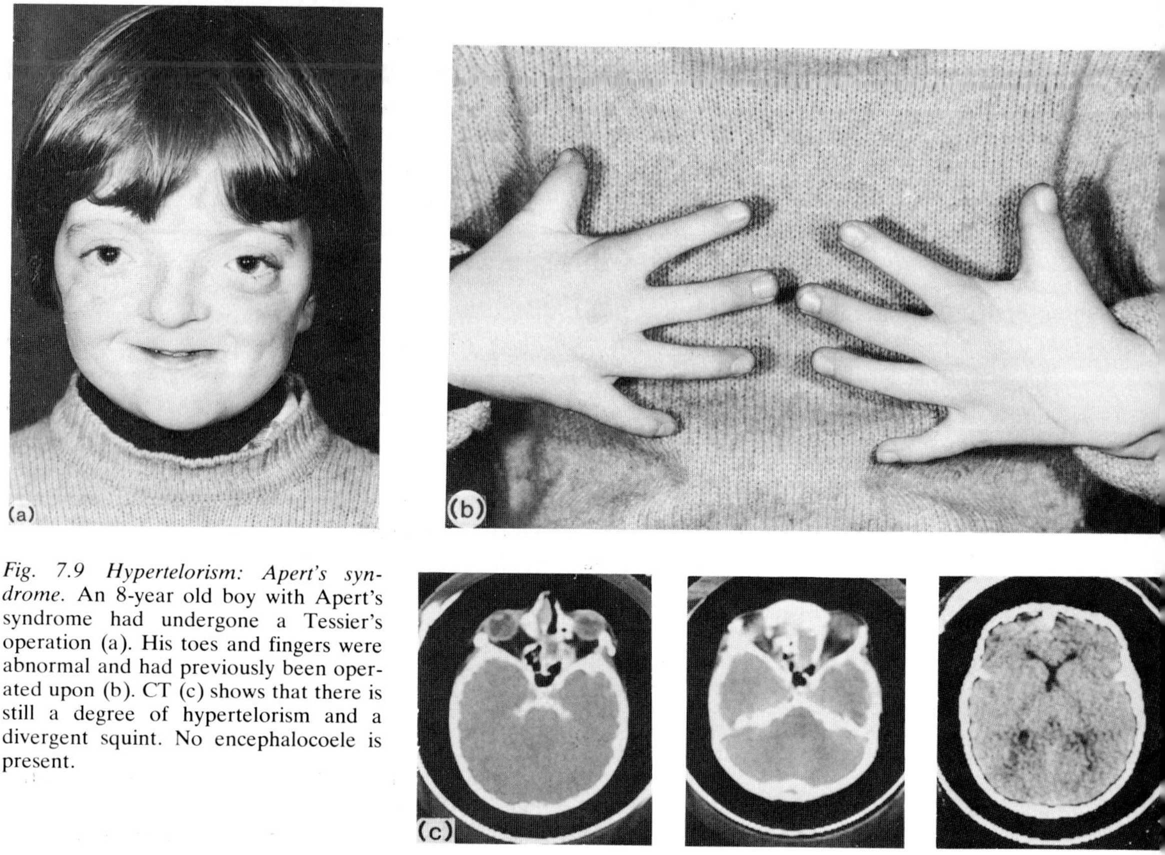

Fig. 7.9 Hypertelorism: Apert's syndrome. An 8-year old boy with Apert's syndrome had undergone a Tessier's operation (a). His toes and fingers were abnormal and had previously been operated upon (b). CT (c) shows that there is still a degree of hypertelorism and a divergent squint. No encephalocoele is present.

sure with lid colobomas, hypoplasia of the malar bones, malformation of the ear, palate, and blind fistulae between the ears and angle of the mouth. Skeletal abnormalities may be seen in addition.

Fibrous dysplasia

This is a congenital disorder of bone, characterized by expansion and abnormal bony texture. Usually seen as a monostotic form, it may occur with multiple bones being involved, in association with precocious puberty (Albright's syndrome). Affection of the skull base and facial bones is classical. The neuro-ophthalmological complications have been systematized by Liakos, Walker and Carruth (1979):

Primary

Depending on the site of involvement:

1. Frontal bone – proptosis and swelling (Fig. 7.10).
2. Skull base – extraocular muscle palsies; trigeminal neuralgia.

Fig. 7.10 *Fibrous dysplasia.* A 20-year old man gave a history of slowly progressive downward displacement and proptosis of the left globe (a) leading to minor vertical diplopia. CT (b) showed massive thickening of the frontal and ethmoid bones, without a focal extension into the orbit, while on a wide window image (c), the typical bone texture of fibrous dysplasia was evident. A central cyst with dense calcification was also visible.

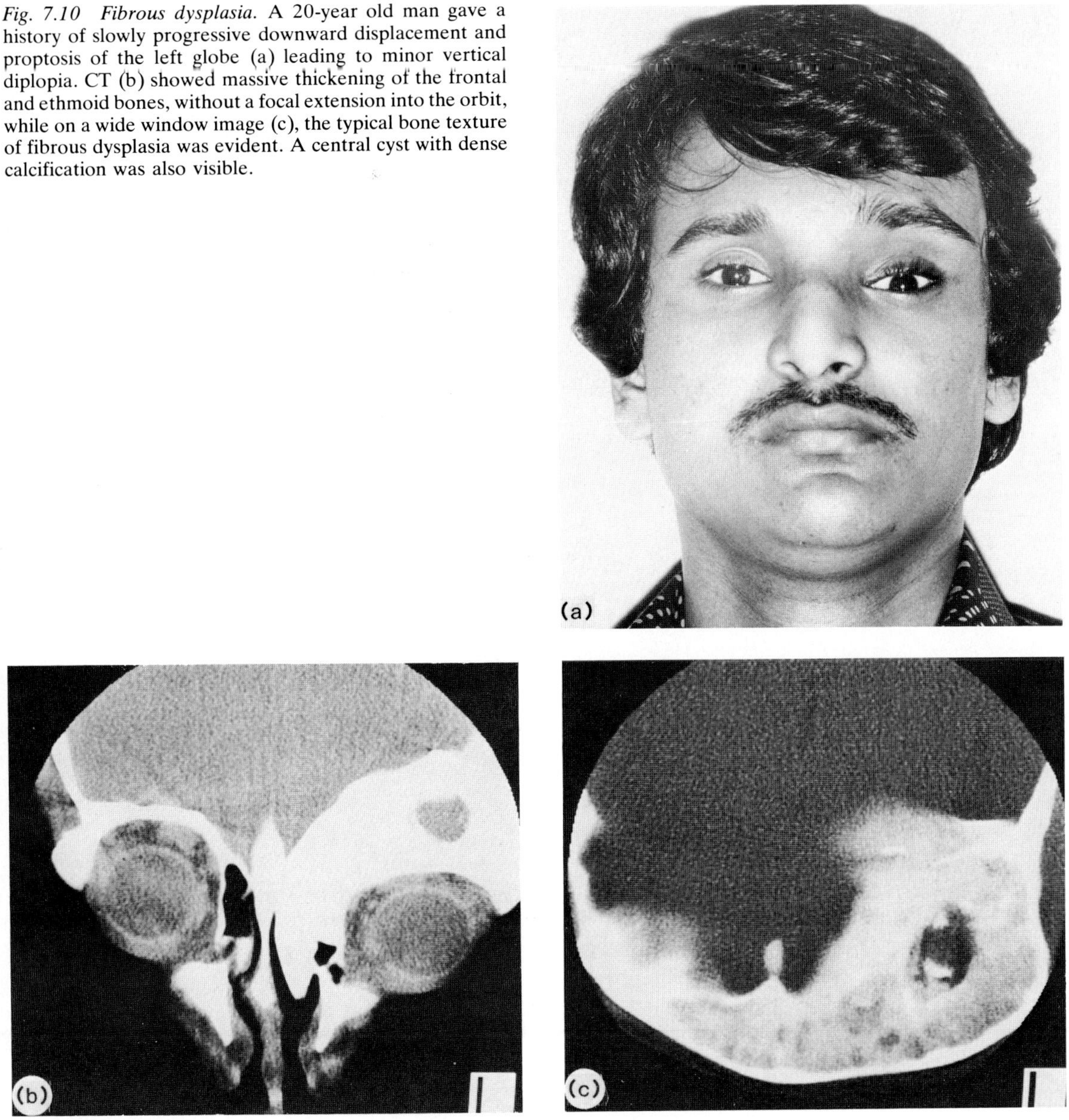

3. Optic canal – visual loss, optic atrophy.
4. Body of sphenoid – chiasmal compression.
5. Maxilla – epiphora.

Secondary

1. Malignant transformation, sarcomatous change.
2. Mucocoele, by obstruction of ostia of sinuses.
3. Ossifying fibroma.

Fig. 7.11 Romberg's hemifacial atrophy. This 38-year old woman gave a seven-year history of wasting of the right side of the face, affecting particularly the maxilla and orbital region. There was marked enophthalmos (a). The eye was involved (b), with marked loss of retinal neurones, a thin retina and degeneration of the pigment epithelium, especially in the peripapillary zone. CT (c) showed the atrophy of the extracranial tissues from the maxilla (1) up to the frontal region (4), where the bone was also markedly thinned (arrow); gross enophthalmos was evident (2).

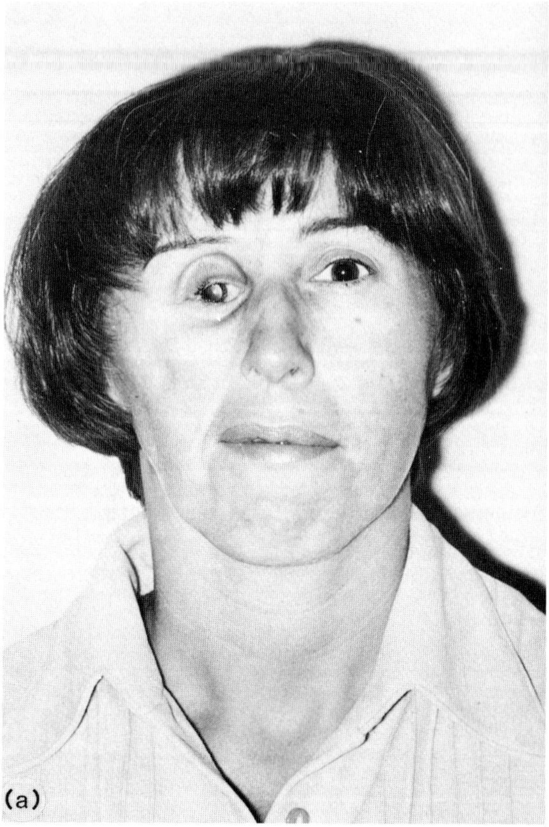

CT examination shows very dense, expanded bone, which may have the classical 'ground glass' featureless texture. Cysts are not uncommonly present. Malignant transformation is manifest by irregular bone destruction or new bone formation, sometimes with extensive soft tissue masses.

Facial hemiatrophy (Romberg's syndrome)

This unilateral dysplasia is more common in females, starting in the first or second decade. It involves one side of the head, with a classical frontal *'en coup de sabre'* cleft of localized alopecia and scleroderma. The progressive type is more common than the congenital form. More widespread unilateral involvement, e.g. of the diaphragm, may occur. Ocular changes are seen in about one third of patients; enophthalmos is typical, and Horner's syndrome, retinal abnormalities and phthisis bulbi may be seen (Fig. 7.11). Subcutaneous injections of medical grade silicone fluid have been used for cosmetic treatment (Muchnick *et al.*, 1979).

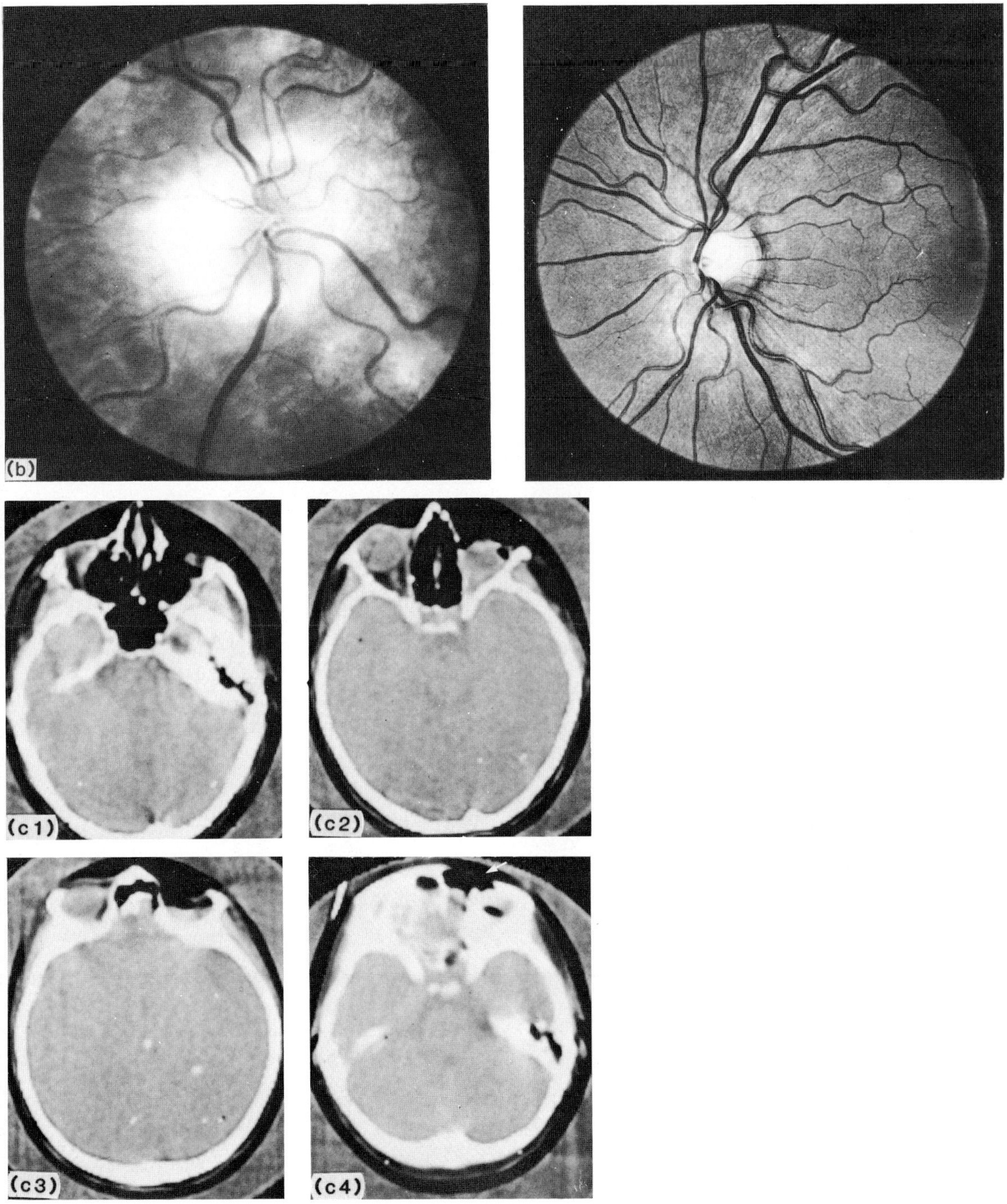
(b)
(c1)
(c2)
(c3)
(c4)

7.3 THE PHAKOMATOSES

These conditions are related clinically, because they all manifest diagnostic cutaneous signs, histologically, because they consist of tissue normally present but with an abnormal orientation (hamartomas), and finally and most importantly because some of them are genetically inherited on a dominant basis. The group includes:

1. Neurofibromatosis.
2. Tuberous sclerosis.
3. Sturge-Weber syndrome and variants.
4. Angiomatosis retinae and cerebellae (von Hippel-Lindau disease).
5. Ataxia telangiectasia (Louis-Bar syndrome).

Neurofibromatosis (Von Recklinghausen's disease)

This dominantly-inherited phakomatosis provides a wide assortment of clinical phenomena transversing all discplines, but usually presenting to ophthalmologists, neurologists, endocrinologists and dermatologists. The hamartomatous lesions may occur in any part of the body.

Cutaneous manifestations

The characteristic feature is the café au lait spot, which is a flat pigmented lesion with a clear margin, usually present on the trunk; five lesions are considered necessary to confirm the diagnosis. Small, soft, elevated lesions due to peripheral neurofibromata are also present. Plexiform neuroma usually involves the first division of the Vth cranial nerve.

Bone lesions

These have been mentioned previously. Absence of the sphenoid wings on the one side is the commonest abnormality and allows transmission of the cerebral pulse to the orbits. Facial asymmetry and cranial hemihypertrophy are well recognized. Osteosclerosis and/or rarification may also occur, and there appears to be an increased incidence of fibrous dysplasia.

CT appearances

The eye is occasionally enlarged and CT is a useful means of confirming that the apparent exophthalmos is a manifestation of an enlarged globe rather than proptosis due to a concomitant optic nerve tumour. Generalized enlargement of the orbit with buphthalmos is uncommon; but maybe on CT the eye elongated.

Enlargement of the optic nerve is most commonly the result of an optic nerve glioma, and meningioma has also been described but it does not fall within our experience. When the enlargement is bilateral, optic chiasm glioma with forward extension is a possibility; bilateral distension of the nerve sheath secondary to papilloedema should be evident clinically.

Ophthalmological manifestations

Orbit. Proptosis may be present, and if neurofibromatosis is suspected the globe and lid should be carefully scrutinized for pulsation. This can often be demonstrated with the applanation tonometer and is due to partial or complete absence of the greater wing of the sphenoid. Orbital tumours include optic nerve gliomas, plexiform neuromas within the orbit, and rarely an orbital meningioma. Anomalies of the shape of the orbit may render one eye more prominent.

Ocular features (Kobrin *et al*., 1979). The globe may be enlarged due to congenital glaucoma, and pathognomonic neurofibromata may be seen on the iris. The corneal nerves may be thickened and the fundus may show pigment naevi. The entity of a retinal phakoma has been reported, but these consist of pallid elevations of the peripapillary retina and choroid rather than the astrocytic hamartoma associated with tuberous sclerosis.

Optic disc changes reflect intracranial or optic nerve involvement.

Ocular motor abnormalities similarly are due to cerebral, brainstem or orbital lesions.

Endocrine abnormalities

Lesions in the hypothalamus may cause precocious puberty, polyuria and polydypsia, growth abnormalities or slipped femoral epiphyses. The association with phaeochromocytoma and other polyglandular syndromes, if suspected, necessitates a full endocrinological assessment.

Glial tumours

These may occur in any situation; most characteristic is the optic chiasm glioma.

Meningiomas

These have been recorded, indistinguishable pathologically from other meningiomas, but more frequently multiple, patients with neurofibromatosis constituting about 50% of cases of multiple meningioma.

Hamartomatous lesions

These may arise in the suprasellar region or elsewhere in the brain and may occur in the pineal region to produce aqueduct stenosis, which has an increased incidence.

Cerebral malformations

These range from cellular heterotopia and microgyria to meningocoele, and manifestations of dysraphism and syringomyelia. Premature cerebral atrophic changes are not rare.

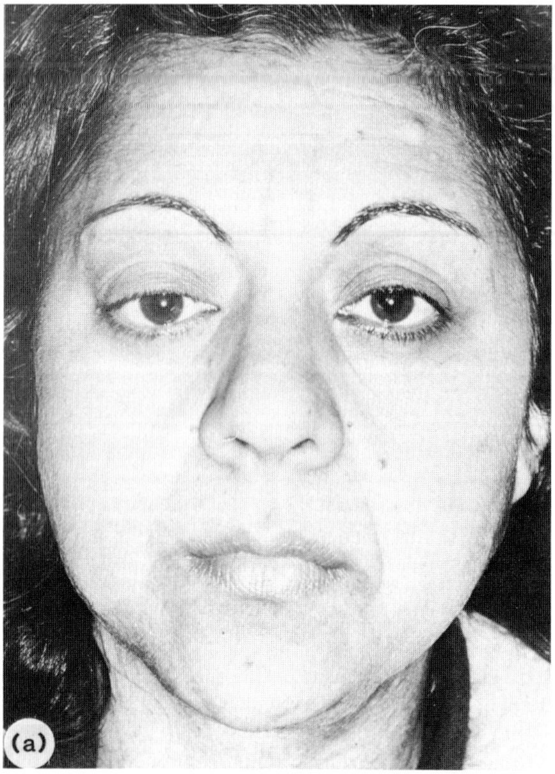

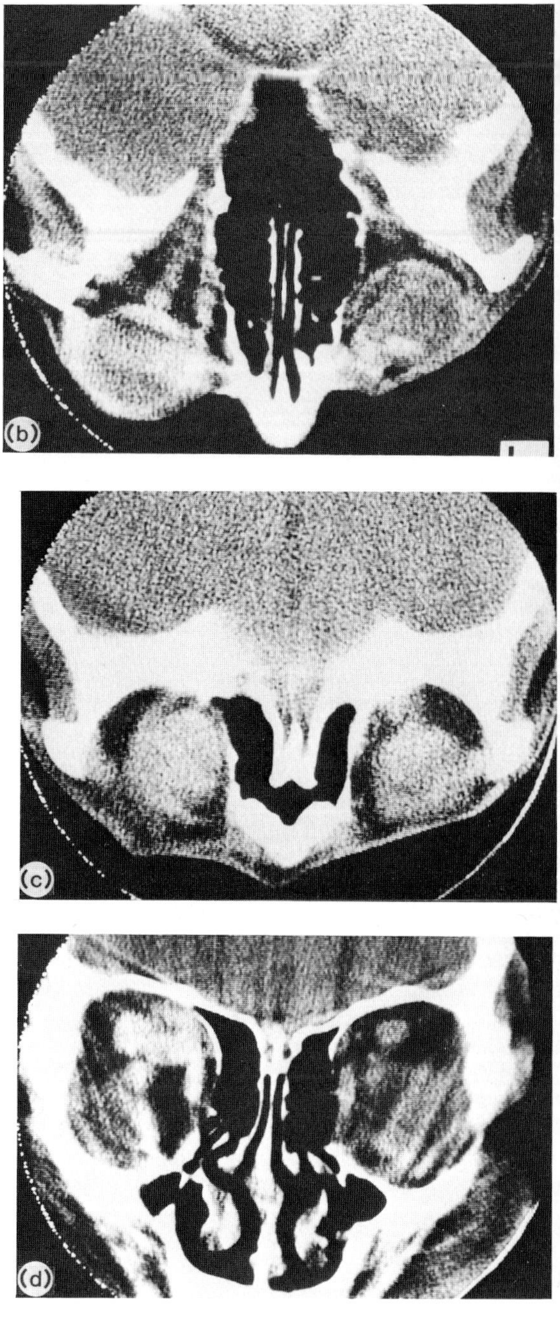

Fig. 7.12 Neurofibromatosis with proptosis due to orbital tumour. This 42-year old woman with known neurofibromatosis complained of diplopia and right proptosis. The right globe was also depressed (a). A mid-orbital axial section (b) showed merely anteroinferior displacement of the globe; the optic nerve appeared stretched. Further sections (c,d) revealed a rounded mass in the superomedial quadrant of the orbit; its relationship to the muscle cone was not clear. Operation was refused.

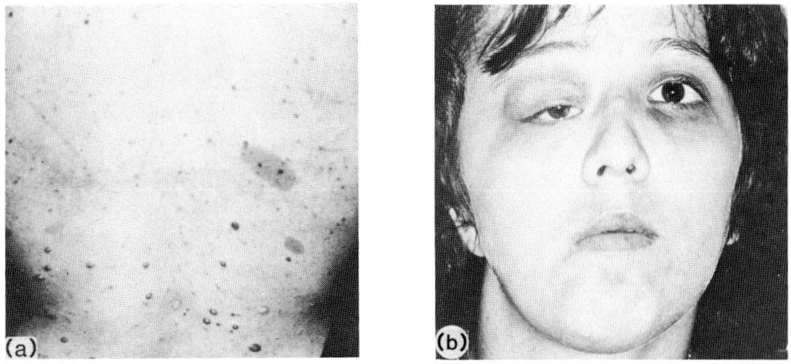

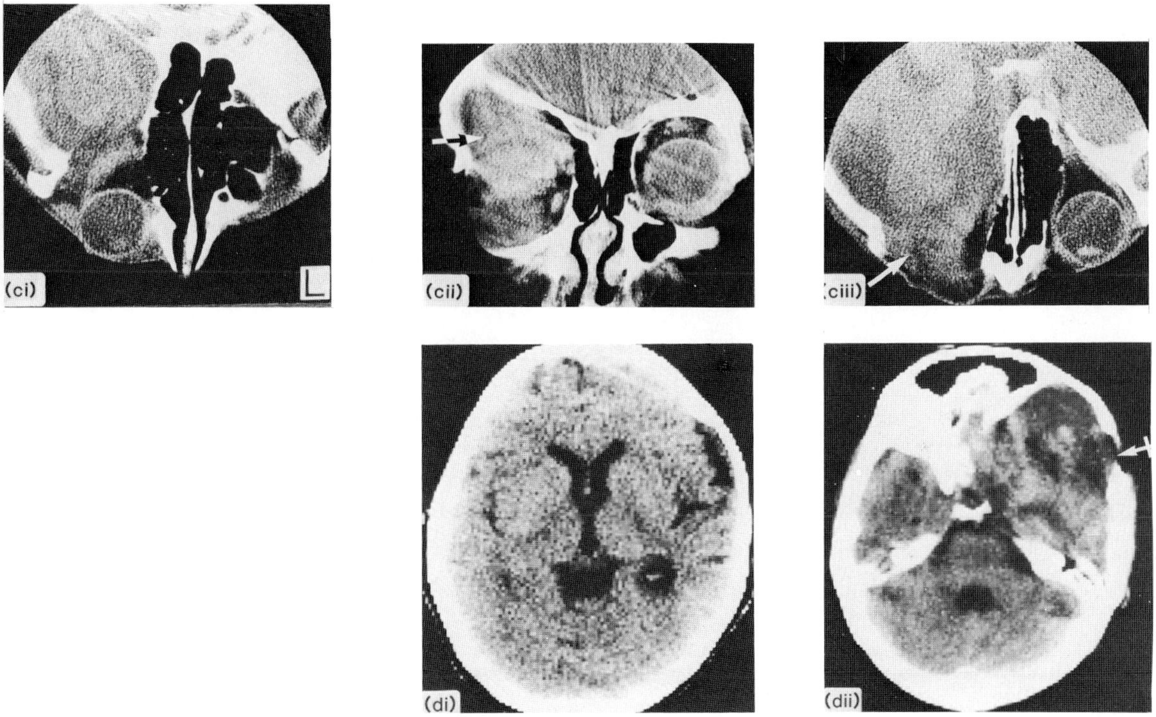

Fig. 7.13 Neurofibromatosis with proptosis due to sphenoid dysplasia. A 23-year old woman with known neurofibromatosis (a) gave a long history of right proptosis. The right eye was pushed forwards and downwards and there was a pulsatile swelling superolateral to it (b). The latter was shown by orbital CT (c) to be due to a dysplastic temporal lobe (arrows), herniated through a defect in the sphenoid bone. The defect was very extensive, affecting the cranial vault, as shown by cranial CT (d, crossed arrow) which also demonstrated the extent of the dysplasia of the cerebral hemisphere.

Other intraorbital tumours may present (Fig. 7.12). A plexiform neuroma, as described above, may be manifest at CT as enlargement of one or more of the extraocular muscles, combined with thickening of the skin and underlying soft tissues in the palpebral region and temporal fossa. Similar changes in the extraorbital tissue can, however, be the result of hemihypertrophy. Cutaneous or subcutaneous neurofibromata may be visible as rounded nodules of slightly increased (or decreased) attenuation relative to the surrounding tissues.

The dysplastic bone changes are characteristic, with asymmetry of the orbits, unilateral expansion of the middle cranial fossa and a more or less extensive ipsilateral defect in the sphenoid wings, through which the temporal lobe projects into the orbit. In such cases the orientation of the globe and therefore the course of the optic nerve may be quite abnormal.

The combination of buphthalmos, plexiform neuroma and sphenoid dysplasia, with or without an optic nerve lesion, is pathognomonic (Fig. 7.13).

Intracranial abnormalities have been listed above; their CT appearances are described elsewhere, and are generally not as characteristic as the orbital lesion. Unusually dense calcification in the choroid plexus of one or, less frequently, both lateral ventricles, which may be hypertrophied, does however appear to be a typical feature, although its cause is not known. It has been attributed to a meningioma arising in the choroid plexus, but the non-progressive course would not favour this suggestion.

Cranial hemihypertrophy, affecting both the bone (principally the middle table) and the paranasal sinuses is another typical but less common anomaly.

Tuberous sclerosis (Bourneville's disease; epiloia)

This dominantly-inherited condition of variable penetrance is to be suspected in children with mental deficiency, convulsive seizures and depigmented lesions on the skin (macular vitiligo). In older children and adults the classical feature is adenoma sebaceum, which may be telangiectatic, and occurs on the face in a butterfly distribution. Other features include a shagreen patch on the back, and subungunal fibromata.

Ocular features are restricted to the fundus and present two main appearances:

1. Mulberry-like lesions at the disc or in the posterior pole which are elevated, globular and resemble large drusen. Fluorescein angiography shows an abnormal capillary pattern in the lesions. These lesions histologically represent astrocytic hamartomas.
2. Small, oval and circular peripheral white or grey areas (Fig. 7.14).

Cerebral changes include macrogyria, microgyria, and corpus callosum defects. Glial nodules develop, mainly in the cerebrum, and small subependymal 'tubers' which calcify, are characteristic. Cortical atrophic lesions are also present, and syringomyelia has been described. The glial nodules tend to enlarge and become manifest tumours, although their degree of invasiveness is variable. Characteristically, tumour formation occurs in the third ventricular region, with the development of obstructive hydrocephalus (Fig. 7.14).

Kingsley (1977, personal communication) reviewed a series of 19 patients from the National Hospital and the Hospital for Sick

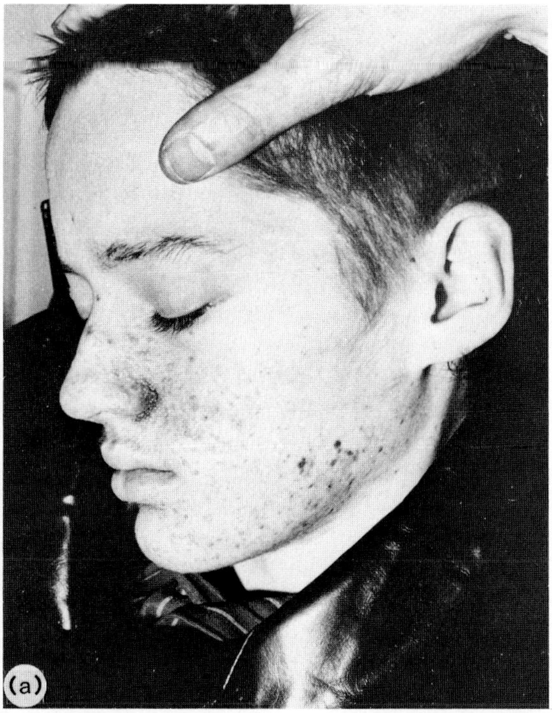

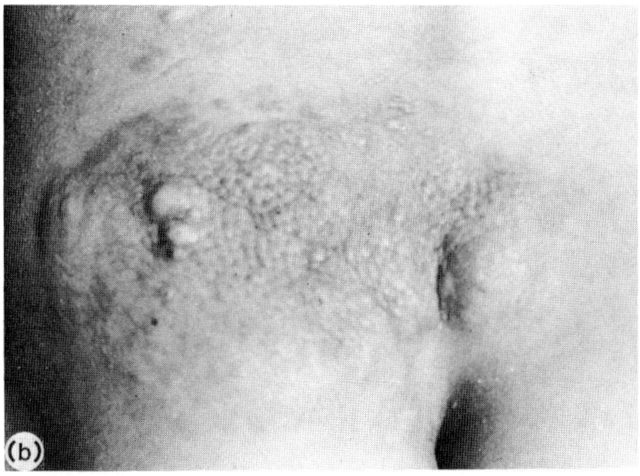

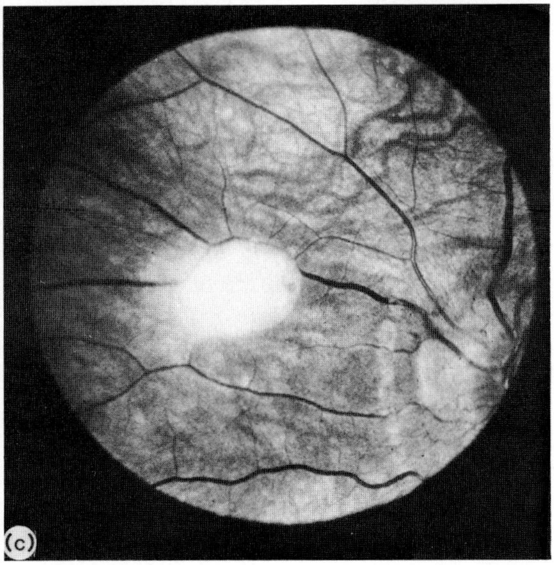

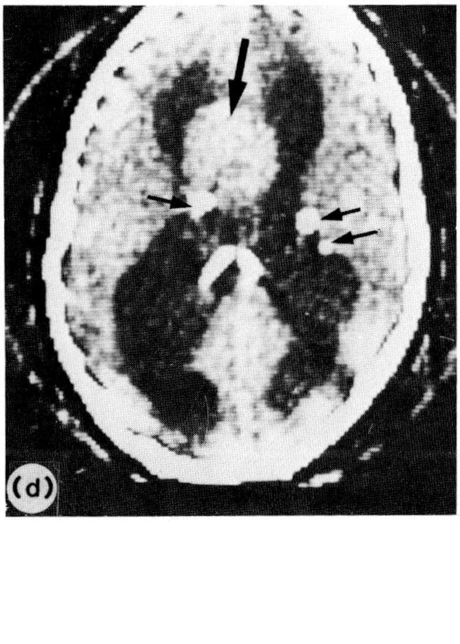

Fig. 7.14 Tuberous sclerosis. A boy aged 11, with a long history of epilepsy and mental retardation showed typical adenoma sebaceum (a) and a shagreen patch in the left loin (b). He was developing signs of raised intracranial pressure, and fundoscopy showed bilateral papilloedema and classical phakomata (c). CT (d) in addition to calcified periventricular tubers (small arrows), showed a smooth, rounded tumour at the foramen of Monro (arrow), causing marked hydrocephalus.

Children, Great Ormond Street. Calcification was visible on the plain skull radiographs in only one of 12 children less than 8 years old, and three aged less than 11 months did not show cutaneous lesions. CT, however, showed periventricular tubers in all these patients. One child with frontal calcification had no detectable tubers at 3 months, but re-examination at 10 months showed formation of a definite tuber. Four of the five patients over 10 years of age had tumours and raised intracranial pressure. Similar CT results were obtained in part of a large series of Lee and Gawler (1978), who also noted that three of 12 patients had parenchymal tubers. About 10% of the patients also showed cortical or subcortical atrophic lesions.

The importance of CT in the early diagnosis of this condition is evident both as regards the management of epilepsy and the future surveillance of the patient, and genetic counselling; tuberous sclerosis has an autosomal dominant mode of transmission.

Sturge-Weber syndrome

This sporadic syndrome produces a characteristic skin appearance, and there are additional ophthalmic and neurological features.

Cutaneous features

Skin involvement produces the familiar 'port wine' naevus, which is due to dilated vascular channels with flattened endothelial cells; it is present at birth and involution does not occur. Cerebral involvement is much more common when the forehead and upper lid are involved. Similar lesions have been reported on other parts of the body, and the associated involvement of the limbs is interesting (Klippel-Trenaunay syndrome).

Ocular features

Glaucoma occurs more commonly when the upper lid and conjunctiva are involved and may be present at birth. Choroidal angioma is feature which, because of the diffuse involvement, may be difficult to detect ophthalmoscopically unless comparison is made with the other eye. The choroidal angioma is flat and may rarely become elevated to produce a retinal detachment. The retinal veins may be tortuous and orbital involvement is rare.

CNS involvement

Cerebral involvement usually occurs on the same side as the cutaneous lesion and produces the characteristic symptom of Jacksonian epilepsy. The leptomeninges (and sometimes the dura mater) are the site of an angiodysplasia, which overlies an atrophic cerebral lesion. Calcium is often deposited in the latter to produce typical 'tram-line' X-ray features and this characteris-

Fig. 7.15 *Sturge-Weber syndrome.* A girl aged 11 had a mild left hemiparesis and severe epilepsy (a). There was a 'port wine' stain on the left side of her face, involving the left cheek but extending to the upper lid and to the mandible. The intraocular pressure was elevated in her left eye. (b) The fundi showed normal retinal vessels, but the choroidal colour was more marked in the left than the right, due to choroidal angioma. (Note the facial angioma does not correspond to the Vth nerve territory). (c) In addition to the classical 'tramline' calcification in the occipital lobe, the skull film showed calcification in a chronic extracranial haematoma (arrow). (d) With normal CT window factors, the calcification appeared amorphous, but a wide-window image (in the positive mode) revealed the typical texture. The vault was smaller, but slightly thicker, on the same side. (e) Sagittal and coronal reconstructions, showing the extent of the lesion.

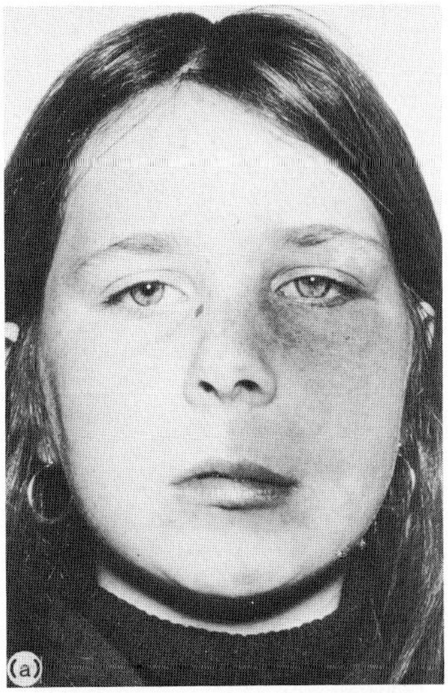

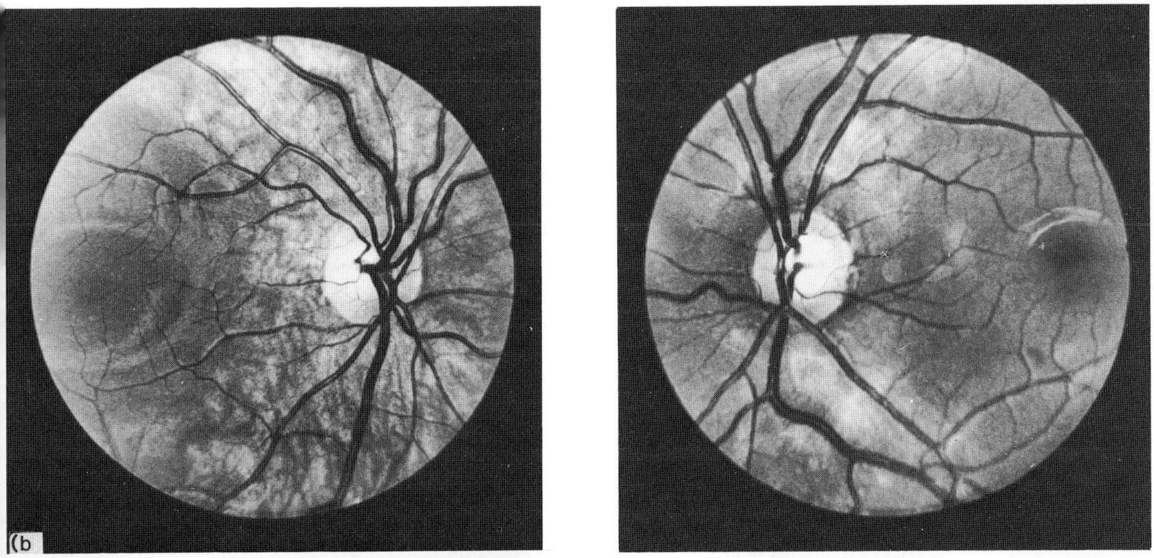

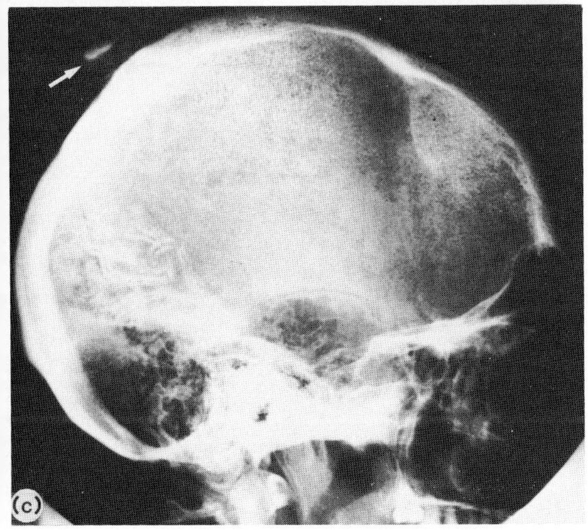

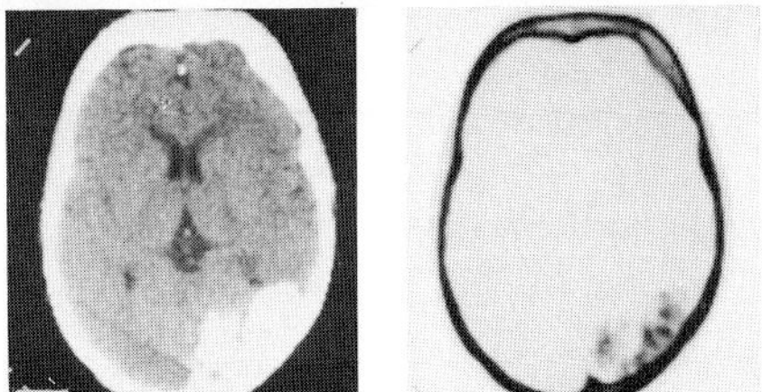

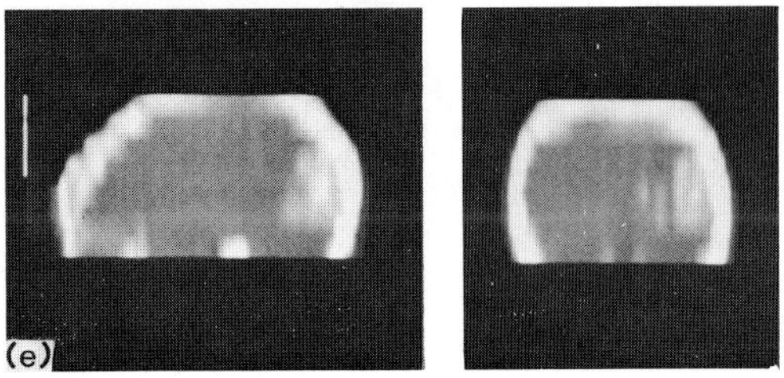

tically occurs in the occipital region. The cerebral hemisphere on the side of the lesion is often poorly developed to produce contralateral hemiatrophy, but hemihypertrophy is not, however, rare. The meningeal vascular and cerebral atrophic lesions are often confused.

The condition may occur in incomplete forms and in addition the palate, gums and soft tissues may be affected, with occasional angiomas elsewhere in the body (e.g. abdomen).

CT examination

CT usually shows no evidence of the cutaneous lesion, but may show thickening of the extracranial soft tissues and exaggerated enhancement with intravenous contrast medium when the angioma is massive. Phleboliths are rarely present.

In the orbital region, thickening of the eyelids and soft tissue masses in the retrobulbar space may be evident, as may enlargement of the globe compared to its fellow. Visualization of the choroidal angioma has been described by Guibert-Tranier, *et al.* (1979), as thickening of the posterior rim of the globe, indistinguishable from malignant melanoma; rarely, the angioma is calcified.

The cerebrum shows focal calcification, superficially in the cortex, and usually occipital, although an entire hemisphere may be involved. Bilateral calcification is occasionally present. It is usual for calcification to appear at normal window settings as amorphous areas of high attentuation, and a wide, high level window is required to display its classical curvilinear form (Fig. 7.15). As in other contexts, CT is considerably more sensitive than plain radiography and Kingsley (1977, personal communication) found calcification on CT which was not visible on plain radiographs in 25% of his cases; he also noted 20% in whom there was bilateral calcification with a unilateral naevus. This latter observation can be of crucial importance if hemispherectomy is being considered because of intractable epilepsy. Up to 10% of patients may show posterior fossa calcification. Increase in attenuation with contrast medium may be observed around the calcified areas.

The other changes to be seen on cranial CT depend on the relative contributions of cerebral and cranial hemihypertrophy or atrophy. Atrophic changes are more common; the affected hemisphere is smaller than its fellow, the sulci and fissures are more prominent, and the lateral ventricle is enlarged, as is the overlying subarachnoid space. The midline structures are shifted towards the affected side, where the cranium is at once smaller and thicker, the diploic space being particularly prominent; the paranasal sinuses are enlarged on the same side. When hemihypertrophy is present, the abnormal hemisphere is, paradoxically, the larger of the two, with a small lateral ventricle; the cranial vault is thicker but also larger.

A number of other phakomatoses have been described as occurring in association with the Sturge-Weber syndrome, i.e. neurofibromatosis, tuberous sclerosis, the von Hippel-Lindau syndrome, the naevus of Ota and Ito and melanotic phakomatosis. These may be manifest on physical and radiological examination. Hofeldt *et al.* (1979) described the CT findings in two cases of orbitofacial angiomatosis, believed to represent a *forme fruste* of the Sturge-Weber syndrome. Both patients had the typical naevus; one also had a well-capsulated, cystic retrobulbar mass, showing marked contrast enhancement, while in the second a similar mass extended through the superior orbital fissure to involve the middle cranial fossa. The brain itself was normal in both.

Von Hippel-Lindau disease

Von Hippel first described the clinical entity of the retinal angioma, and this was followed by Lindau's establishment of the association between the retinal lesion and similar lesions situated in the cerebellum. In addition, malignant tumours were recognized in other parts of the body, such as the kidney. The condition is inherited as an autosomal dominant.

Ocular features

The retinal lesion commences as a minute capillary anomaly which enlarges to form a pale circular or oval elevation. The lesion may be detected on routine ophthalmoscopy by the characteristic enlarged feeding arterioles and venules. Fluorescein angiography shows a rapid flow through these vessels with marked leakage. The lesion may be bilateral, multiple, and situated on the optic disc or more commonly in the mid-periphery. Progressive enlargement leads to exudation (often massive), vitreous haemorrhages and, ultimately, retinal detachment. Pathologically the lesion represents a capillary angioblastoma.

CNS features

Lesions similar to those in the retina may afflict the cerebellar circulation and may be multiple. As many as eleven lesions have been detected at craniotomy. Presenting features include subarachnoid haemorrhage, raised intracranial pressure and cerebellar signs. Lesions also occur in the spinal cord and less commonly in the cerebrum.

CT shows the haemangioblastomas as rounded areas of brain attenuation or slightly above, often with a surrounding low attenuation cyst. Contrast enhancement is usually very marked; it may involve the whole lesion, or a mural nodule. Angiography is more reliable for the detection of small lesions (Wilson and Moseley, 1977) (Fig. 7.16).

Fig. 7.16 von Hippel-Lindau disease. A boy of 14 presented with signs of a cerebellar lesion. There was no papilloedema, but an angioma was present at the right disc margin (a, colour photograph and fluorescein angiogram). CT (b,c) showed large, rounded areas of low attenuation in the left temporal lobe and the right cerebellar hemisphere, with marked nodular contrast enhancement. Angiography (d,e) subsequently revealed multiple cerebellar tumours.

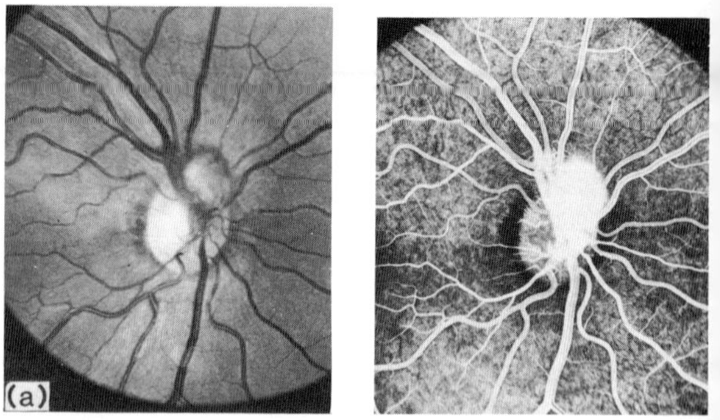

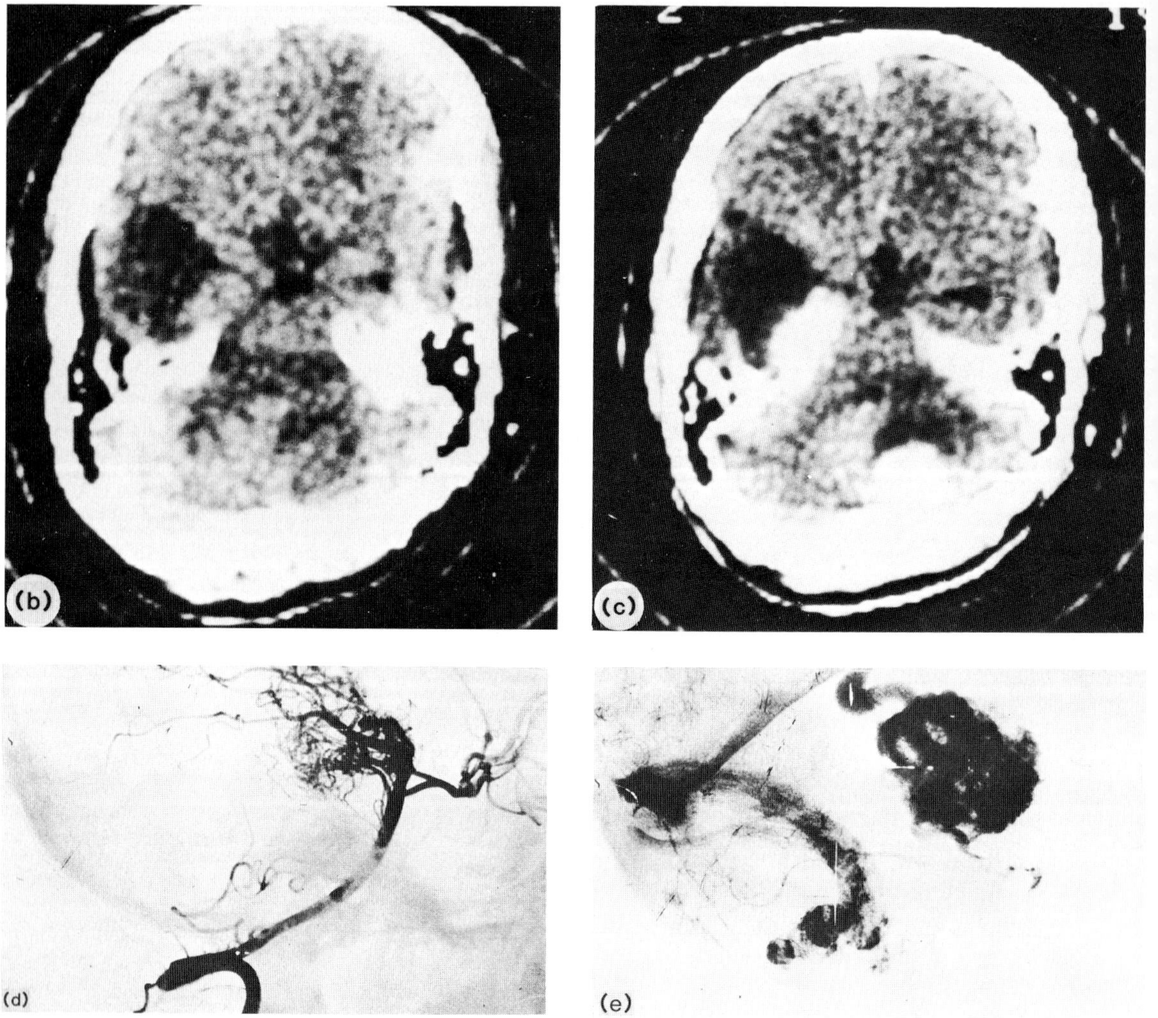

Ataxia telangiectasia

Dilated conjunctival vessels and erythematous areas in the skin flexures should be searched for in any child with a cerebellar syndrome. CT shows no abnormality (Kingsley, 1977), or demonstrates cerebellar atrophic features.

7.4 CONGENITAL VASCULAR LESIONS

Arteriovenous malformations of the orbit have two main forms: orbital angioma, with rapid arteriovenous shunting, which is relatively uncommon; and orbital varix, or venous angioma, where shunting is not a prominent feature, and which is a common cause of proptosis, particularly of episodic or gravity-dependent type.

Angiomatous malformations

The combination of retinal, facial, orbital and cerebral arteriovenous anomalies presents an impressive, though rare, clinical appearance. The term retinocephalic vascular malformation (Théron *et al.*, 1974) has the advantage of verisimilitude but the historical descriptions by Bonnet *et al.* (1937) and Wyburn-Mason (1943) have provided attractive eponymous attributions. The existence of the association of midbrain and retinal arteriovenous anomalies described by Wyburn-Mason has not been clinically established, and a review of case notes of some of his original patients does not lead us to alter this view.

The retinal appearances are important in diagnosis and provide a clue to the more extensive involvement of the face and brain, which in certain cases extends from the retina to the occipital cortex. A review of the angiographic features was provided by Théron *et al.* (1974).

The CT features will depend on the localization and severity of the various lesions. The posterior portion of the globe may appear thickened externally and show an abnormal degree of enhancement with intravenous contrast medium. Apparent thickening and irregularity of the optic nerve can be shown with high resolution CT to be the result of a leash of fine vessels twined around the nerve sheath; these also show marked enhancement (Fig. 7.17). In severe cases, most of the retrobulbar space is occupied by these vessels (which cannot be identified specifically as either arteries or veins).

Also in this condition, or as an isolated anomaly, the scalp or facial vessels may be malformed, often with bizarre results, since the draining veins are not contained by the enclosing skull or bony orbit. A cutaneous component is often manifest as thickening of the extracranial soft tissue around the orbit with a nodular or tubular appearance, with intense enhancement by intravenous contrast medium.

Fig. 7.17 Orbito facial angioma. This 17-year old boy had been treated as a child by cautery of a cutaneous angioma on the left cheek, now apparent only in minor scarring and telangiectasia (a). He complained of impaired vision in the left eye; acuity was 6/18. Fluorescein angiography showed a massive retinal arteriovenous malformation (b). At CT (c) the outer layer of the left globe appeared thicker than that of the right; there was also thickening of the eyelid and external ocular muscles. The optic nerve at first appeared thickened, but it became apparent that this was due to vessels surrounding it (arrows). (d) Carotid angiography (1) confirmed the presence of an angioma, mainly around the optic nerve, but also involving the other orbital soft tissues (arrow) and draining to the cavernous sinus (open arrowheads). There was no intracranial extension (2), but abnormal vascularity was shown in the palatal (crossed arrows) and ethmoidal (arrowheads) territories of the external carotid artery (3).

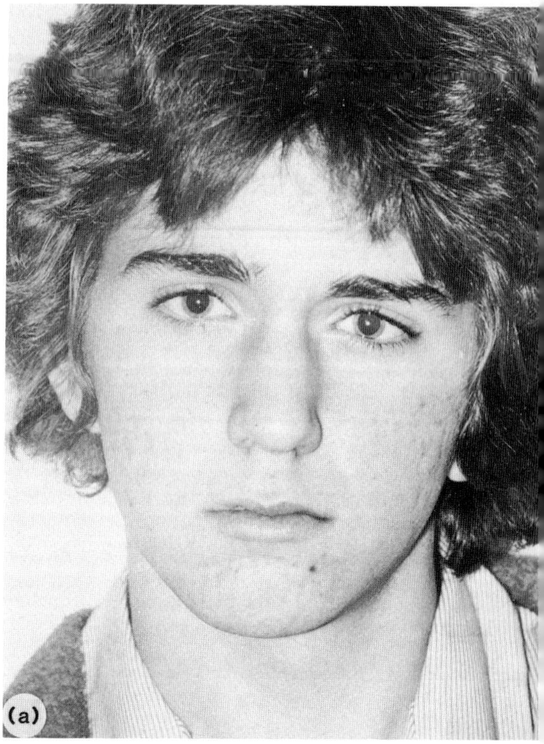

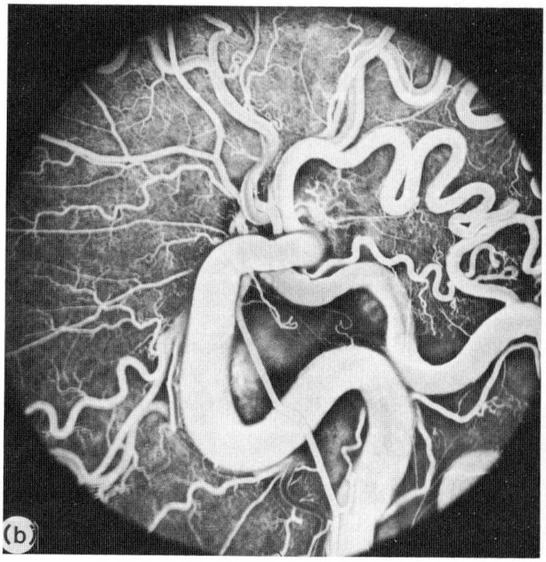

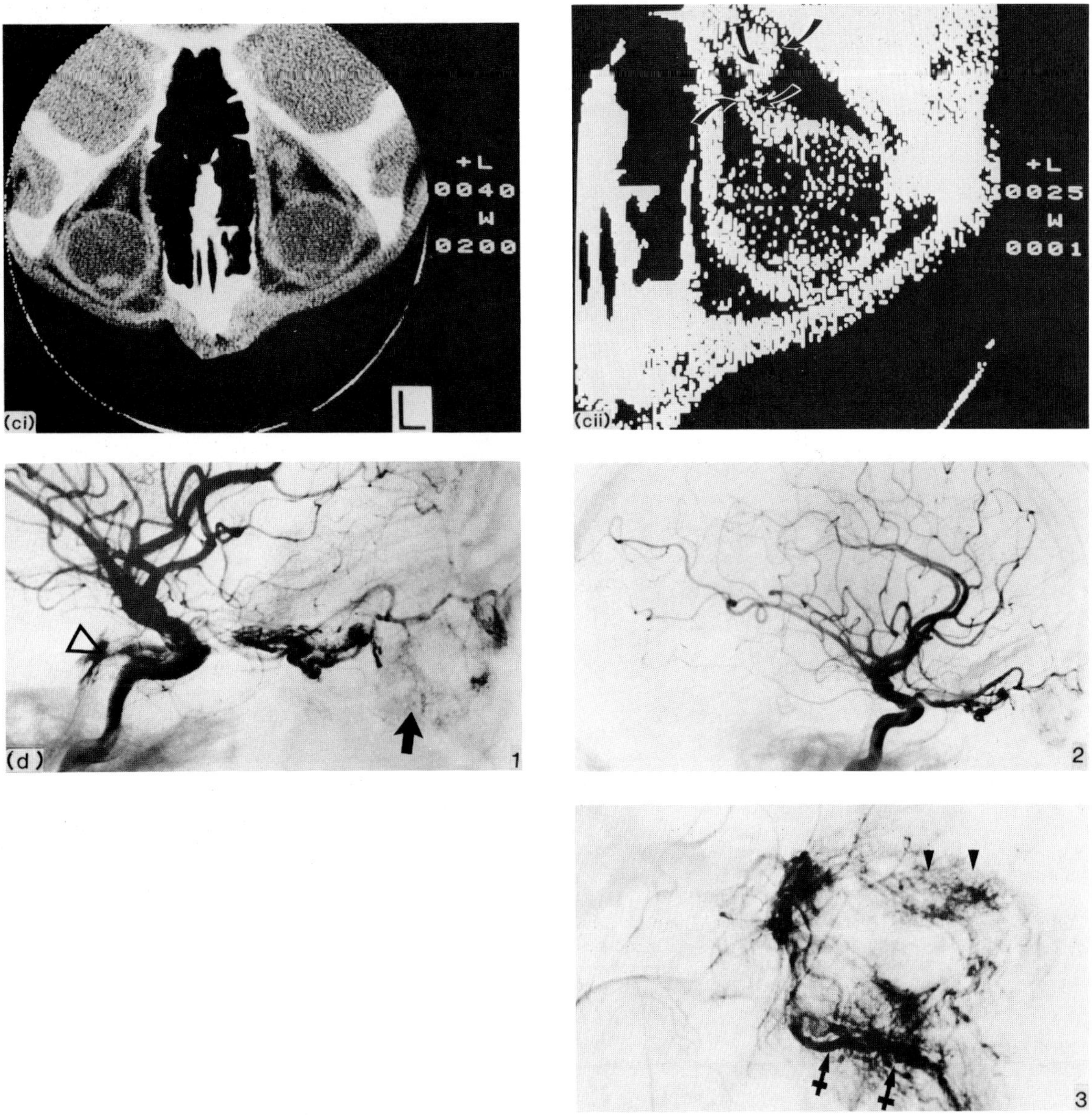

In one of our cases of orbital arteriovenous malformation, a middle-aged woman who presented with acute onset of orbital pain, restricted eye movements and severe diminution of vision in one eye, CT showed apparent slight thickening of the medial rectus on that side, with intense enhancement after intravenous contrast medium. The latter was the radiological clue to the nature of the lesion, confirmed at angiography (Fig. 7.18).

In those cases in which the diagnosis is evident, or rests bet-

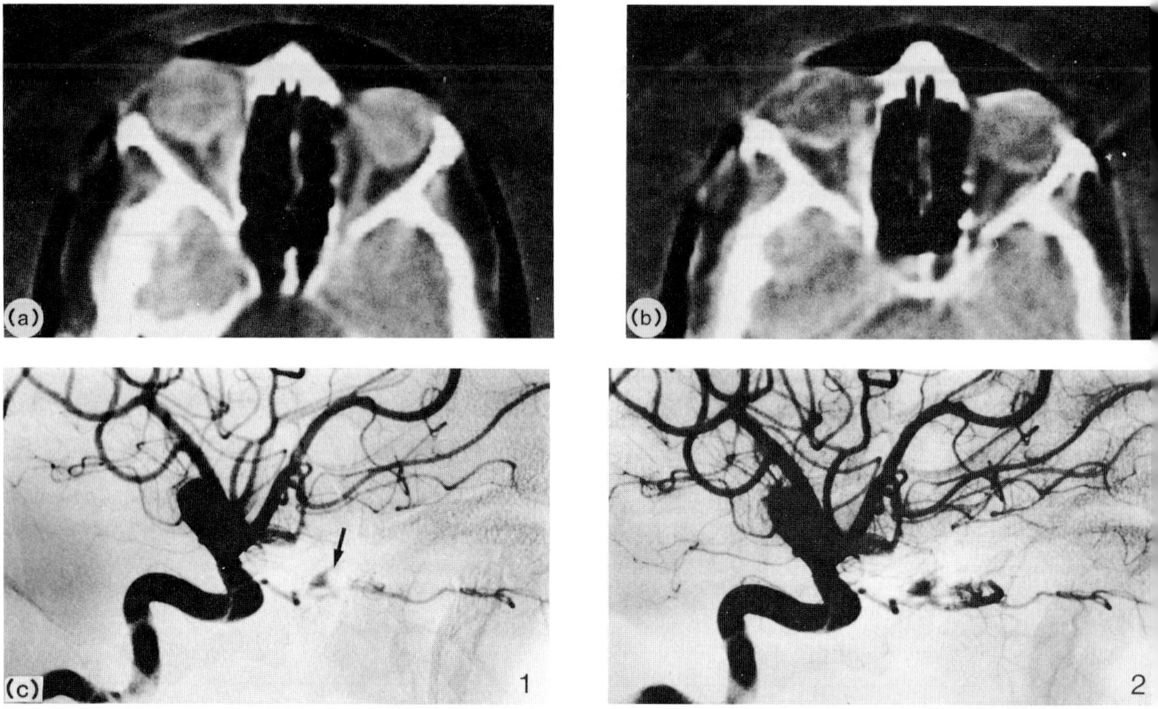

Fig. 7.18 Orbital arteriovenous malformation. A 56-year old woman was woken by acute left orbital pain, and found she could not see with the left eye. Vision was reduced to hand movements, there was proptosis with periorbital swelling and eye movements were limited and painful. There was no bruit. CT (a) confirmed the proptosis; the left medial rectus muscle was prominent, and showed very marked contrast enhancement (b). These findings were thought compatible with acute inflammation, but carotid angiography (c), revealed an arteriovenous malformation (arrow) fed by the ophthalmic artery, with very rapid venous shunting (frame 3 is late arterial phase).

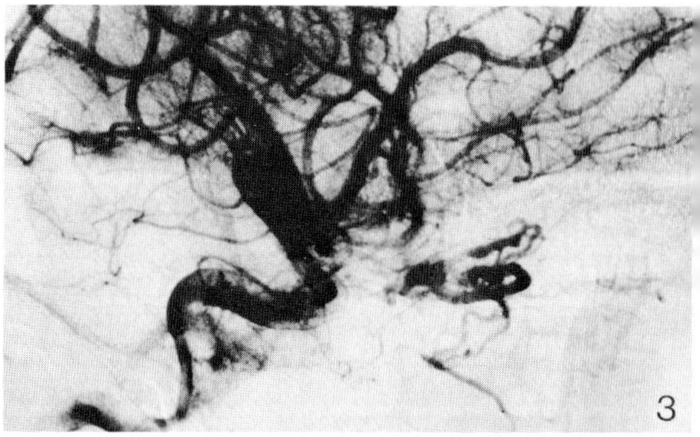

ween arteriovenous malformation and fistula, angiography of the internal and external carotid arteries on both sides is clearly the definitive diagnostic procedure, and may indeed also be therapeutic if embolization proves to be possible. In many cases, however, particularly when the diagnosis is less clear, there is nothing to be lost in carrying out a CT examination prior to angiography: it is non-invasive, and may give useful information. There are a number of patients who present as the result of partial or complete thrombosis, in whom the CT study will show a lesion demonstrated imperfectly or not at all by angiography.

Orbital varices

These are very common lesions (three times as frequent as haemangiomas) which are often classical in their clinical and radiological features, producing intermittent proptosis. Clinical recognition therefore depends on postural examination of the patient with the neck extended, with the head between the knees, and the Valsalva manoeuvre, procedures which may produce proptosis or fullness of the lids. Patients usually present acutely with proptosis due to haemorrhage, thrombosis of draining veins, or some other change in haemodynamic status.

Pathologically, there is a difference between venous angiomas which are benign neoplasms of redundant newly formed channels, and the orbital varix which is a congenital or acquired dilatation of venous channels (Jakobiec and Jones, 1979).

In conjunction with the typical clinical features, plain radiographs showing phleboliths establish the diagnosis beyond reasonable doubt. In the large majority of cases no specific treatment is possible, but superficial cosmetic surgery is sometimes recommended.

If a CT examination is to be carried out, it may be particularly helpful to perform the study with the patient prone, and with the feet raised, if this is feasible with the available apparatus. If for some reason this is not possible, then a Valsalva manoeuvre sustained during a fast scan will also have the effect of engorging the orbital veins. The scan should show the dilated retrobulbar veins as serpiginous or linear structures replacing the orbital fat, possibly with one or more small rounded calcific areas, representing phleboliths, within them (Fig. 7.19). Intravenous contrast medium causes a considerable, more or less homogeneous increase in attenuation. It is very uncommon for there to be any intracranial abnormality (Fig. 7.20).

Opacification of orbital varices at orbital phlebography is not infrequently unsatisfactory, because of limited filling of the capacious, slow flow system. Despite this, it is often stated that demonstration of varices is one of the principal indications for phlebography. For the reasons stated above, and because of the clear confirmation of the diagnosis possible by CT, invasive studies would rarely seem to be indicated in this condition.

Hereditary haemorrhagic telangiectasia
(Rendu-Weber-Osler disease)

Cutaneous and visceral lesions are the hallmark of this condition. However, both the eyes and the brain may rarely be affected.

Ocular changes reported include tortuosity and segmental dilatation of the retinal veins. Retinal or vitreous haemorrhage may occur, and ischaemic changes may be seen.

Telangiectasia of the brain is not uncommon, but is not detectable at CT, although it may be manifest as cerebral or subarachnoid haemorrhage. However, there would appear to be an

Fig. 7.19 Orbital varices. A 27-year old woman presented with a history of fluctuating left proptosis, which was increased by jugular vein compression. Skull films (a) showed typical phleboliths (small arrows) in the left orbit, which was expanded; the roof had an abnormal scalloped appearance (open arrow). At carotid angiography (b), the arterial phase was normal but abnormally large vessels were seen in the late venous phase (arrows). At CT (c) the retrobulbar space was largely filled by serpiginous vessels, the phleboliths (arrowheads), with a vessel joining them, being clearly visible. There was massive contrast enhancement (d).

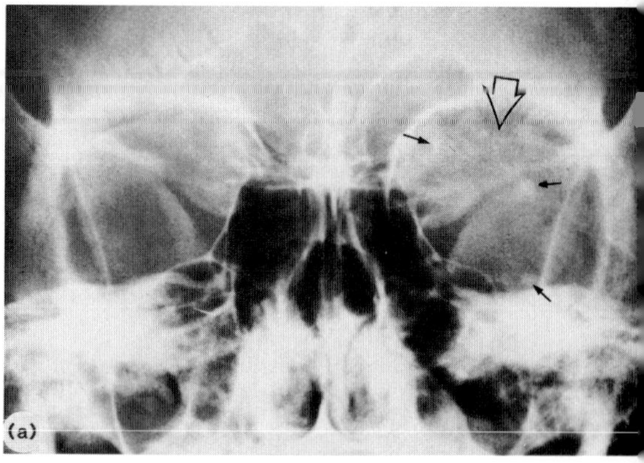

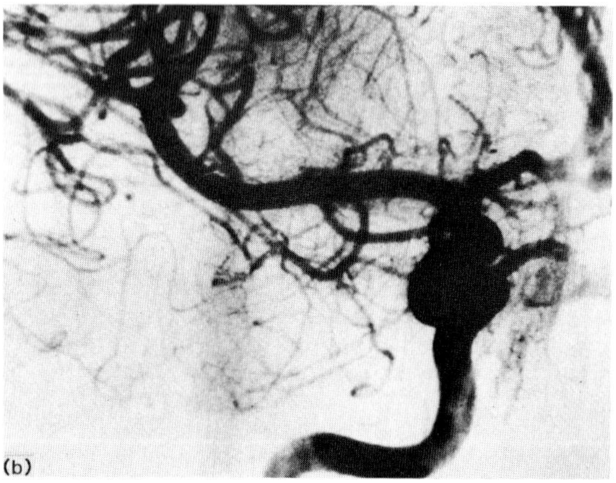

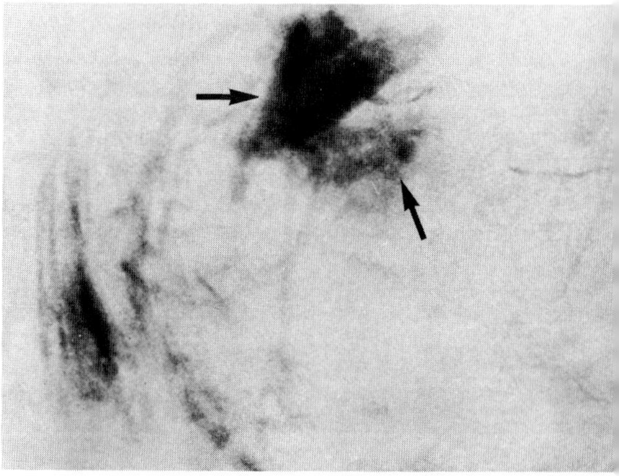

increased incidence of cerebral angioma in this condition (Tress and Moseley, 1977), and since patients' neurological symptoms may be secondary to such a treatable lesion rather than to telangiectasia, CT examination is indicated in suggestive cases.

Up to 50% of patients with this disorder may have pulmonary arteriovenous fistulae; secondary infection of these lesions, with metastatic cerebral abscess, is well recognized.

Angioma serpiginosum

We have studied a patient with a unique, but *progressive* capillary angiomatous condition in whom the skin lesion resembles the Sturge-Weber syndrome, but differs in blanching on pressure and pursuing a progressive course. Since the original description (Gautier-Smith *et al*., 1971) the retinal, cerebral, and cutaneous lesions have progressed. In addition an orbital angiomatous abnormality has now developed (Fig. 7.21).

Retinal and cerebral lesions

The foregoing descriptions of retinal lesions with cerebral

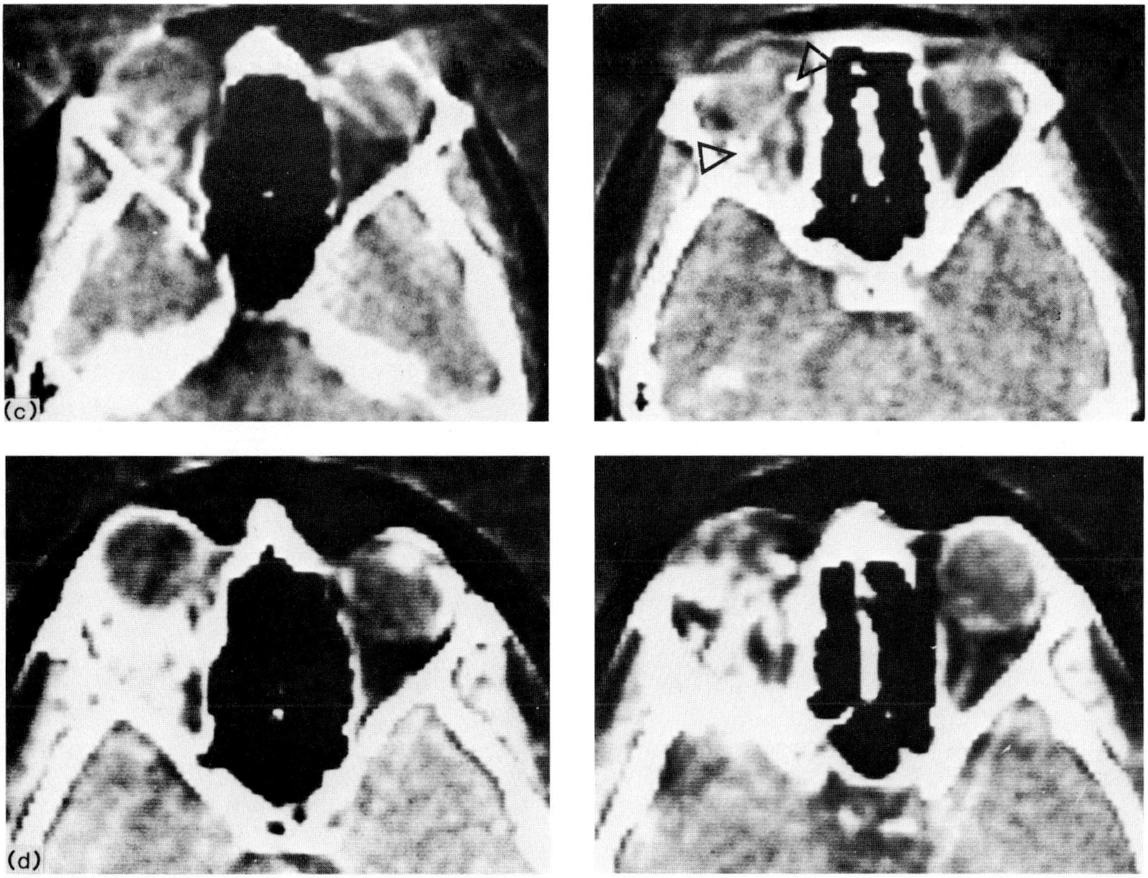

involvement is probably incomplete and recognition of a retinal vascular malformation should alert the clinician to associated cutaneous or neurological lesions. We have seen one patient, for example, with a cavernous haemangioma of the optic disc, presenting a characteristic grape-like appearance on fluorescein angiography, and an associated parietotemporal lesion. Cutaneous lesions have also been described in association with disc or retinal lesions, and reports of a familial tendency may link this condition with the phakomatoses.

7.5 HEREDODEGENERATIVE DISORDERS OF THE CENTRAL NERVOUS SYSTEM

These disorders may be subdivided into those involving the cerebral tracts or white matter (leukodystrophies) and those involving principally the ganglion cells or grey matter.

Fig. 7.20 Intracranial dural arteriovenous fistula. This 9-year old boy had suffered grand mal epilepsy since 1 year of age. Two months before the CT study he had a minor head injury, and two weeks later sudden left orbital pain, with vertical diplopia. Examination confirmed proptosis and depression of the left eye (a) unaffected by jugular compression. There was a 'machinery' bruit, loudest over the left eye. Orbital CT (b,c), showed a large dense mass in the position of the left superior ophthalmic vein, which was also prominent (small arrows). Cranial scans demonstrated left cerebral hemiatrophy and suggested prominent vessels in the interhemispheric fissure. Carotid angiography revealed these to be due to a dural arteriovenous malformation fed on both sides by middle meningeal arteries (d, arrowheads indicate superficial temporal artery branches) and an anterior falcine branch (e, crossed arrow) arising from a hypertrophied ophthalmic artery (arrow). There was no visualization of the cavernous sinus or superior ophthalmic veins, and it seems probable that the orbital abnormalities were due to venous thrombosis.

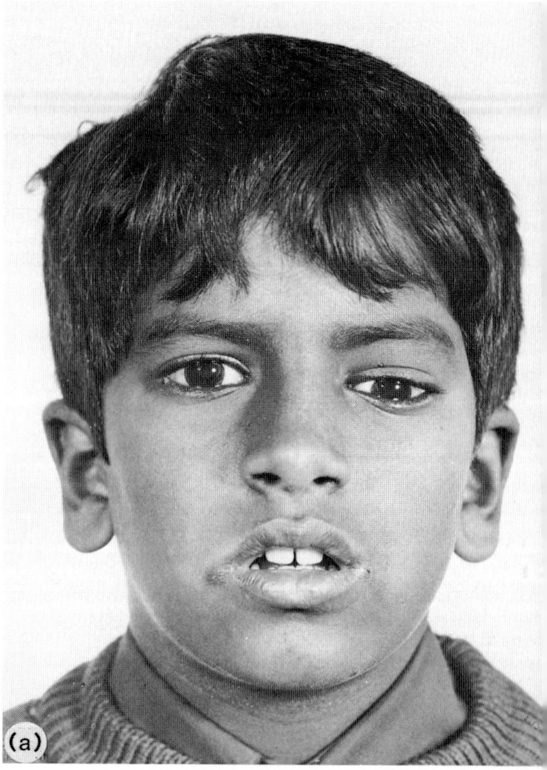

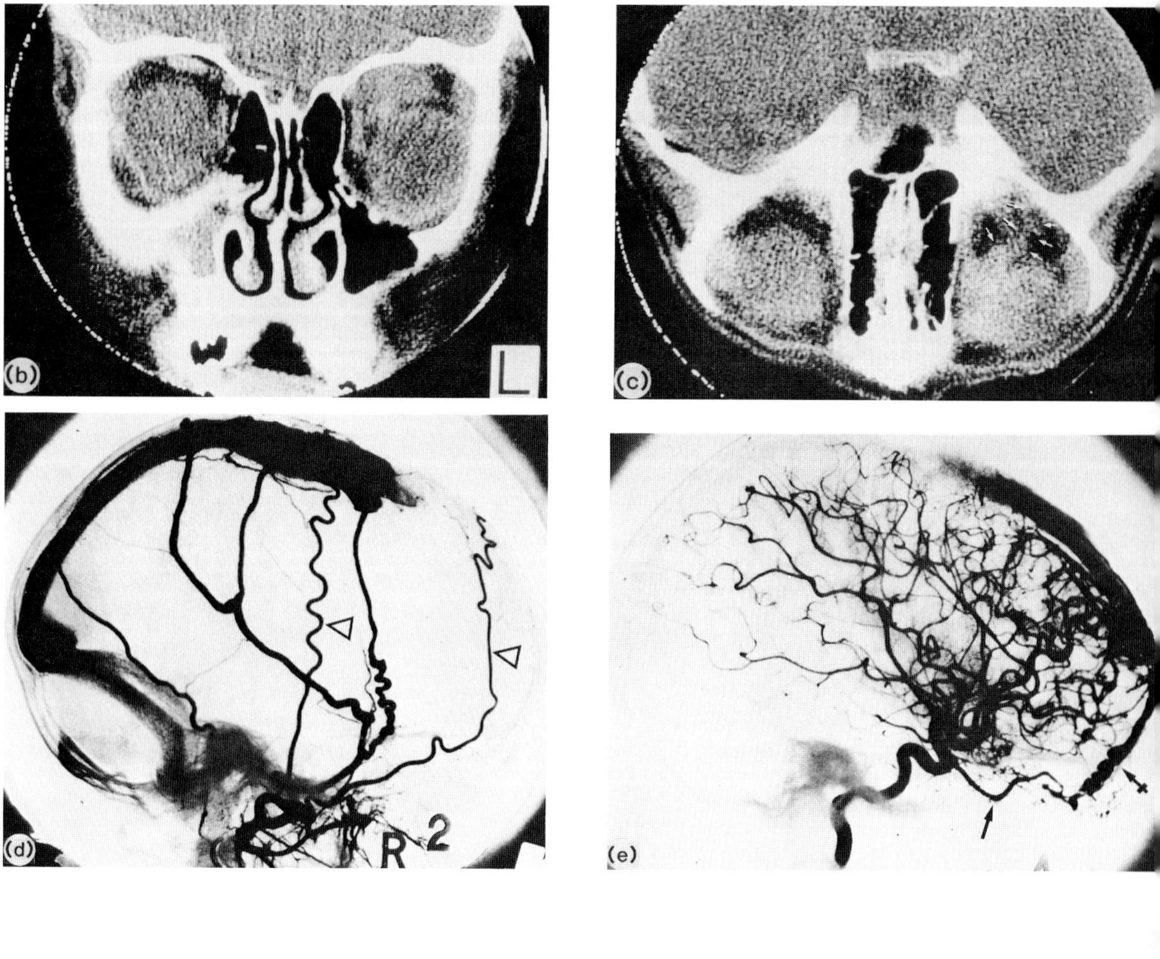

Fig. 7.21 Angioma serpiginosum. Although normal at birth, this patient's right leg was noted to have an angiomatous lesion at 1 year of age. The lesion has been progressive, involving the trunk and the right axilla. The right arm is weak, with wasting in the C5 and C6 nerve distribution (a). Movements of the right eye, other than abduction, are limited. The right pupil is dilated and unreactive (b). There are numerous discrete capillary angiomata in the right retina (c, fluorescein angiogram). Orbital CT (d) showed the divergent squint, and irregular soft tissue masses (arrows) thought to represent further angiomata. The neurological deficits are presumably the result of angiomatous involvement of cranial and spinal nerves. (Previously published by Gautier-Smith, P.C., Sanders, M.D. and Sanderson, K.V. 1971).

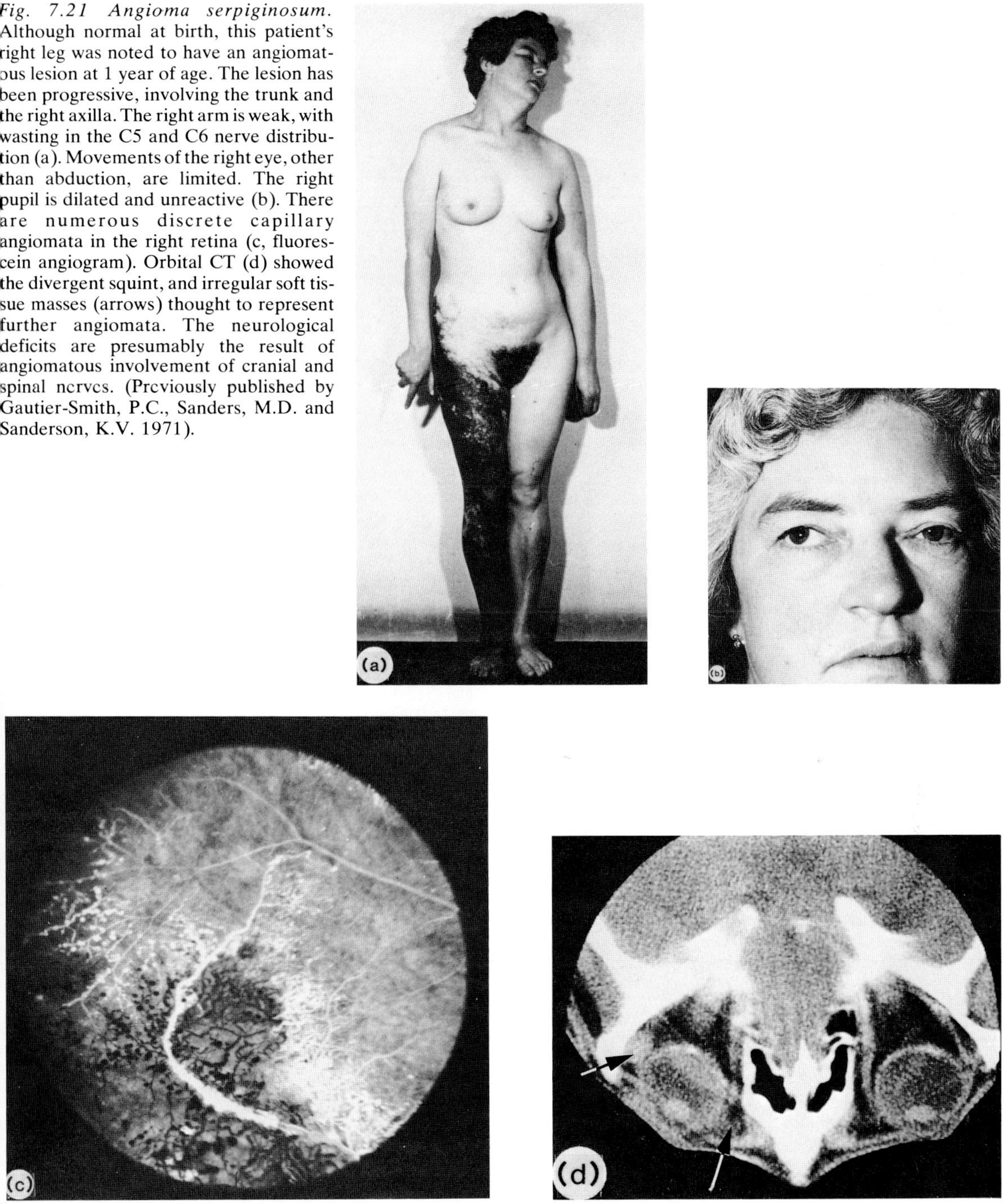

White matter disorders

These may be either myelinoclastic, where normal myelin is broken down, or dysmyelinating, where abnormal myelin is produced, and these are termed the leukodystrophies. They are usually inherited as a recessive condition.

Metrachromatic leukodystrophy
Early development is often normal but at about two years difficulty with the limbs develops, with progressive hypotonia, ataxia and weakness, leading to spastic paraplegia. Loss of vision, bilateral optic atrophy and pigmentary retinopathy (Libert *et al.*, 1979) are seen. Cerebroside sulphate is stored due to an abnormality in the enzyme cerebroside sulphatase. Death occurs within several years of onset.

This is the most common disorder and characterizes the white matter degenerative conditions, though biochemical investigations and isolation of the enzymatic abnormality are replacing the series of eponymous names used to describe these conditions.

CT shows low attentuation in the cerebral white matter, often most marked in the centrum semiovale. The optic radiations tend to be spared until the late stages.

Adrenoleukodystrophy
This is an X-linked disease which usually becomes manifest between four and ten years of age. Cerebral changes of defective myelination are associated with adrenal insufficiency. Affected boys often show poor school or social performance and are found to have severe cortical visual loss. The fundi are normal in the early stages, with normal pupillary responses. CT shows more or less symmetrical low attenuation in the white matter of the occipital lobes and the adjacent parts of the parietal and temporal lobes. Intravenous contrast medium may produce marked enhancement at or near the periphery of the abnormal areas; this is thought to indicate a breakdown of the blood-brain barrier, and decreases with steroid therapy (Fig. 4.38, p.138). It is less commonly seen in other forms of leukodystrophy, e.g. Alexander's disease. In advanced cases the zones of low attenuation become more widespread and are associated with atrophy and enlargement of the occipital horns – a true hydrocephalus '*ex vacuo*'. The relationship of adrenoleukodystrophy to Schilder's disease or sudanophilic diffuse cerebral sclerosis is not clear; they may all be variants of the same disease.

Other leukodystrohies Early involvement of the optic radiations also typifies *Krabbe's disease (globoid cell leukodystrophy)*; as in adrenoleukodystrophy, advanced cases show widespread white matter involvement and atrophic changes. The related condition of *spongiform degeneration (Canavan's disease)*, produces the most striking CT pictures, with enlargement of the brain and

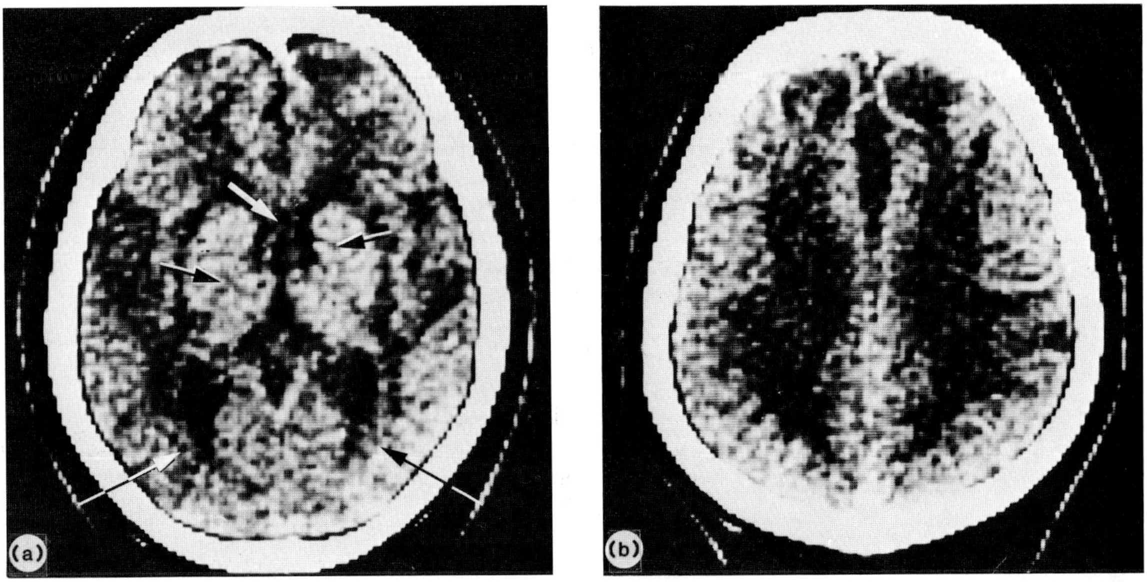

Fig. 7.22 Spongiform degeneration. One of two siblings, aged 9, suspected of having hydrocephalus, because of global retardation and a large head. The brain is large, but the skull vault is thick. The attenuation coefficients of the white matter are grossly reduced, but the internal capsule is spared (arrows) and the region of the optic radiations is relatively normal (long arrows). There is cortical atrophy, but the ventricles are not enlarged. There is a cavum of the septum pellucidum (single arrow). Brain biopsy in the sibling showed spongiform degeneration.

skull, and marked low attenuation throughout not only the white matter (often sparing the internal capsule (Fig. 7.22)), but also in the basal ganglia, thalamus and brain stem. The radiations are not involved except in a rapidly progressive infantile type (Kendall, 1979). *Alexander's disease* also produces mega-encephaly, but the low-attenuation areas are characteristically more prominent in the frontal lobes. *Pelizaeus-Merzbacher disease*, though rare, is of interest to the clinician because of wandering eye movements which may resemble nystagmus; CT is usually normal.

The gangliosidoses

These disorders usually present with epileptiform seizures and myoclonic jerks in young children, and progressive mental and motor degeneration proceeds to an early death. Neuro-ophthalmic signs contribute to diagnosis, particularly in the Tay-Sachs group. A cherry red spot may be seen in Tay-Sachs disease, Sandoff's disease, generalized gangliosidosis, in GM_1 gangliosidosis and cherry red spot myoclonus syndrome. Recognition of the cherry red spot is important; in the later stages ocular movements become reduced to voluntary, pursuit and oculovestibular stimuli.

Batten's disease

Batten's disease may present to the ophthalmologist as visual loss, due to a pigmentary retinopathy prior to the development of other neurological signs. It may occur at different ages: (a) infantile; (b) Bielschowsky (1–4) years; (c) Spielmeyer-Vogt (6–14 years); and (d) Kuf (adults), although this is disputed and has never been seen by the authors.

Niemann-Pick disease

Sphingomyelin is stored and may occur in the CNS, or in visceral organs. A cherry red spot may be seen in the acute neuropathic type A. Several subdivisions of the condition exist.

Gaucher's disease

This progressive neurological degenerative condition is due to the accumulation of cerebroside, and hepatosplenomegaly is a feature. In adults a horizontal supranuclear ophthalmoplegia has been described. The fundi are usually normal, but a cherry red spot is described.

CT

The cerebrum may be small and atrophic, normal in size, or more rarely, enlarged due to swelling of the cells; there may be ventricular dilatation. This variability is echoed in the CT findings, since while some workers have reported megalencephaly and widespread low attenuation affecting both white matter and cortex in Tay-Sachs disease, others have found no abnormality.

Cherry red spot myoclonus syndrome

This condition combines a cherry red spot with myoclonus and cerebellar signs. Ocular motor signs are important in clinical diagnosis with periodic alternating nystagmus and down-beat nystagmus. CT showed no abnormality in the cases we have examined.

Subacute necrotizing encephalomyelopathy (Leigh's disease)

This is a grey matter disease of autosomal recessive inheritance, commoner in males than females, in which the essential abnormality is necrosis of the spinal cord, brain stem, basal ganglia and optic pathways. The infantile form is usually manifest by 1–2 years, the children showing marked nystagmus and optic atrophy. Death ensues from respiratory failure. Children with the juvenile form are retarded and show in addition ataxia and extrapyramidal features. The CT appearances were described by Hall and Gardner-Medwin (1978): in the infantile form, areas of low attenuation in the putamen, globus pallidus, hypothalamus and the head of the caudate nucleus; in the juvenile form, cerebellar atrophy and cavitation in the putamen, similar to that seen in some cases of postencephalitic Parkinsonism. Some patients show changes confined to the putamen.

Subacute sclerosing panencephalitis

This is an inflammatory condition due to the measles virus acting as a slow virus and is characterized by myoclonic seizures. Ocular features include disc oedema, characteristic pigmentary macular changes and a pigmentary retinopathy. White matter low-attenuation and atrophic changes of variable extent have been noted at CT (Kendall, 1979); contrast enhancement is uncommon.

The mucopolysaccharidoses

A number of defects of mucopolysaccharide metabolism have been identified, which are inherited as autosomal or sex-linked recessives. They are usually divided as follows:

MPS	I	– Hurler's disease (gargoylism)
MPS	II	– Hunter's disease
MPS	III	– Sanfilippo disease
MPS	IV	– Morquio-Brailsford disease
MPS	V	– Scheie's disease
MPS	VI	– Maroteaux-Lamy disease

Further subdivisions are recognized, although it has been suggested that the basic defect is the same in all types, variations in clinical and biochemical anomalies resulting from differing enzyme deficiencies. Ocular features are of clinical significance although they may not be the most striking clinical feature. The CT findings have recently been summarized (Kendall, 1979).

Hurler's syndrome

This is the clinical archetype, affected individuals showing the most severe and widespread defects. They are dwarfed, of low intelligence, frequently hydrocephalic and usually die before the age of 20. Corneal clouding is the major ocular feature (seen also in MPS IV, V and VI), but in addition tapetoretinal degeneration has been described, with optic disc oedema in some cases. The pathogenesis of the disc oedema has not been established.

CT is often normal, but hydrocephalus, attributed to infiltration of the meninges may be seen, especially in MPS I. Meningeal infiltration may also result in the development of arachnoid cysts, seen at CT as rounded, well-defined areas of low attenuation lying in relation to the basal cisterns or cortical subarachnoid space. Such cysts may become space-occupying, compressing the brain and thinning the overlying bone. There may be evidence of cerebral atrophy. In some cases of MPS I, II, III and VI, characteristic irregular areas of low attenuation are seen surrounding the lateral ventricles, especially when there is hydrocephalus (Fig. 7.23). Since more widespread low attenuation, similar to that seen in the leukodystrophies, may be present, it is not certain whether the low attenuation areas represent zones of leukomalacia or whether they are periventricular lucencies as

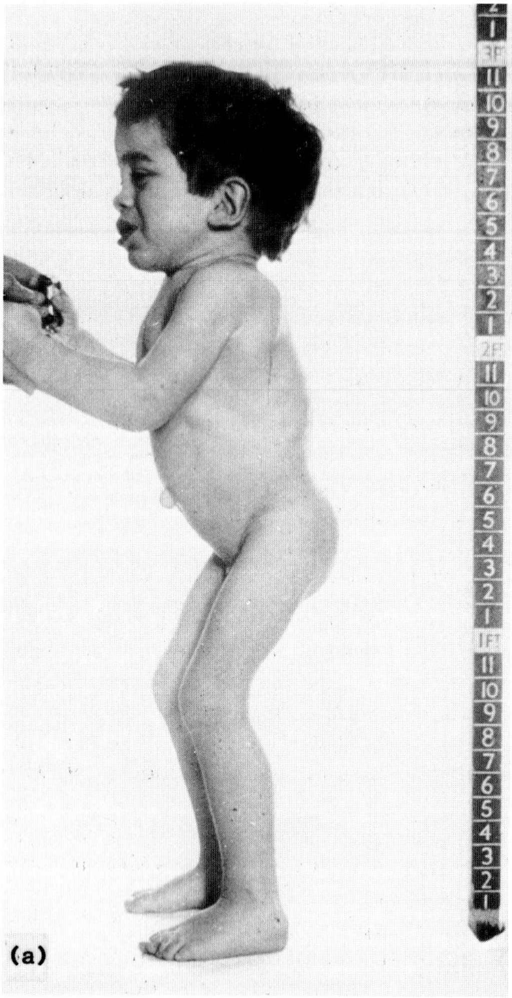

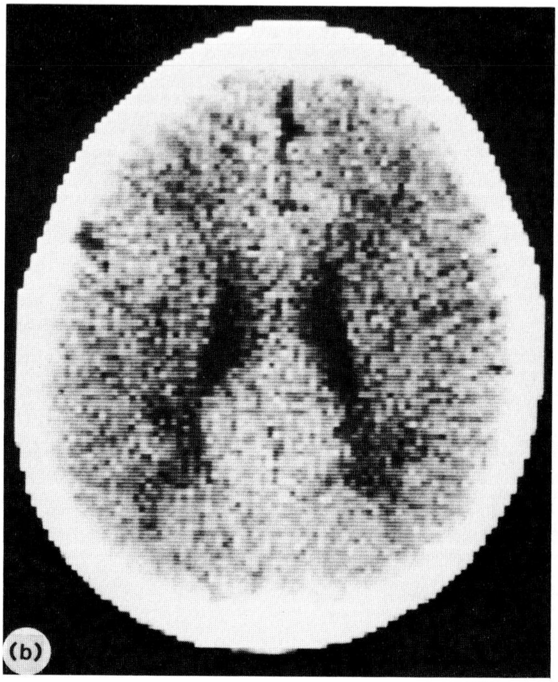

Fig. 7.23 Hurler's syndrome. (a) Typical physical features, including macrocephaly (see text). (b) CT shows megalencephaly, but the ventricles are not enlarged. Symmetrical, irregular areas of low attenuation are seen in the periventicular white matter, most marked posteriorly.

seen in hydrocephalus (Chapter 5). It may even be the case that the abnormal areas represent the combined effect of cerebral infiltration and transependymal passage of cerebrospinal fluid.

Progressive external ophthalmoplegia (Kearns-Sayre syndrome)

This rare condition, previously considered a form of ocular myopathy, is of interest because of the generalized nature of the disorder, which includes atypical pigmentary degeneration of the retina, heart block, generalized weakness, ataxia, hearing loss and defective or delayed sexual and skeletal maturation, with microcephaly. There is usually progressive, symmetrical loss of all ocular movements in combination with bilateral ptosis. Diagnosis is confirmed by skeletal muscle biopsy, and microscopy shows typical 'ragged red fibres', which on electron microscopy represent abnormal mitochondrial patterns. There appears to be an association with abnormal parathyroid function.

CT findings have been reported by Bertorini *et al*., (1978) and Seigel *et al*. (1979). The classical observation is of widespread leukoencephalopathy, i.e. bilateral, symmetrical, irregular low attenuation in the white matter of the cerebrum and cerebellum, involving also the thalamus and brain stem, with enlargement of all the ventricles and atrophy, as shown by increased size of the sulci and basal cisterns. Severity of the CT changes correlates with clinical involvement, and only a minority of the patients showed the full range of abnormalities. Calcification of the basal ganglia, thalamus and even of the cerebral substance was present in almost half of the patients in one series, but in none of those in the other. Of the 22 patients in the two series, eight had normal scans; most of these were adults, who were not severely affected. The few adult cases we have had the opportunity to examine, also had normal scans or showed mild atrophy.

Idiopathic hypoparathyroidism

This may produce a variety of ocular signs: lenticular opacity is the most common abnormality, while papilloedema, photophobia, keratoconjunctivitis and blepharospasm are much less frequently encounted (Blake, 1976). In both hypoparathyroidism and pseudohypoparathyroidism, CT may show calcification in basal ganglia, the dentate nucleus of the cerebellum and, rarely, in the cerebral white matter. As noted above, these conditions may coexist with oculocraniosomatic disease.

Cockayne's syndrome

This is an autosomal recessive form of dwarfism with some clinical features in common with oculocraniosomatic disease, e.g. retinal pigmentary changes, deafness, ataxia and microcephaly. The CT findings are also similar, but as in Hurler's syndrome, the picture may be complicated by associated normal pressure hydrocephalus, with periventricular lucencies.

Lowe's syndrome (oculocerebrorenal disease)

In this, one of the aminoacidoses affecting males in which bilateral microphthalmia and cataracts are typically present, poorly defined low-attenuation areas may also be seen in the cerebral white matter.

REFERENCES

Bertorini, T., Engel, K., Di Chiro, G. and Dalakas, M. (1978),

Leukoencephalopathy in oculocraniosomatic neuromuscular disease with ragged-red fibres. *Archs. Neurol.*, **35**, 643–7.

Blake, J. (1976), Eye signs in idiopathic hypoparathyroidism. *Trans. Ophthal. Soc. U.K.*, **96**, 418–51.

Bonnet, P., Dechaume, J. and Blanc, E. (1939), L'anévrysme cirsoide de la retine. *J. Med. Lyon*, **18**, 165–78.

Bull, J.W.D. (1967), The corpus callosum. *Clin. Radiol.*, **18**, 1–18.

De Morsier, G. (1956), Etudes sur les dysraphies crânio-encéphaliques. III Agénésie du septum lucidum avec malformation du tractus optique. La dysplasie septo-optique. *Schweizer. Arch. Neurol. Psychiat.*, **77**, 267–92.

Frisen, L. and Holmegaard, L. (1978), Spectrum of optic nerve hypoplasia. *Br. J. Ophthal.*, **62**, 7–15.

Gautier-Smith, P., Sanders, M.D. and Sanderson, K. (1971), Ocular and nervous system involvement in angioma serpiginosum. *Br. J. Ophthal.*, **55**, 433–43.

Guibert-Tranier, F., Piton, J., Calabet, A. and Caillé, J.M. (1979), Orbital syndromes – CT analysis of 100 cases. *Comput. Tomog.*, **3**, 241–65.

Hall, K. and Gardner-Medwin, D. (1978), CT scan appearances in Leigh's disease. *Neuroradiology*, **16**, 48–50.

Hofeldt, A.J., Zarer, C.R., Jakobiec, F.A., Behrens, M.M. and Jones, I.S. (1979), Orbitofacial angiomatosis. *Archs Ophthal.*, **97**, 484–8.

Jakobiec, F.A. and Jones, I.S. (1979), Introduction to ultrastructure, inflammation, and neoplasia. In: *Diseases of the Orbit* (eds. I.S. Jones and F.A. Jakobiec), Harper and Row, Maryland, USA.

Kendall, B.E. (1979), Symmetrical white matter low attenuation. *X-tract*, **7**, 3–14.

Kingsley, D.P.E. (1977), C.A.T. in the phakomatoses. In: *First European Seminar on Computerised Axial Tomography in Clinical Practice*. (eds. G.H. Du Boulay and I.F. Moseley), Springer, Berlin, pp. 174–81.

Kobrin, J.L., Blodi, F.C. and Weingeist, T.A. (1979), Ocular and orbital manifestations of neurofibromatosis. *Surv. Ophthal.*, **24**, 45–51.

Lebuisson, D., Aron, J.J., Di Constanzo, P., Aron-Rosa, D. and Coudere, J.L. (1979), Hypoplasie de la tête du nerf optique. *J. Fr. Ophtalmol.*, **2**, 11–22.

Lee, B.C.P. and Gawler, J. (1978), Tuberous sclerosis. Comparison of computed tomography and conventional neuroradiology. *Radiology*, **127**, 403–97.

Liakos, G.M., Walker, C.B. and Carruth, J.A.S. (1979), Ocular complications in craniofacial fibrous dysplasia. *Br. J. Ophthal.*, **63**, 611–16.

Libert, J., Van Hoof, F., Toussaint, D., Roozitalab, H., Kenyon, K.R. and Green, W.R. (1979), Ocular findings in metrochromatic leukodystrophy. *Archs Ophthal.*, **97**, 1495–1504.

Limnaios, E.E., Panayiotopoulos, C.P., Theodosiadis, G., Economou, M. and Papapetropoulos, T. (1979), Ophthalmological features of Aicardi's syndrome. *Br. J. Ophthal.*, **63**, 713–17.

Lindenberg, R. (1967), Malformations of the brain of interest to neuro-ophthalmologists In: *Neuro-Ophthalmology*, (ed. J.L. Smith), Mosby, St. Louis.

Muchnick, R.S., Aston, S.J. and Rees, T.D. (1979), Ocular manifestations and treatment of hemifacial atrophy. *Am. J. Ophthal.*, **88**, 889–97.

Sanders, M.D. and Brook, C.G.D. (1974), Septo-optic dysplasia. *Trans. Ophthal. Soc. U.K.*, **94**, 197–202.

Siegel, R.S., Seeger, J.F., Gabrielsen, T.O., Allen, R.J. (1979), Computed tomography in oculocraniosomatic disease. *Radiology*, **130**, 159–64.

Théron, J., Newton, T.H. and Hoyt, W.F. (1974), Unilateral retinocephalic vascular malformations. *Neuroradiology*, **7**, 185–97.

Tress, B.M. and Moseley, I.F. (1977), Cleidocranial dysostosis, hereditary haemorrhagic telangiectasia and epilepsy: a rare association. *Neuroradiology*, **12**, 233–6.

Wilson, J.L. and Moseley, I.F. (1977), A diagnostic approach to cerebellar lesions. In: *First European Seminar on Computerised Axial Tomography in Clinical Practice* (eds. G.H. Du Boulay and I.F. Moseley), Springer, Berlin, pp.123–33.

Wyburn-Mason, R. (1943), Arteriovenous aneurysms of midbrain and retina, facial naevi and mental changes. *Brain*, **66**, 163–203.

8 · The relationship of CT to other methods of investigation

'It may not be the business of the radiologist to dictate to the clinician what diagnostic information he should have before deciding on treatment of any given patient, but it is his duty to make him aware of the best ways of obtaining that information' (Moseley, 1977). We have previously pointed out that investigations have a double role: establishment of the diagnosis and the provision of as much information as is required for safe, adequate treatment (Moseley *et al.*, 1979). The decision to use various diagnostic modalities in the investigation of a given patient will be determined by these principles.

Reference has been made in the appropriate sections to radiological and non-radiological investigations which provide the maximum diagnostic yield. The purpose of this final chapter is threefold: to indicate those areas in which CT is of limited value or reliability, those in which other modalities can or should be employed, and to outline the authors' own diagnostic approach to various common problems.

8.1 OTHER MODES OF RADIOLOGICAL INVESTIGATION EMPLOYED IN NEURO-OPHTHALMOLOGY

These include plain skull radiography (supplemented if necessary by tomography), orbital phlebography, cerebral angiography and pneumography. Such techniques as contrast orbitography must now be considered as of historical interest only.

Plain radiographs

These can make positive contributions to the diagnosis of orbital disease (Lloyd, 1975) and should probably precede CT in the investigative sequence of patients suspected of having mass lesions in the orbit. *Calcification* may indicate the presence of phleboliths within orbital varices. *Malformations* of the orbital walls in, for example, neurofibromatosis (Chapter 7) can be clearly displayed by plain radiographs, rendering further investigation unnecessary unless a concomitant lesion such as an optic nerve glioma is suspected clinically. The *abnormal bone texture* in such conditions as fibrous dysplasia, Paget's disease or meningioma, is probably best assessed on plain films. Generalized *enlargement of the orbit* is non-specific, but focal erosive changes as a result of, for example, lacrimal gland or paranasal sinus tumours or mucocoeles, shown simply by plain radiographs, play an important part in establishing the differential diagnosis. Inflammatory disease in the sinuses may also be shown clearly.

Changes in the optic canals can be shown with suitable radiographic projections, but enlargement is relatively non-specific, and does not correlate completely with extension of tumours through the canal.

Plain lateral and posteroanterior radiographs of the skull, the former centred on the pituitary fossa, are mandatory in any patient with evidence of chiasmal compression. 'Coned films' are unnecessary, since their diagnostic quality should be no higher than those of properly exposed full-size films, if the latter are not substandard.

There is, we belive, considerable misunderstanding of the role of tomography of the sella turcica in patients with compression of the chiasm (or of the optic nerve or tract). *If it is evident that the sella is enlarged*, plain films in the two recommended orthogonal planes are usually adequate for assessment; a submentovertical view may be added. The only possible role for tomography is to define the anatomy of the sphenoid sinus and its septa, should the surgeon require this information before employing the transsphenoidal approach. *If the sella is not clearly abnormal*, CT should be carried out, since chiasmal compression by a pituitary tumour which has not enlarged the sella turcica is extremely uncommon. The foregoing remarks apply particularly to patients suspected of having pituitary tumours causing neurological (visual or ocular motor) deficits. However, sellar tomography need not be regarded as a routine procedure in the endocrine clinic: it should certainly not precede lateral and frontal plain films *and* full endocrine assessment. Since many microadenomas can be detected in this way, the endocrine radiologist should be expert in evaluating the sella turcica from plain films, rather than relying on routine tomography.

Careful examination of the base of the skull in patients with ocular motor problems may require a combination of plain films, conventional tomograms and CT.

Plain films have relatively little to add in the assessment of cerebral lesions causing visual loss, papilloedema or disordered eye movements.

Complex movement orbital tomography (polytomography)

This technique has been used to show changes in the orbital walls, providing indirect information as to the presence of an expanding lesion. It also gives limited visualization of the intraorbital soft tissue structures, lying in the orbital fat. Complex motion tomography is of course essential, and this entails high radiation dose to the eye. Isherwood *et al.* (1978) compared this technique with other neuroradiological procedures, and found the lens dose, 12 rad, to be six times that of pneumoencephalography and more than 1.5 times that of cerebral angiography. The cataractogenic dose in mice is 15 rad, but there are very marked interspecies variations in sensitivity. CT dosage is relatively high per section (1–5 rad) but the beam is finely collimated, so that irradiation of adjacent structures is minimized.

With the introduction of high resolution CT, which shows both bone and soft tissue changes with great fidelity, but without increased X-ray dose, the utility of hypocycloidal tomography in orbital disease would seem to have largely disappeared. Lloyd (1979) showed that its diagnostic accuracy was markedly lower than that of standard resolution CT, regardless even of differential diagnostic considerations, while Mancuso *et al.* (1978) reached similar conclusions with respect to sinus disease and orbital involvement; these findings, combined with the high radiation dose, render it no longer the examination of choice.

Ultrasound

'The use of ultrasound for orbital soft-tissue diagnosis has become less necessary with the development of CT scanning, which generally shows the location and shape of soft-tissue masses more obviously' (Lloyd, 1979). Prior to the introduction of CT, ultrasound was a valuable method of investigating the orbit, although it requires very skilled recording and interpretation, and remains, in the case of C-scanning, rather unpleasant for the patient. An early comparative study of ultrasound and CT diagnosis of the cause of proptosis in 532 cases (Dallow *et al.*, 1976) suggested that ultrasound was still superior to CT; with further development of CT techniques, this is no longer the case.

According to one of the leading authorities on orbital ultrasound (Ossoinig, 1977), the technique is valuable for measurement of the optic nerve, the extraocular muscles and the axial dimension of the eye, for the differentiation of retrobulbar lesions and for demonstration of intraocular abnormalities. The first of these three uses is clearly redundant in the CT era, while Ossoinig's own data (1977) suggest that for clear differentiation of orbital tumours ultrasound is not superior to CT, since the lesions mentioned have grossly different morphological characteristics (Table 8.1). There can, however, be no doubt that ultrasound remains of use in the assessment of intraocular abnormalities, e.g. in the detection of the cause of secondary retinal detachment. Ossoinig claims that vitreous opacities of 0.05 mm or more can be demonstrated (an aspect of particular importance with the expansion of vitreous surgery) as can ocular fundus lesion lesions no more than 1.5 mm thick and elevated 0.75 mm. It is doubtful whether most workers would aspire to

Table 8.1 Ultrasound differentiation of retrobulbar lesions by reflectivity: % of spike height at tissue sensitivity (after Ossoinig, 1977).

Reflectivity	*Range %*	*Tissue*
Extremely high	95–100	Normal
High	65–95	Cavernous haemangioma
Medium	40–60	Glioma
Low	5–40	Lymphoma
Extremely low	0–5	Serous cyst

such finesse. Ultrasound may also have a place in determining the nature of optic nerve lesions (Skalka, 1972; Aubin and Vignaud, 1978; Lloyd, 1979).

The chief merit of ultrasound is that in the levels used diagnostically it is apparently without risks such as those of X-irraditation. However, even in expert hands, it currently has a lower detection rate and gives more false positive results than CT (Lloyd, 1979).

Radio-isotope techniques

Isotope scanning and gamma camera techniques have been widely applied to preliminary diagnosis of intracranial and orbital lesions and extracranial vascular disease.

Grove (1975) discussed the use of such studies in the diagnosis of orbital lesions, using combinations of three different isotopes: technetium-99 m, 197-Hg chlormerodrin and gallium. Even with such complex methods, the results were of little value in differential diagnosis.

That CT has replaced isotope scanning for the demonstration and differential diagnosis of intracranial lesions is evidenced by the statistics from our own hospital: in 1973, prior to the introduction of CT, approximately 2000 isotope studies were being performed each year; in 1980 the rate is less than 80 per year. Isotope techniques were always rather unsatisfactory for elucidation of chiasmal compression (Clavería *et al.*, 1973).

Thermography

The technique of thermography has been employed for the investigation of orbital lesions (Bourjat and Gautheric, 1975), but with limited differential diagnostic capability, hyperthermy indicating acute inflammation or malignant neoplasm, absence of hyperthermy suggesting endocrine exophthalmos or a deep and/or weakly thermogenous neoplasm. It would appear to have little or no part to play in the CT era.

Orbital phlebography

Phlebography is an invasive technique with an accepted failure rate and slight, but definite morbidity (Safer and Guibor, 1975). Direct radiation to the eyes is inevitable, and may be considerable if anteroposterior, submentovertical and lateral magnification series are obtained. The dose can be reduced significantly by placing the X-ray tube beneath the head, but this presents practical difficulties.

An early report comparing phlebography and CT for the diagnosis of mass lesions indicated that in centres in which CT was available, relatively few patients were subjected to phlebography (Moseley and Bull, 1975).

Lloyd (1979) compared the diagnostic accuracy of CT and phlebography for the demonstration of orbital masses in a series of 100 proven cases. On a yes/no basis, CT was slightly more sensitive, but venography had a significantly higher false negative rate, even in very experienced hands. CT images are easier to interpret and considerably more accurate in terms of differential diagnosis. These results were similar to those of Peeters *et al* (1977) who obtained correct results in 88% of cases using CT and only 68% with orbital phlebography.

Current indications for phlebography would seem to include venous malformations of the orbit (although, since the diagnosis can be established by other means, phlebography should probably be reserved for the few cases in which surgery is being considered); lesions of the cavernous sinus, e.g. meningioma *en plaque*, a diagnosis which is occasionally difficult to establish by other methods, and small lesions at the superior orbital fissure. In some centres, orbital phlebography is used routinely in cases of pituitary adenoma, to assess lateral extent of the lesion prior to surgery. This information can also be gained from CT and carotid angiography, the latter giving considerable additional information, e.g. excluding a parasellar aneurysm.

Arteriography

Carotid and vertebral angiography are highly invasive procedures, frequently carried out under general anaesthesia, with well-documented morbidity. It is therefore obvious that they should not be embarked upon without clear indications.

Variations in the course and branching pattern of the ophthalmic artery within the orbit make arteriography an unsatisfactory method for detection of intraorbital masses. Moseley and Bull (1975) found it unhelpful as compared with CT in primary intraorbital mass lesions, while Peeters *et al.* (1977) obtained correct results in only 50% of cases. In both of these series, a number of patients were not subjected to arteriography, so that the overall contribution of angiography was even smaller than this percentage would suggest.

While these remarks apply to mass lesions within or involving the orbit, it is self-evident that vascular lesions such as arteriovenous malformations and fistulae require angiography:

indeed, it can be argued that CT has little part to play in cases in which the vascular nature of the abnormality is obvious. Angiography may be indicated not only for diagnosis, but for intravascular therapy, e.g. embolization or balloon occlusion.

With lesions in the vicinity of the optic canal and pituitary fossa, angiography and CT have complementary roles, both in terms of diagnosis and preoperative assessment. CT will show a large proportion of the lesions compressing the optic nerve, chiasm or tract or causing ocular motor disturbances. Small aneurysms and other lesions within the cavernous sinus, e.g. granuloma or meningioma, may be demonstrated or suggested by angiography when CT is negative. In the pre-CT era, it was possible to mistake aneurysms for pituitary tumours if angiography was not carried out, an error having possibly disastrous consequences. CT has not eliminated that possibility (Moseley *et al*., 1979), but reduces the number of cases in which confusion can arise: there are many pituitary tumours whose CT appearances could not be mimicked by an aneurysm. However, it would appear that the incidence of associated non-symptomatic aneurysms is increased in patients with pituitary tumours, especially those previously treated by interstitial radiotherapy (Jakubowski and Kendall, 1978). The surgeon should be forewarned of the possible presence of an incidental aneurysm, and angiography is thus desirable in all cases of pituitary tumour. Since the CT differential diagnosis may not be absolute, this rule can probably be extended to suspected craniopharyngiomas and parasellar meningiomas.

The role of angiography in the assessment of cerebral lesions is nowadays a secondary one (Michotey *et al*., 1977). Certain conditions, e.g. leukodystrophy or multiple sclerosis, require CT as the only radiological investigation. In other parenchymal diseases such as tumour or abscess CT is the definitive diagnostic procedure; the surgeon may or may not require angiography prior to operation should the latter be indicated. In cases in which CT suggests a potentially treatable cerebral angioma, angiography is mandatory, while in cerebral haemorrhage and infarction angiography is similarly performed with a view to excluding an underlying treatable cause, such as an aneurysm or a lesion of the cervical carotid artery. The demonstration of the intracranial vascular consequences of, for example, occlusion of the posterior cerebral artery is of academic interest, but little practical value unless vascular microsurgery is planned, since a diagnosis can effectively be made by CT.

Cerebral pneumography

Air encephalography, carried out under local anaesthesia, is unpleasant for patient and operator. There are strong arguments for general anaesthesia if the radiological examination is indicated; even then, the postencephalographic morbidity is high.

The indications for pneumography in centres in which CT is available have contracted very markedly. It is still currently used for the investigation of the sellar region and the brainstem. The present degree of refinement of CT is often insufficient to show the position of the optic chiasm relative to a suprasellar mass. Some surgeons require this information and consider pneumography essential, while others request the investigation rarely or never. Early expansion of the pons by a lesion such as a glioma can be detected more reliably by pneumography, with tomography, than by other methods. It is to be anticipated that both these shortcomings of CT will be short-lived, as the quality of sagittal and coronal reconstructions improves.

Cisternography with water-soluble contrast media

Early reports suggest that cisternography with metrizamide may replace pneumography, and prove more acceptable, despite the well-documented risks of epilepsy with intracranial use of the contrast medium. One of the great advantages of the technique is the possibility of combining conventional radiology and CT studies (Hall and McAllister, 1980).

8.2 INVESTIGATIONAL PROCEDURES

The following paragraphs summarize much that has been mentioned in preceding chapters. They represent the authors' views on the role of CT in the investigation of patients with certain clinical syndromes.

Visual loss

Monocular visual loss

This demands the exclusion of retinal disease, and experienced clinicians will realize that subtle retinal lesions such as acute neuroretinopathy, cone dysfunction syndromes and early tapetoretinal disorders may be diagnostically difficult, requiring fluorescein angiography and neurophysiological data provided by the VER, ERG and EOG. Optic disc anomalies such as pits, buried drusen and hypoplasia may be subtle. If disc swelling accompanies severe visual loss, inflammatory or infiltrative disease of the optic disc should be suspected, whereas in papilloedema vision is well preserved unless atrophy develops.

Localization of visual loss due to lesions of the optic nerve has been revolutionized by CT: the bulbous nerve of an optic nerve glioma is almost pathognomic, as is the dense, slightly enlarged nerve of the optic nerve meningioma. However, granulomatous disease such as sarcoid or tuberculosis may rarely mimic this appearance.

Orbital compression of the optic nerve is similarly best detected by CT. Lesions within the optic canal are rare without concomitant orbital or intracranial involvement and though CT may be diagnostic, this is an area where polytomography of the canal may be necessary. Maximal difficulty is experienced with the infiltrating meningioma arising from the region of the optic canal, where tumour mass may be minimal and the site provides maximum protection from the diagnostic X-ray beam. In this situation, venography may show obstruction of the venous return from the ophthalmic veins or magnification angiography with subtraction may show a pathological circulation.

Optic nerve compression may rarely be produced from below, by lesions such as the sphenoid sinus mucocoele, which should be detected by conventional X-rays, often combined with CT.

Bilateral visual field loss

In bilateral visual field loss, accurate field testing provides the simplest means of localization of the anticipated site of the lesion. Diagnostic tests for pituitary function have become sophisticated and expensive, but provide information which can be useful for management of the endocrine disturbance. The combination of skull films, CT and endocrine assessment may be all that is necessary prior to surgery in parasellar lesions. Particular additional studies may be necessary for planning transphenoidal or intracranial approaches; a carotid angiogram is required by most neurosurgeons, while some demand air encephalography.

Retrochiasmal visual loss is usually caused by large lesions. Lesions of the optic tract may, however, be small, for in this situation the visual sensory fibres are relatively compact. CT is able to localize lesions, and provide diagnostic information in a significant number of cases. Thus, in a patient with an homonymous hemianopia, CT is the primary investigation and more invasive techniques such as angiography may be indicated, if further information is required, as in vascular malformations, or prior to surgery.

Proptosis

Protrusion of the globe occurs when the size of the orbit is reduced or when a mass develops within the confines of the orbit. Slowly growing masses within the orbit may produce sufficient atrophy of fat to avoid protrusion of the globe and therefore resistance of the globe to retropulsion provides an important indication of the presence of an orbital mass. Clinical signs, the age and sex of the patient and a full history may provide sufficient information to arrive at a diagnosis. Skull X-rays may be diagnostic in certain conditions such as lacrimal gland tumours or sphenoidal ridge meningiomas, but do not usually contribute the quantity or quality of information provided by a high resolution CT study. Accurate localization enables the clinician to plan the most advantageous surgical approach, and this information was previously difficult to obtain using angiography, venography c orbital pneumoencephalography. The need for invasive orbit studies is now limited almost solely to vascular abnormalities c the orbit.

Ocular motor abnormalities

Clinical examination usually localizes ocular motor abno malities to the cerebral cortex, the cerebellum, the brainstem c the ocular motor nerves, either in their paths to the cavernou sinus, within the cavernous sinus or within the orbit. In cerebra disturbances ocular movement abnormalities are accompanie by other neurological signs but CT would seem the investigatio of choice. Cerebellar disturbances may also be shown, but i brainstem disorders CT provides less information, and an ai encephalogram may indicate an expanded pons with greate precision. Cavernous sinus lesions may be detected when there i a mass effect although vascular lesions may be demonstrate preferentially by venography or angiography. It may on occasio be difficult when confronted with a gaze palsy or abductor o adductor weakness to determine whether the lesion is orbital o brainstem. CT may show inflammatory changes or thickene muscles which localize the lesion to the orbit.

8.3 CONCLUSION

This brief analysis serves to emphasize the reliance which the clinician places on CT as the preliminary investigation, anc further sophistication of technique will surely enhance this position. Virtually all radiological tests are now complementary tc computerized tomography in neuro-ophthalmology; and this may well apply, in due course, to plain skull radiographs.

REFERENCES

Aubin, M.L. and Vignaud, J. (1978), Computerised tomography of the eye: a study of 62 pathologic cases. *Neuroradiology*, **16**, 456–7.

Bourjat, P. and Gautheric, M. (1975), Unilateral exophthalmos investigated by infrared thermography. In: *Orbital Disorders* (eds. G.M. Bleeker, J.B. Garston, B. Kronenberg and T.K. Lyle), Karger, Basel, pp.278–85.

Clavería, L.E., Du Boulay, G., and Zingesser, L. (1973), Radioisotope scanning of the nervous system: reasons for scanning. *Proc. R. Soc. Med.*, **66**, 823–7.

Dallow, R.L., Momose, K.J., Weber, A.L. and Wray, S.N. (1976), Comparison of ultrasonography, computerised tomography (EMI Scan) and radiographic techniques in evaluation of exophthalmos. *Trans. Am. Acad. Ophthal.*, **81**, 305–22.

Grove, A.S. (1975), Radionuclide evaluation of the orbit. In: *Orbital Disorders* (eds. G.M. Bleeker, J.B. Garston, B. Kronenberg and T.K. Lyle), Karger, Basel, pp.190–1.

Hall, K. and McAllister, V.L. (1980), Metrizamide cisternography in pituitary and juxtapituitary lesions. *Radiology*, **134**, 101–8.

Isherwood, I., Pullan, B.R. and Ritchings, R.T. (1978), Radiation dose in neuroradiological procedures. *Neuroradiology*, **16**, 477–81.

Jakubowski, J. and Kendall, B. (1978), Coincidental aneurysms with tumours of pituitary origin. *J. Neurol. Neurosurg. Psychiat.*, **41**, 972–9.

Lloyd, G.A.S. (1975), *Radiology of the Orbit*. Saunders, London.

Lloyd, G.A.S. (1979), Orbits: computed tomography and ultrasound, In: *Medical Imaging* (ed. L. Kreel), HM + M, Aylesbury, pp.124–7.

Mancuso, A.A., Manafee, W.N., Winter, J. and Ward, P. (1978), Extension of paranasal sinus tumours and inflammatory disease as evaluated by CT and pluridirectional tomography. *Neuroradiology*, **16**, 449–53.

Michotey, P., Moseley, I.F., Lecaque, G. and Palmieri, P. (1977), The comparative value of various neuroradiological investigations in the diagnosis of intracranial optic pathway lesions. In: *First European Seminar on Computerised Axial Tomography in Clinical Practice*. (eds. G.H. Du Boulay and I.F. Moseley), Springer, Berlin, pp.147–53.

Moseley, I.F. (1977), La contribution de la tomodensitométrie au diagnostic des lesions intracraniennes. *Revue Prat.*, **27**, 2237–52.

Moseley, I.F. and Bull, J.W.D. (1975), Computerised axial tomography, carotid angiography and orbital phlebography in the diagnosis of space occupying lesions of the orbit. In: *Advances in Cerebral Angiography* (ed. G. Salamon), INSERM/Springer, Berlin, pp.361–9.

Moseley, I.F. Sanders, M.D., Karoutas, G. and Radü, E.W. (1979), CT scan in neuro-opthalmology, In: *Topics in Neuro-Ophthalmology* (ed. H.S. Thompson), Williams and Wilkins, Baltimore, pp.302–17.

Ossoinig, K. (1977), Echography of the eye, orbit and periorbital region. In: *Orbital Roentgenology*. (ed. P.H. Arger), Wiley, New York, pp.224–69.

Peeters, F., Korger, R., Verbeeten, B. and Versteege, C. (1977), The value of computer tomography, orbital venography and carotid angiography in the diagnosis of exophthalmos. *Radiol. Clin.*, **46**, 430–8.

Safer, J.N. and Guibor, P. (1975), Ocular complications of orbi-

tal venography. *Radiology*, **114**, 647–8.
Skalka, H. (1978), Perineural optic nerve changes in endocrine orbitopathy. *Archs Ophthal.*, **96**, 468–73.

Index